Advances in Nanoscience and Nanotechnology

Series Editors-in-Chief

Sabu Thomas, PhD

Dr. Sabu Thomas is the Director of the School of Chemical Sciences, Mahatma Gandhi University, Kottayam, India. He is also a full professor of polymer science and engineering and Director of the Centre for nanoscience and nanotechnology of the same university. He is a fellow of many professional bodies. Professor Thomas has authored or co-authored many papers in international peer-reviewed journals in the area of polymer processing. He has organized several international conferences and has more than 420 publications, 11 books and two patents to his credit. He has been involved in a number of books both as author and editor. He is a reviewer to many international journals and has received many awards for his excellent work in polymer processing. His h Index is 42. Professor Thomas is listed as the 5th position in the list of Most Productive Researchers in India, in 2008.

Mathew Sebastian, MD

Dr. Mathew Sebastian has a degree in surgery (1976) with specialization in Ayurveda. He holds several diplomas in acupuncture, neural therapy (pain therapy), manual therapy and vascular diseases. He was a missionary doctor in Mugana Hospital, Bukoba in Tansania, Africa (1976-1978) and underwent surgical training in different hospitals in Austria, Germany, and India for more than 10 years. Since 2000 he is the doctor in charge of the Ayurveda and Vein Clinic in Klagenfurt, Austria. At present he is a Consultant Surgeon at Privatclinic Maria Hilf, Klagenfurt. He is a member of the scientific advisory committee of the European Academy for Ayurveda, Birstein, Germany, and the TAM advisory committee (Traditional Asian Medicine, Sector Ayurveda) of the Austrian Ministry for Health, Vienna. He conducted an International Ayurveda Congress in Klagenfurt, Austria, in 2010. He has several publications to his name.

Anne George, MD

Anne George, MD, is the Director of the Institute for Holistic Medical Sciences, Kottayam, Kerala, India. She did her MBBS (Bachelor of Medicine, Bachelor of Surgery) at Trivandrum Medical College, University of Kerala, India. She acquired a DGO (Diploma in Obstetrics and Gynaecology) from the University of Vienna, Austria; Diploma Acupuncture from the University of Vienna; and an MD from Kottayam Medical College, Mahatma Gandhi University, Kerala, India. She has organized several international conferences, is a fellow of the American Medical Society, and is a member of many international organizations. She has five publications to her name and has presented 25 papers.

Dr. Yang Weimin

Dr. Yang Weimin is the Taishan Scholar Professor of Quingdao University of Science and Technology in China. He is a full professor at the Beijing University of Chemical Technology and a fellow of many professional organizations. Professor Weimin has authored many papers in international peer-reviewed journals in the area of polymer processing. He has been contributed to a number of books as author and editor and acts as a reviewer to many international journals. In addition, he is a consultant to many polymer equipment manufacturers. He has also received numerous award for his work in polymer processing.

© 2013 by
Apple Academic Press Inc.
3333 Mistwell Crescent
Oakville, ON L6L 0A2
Canada

Apple Academic Press Inc.
1613 Beaver Dam Road, Suite # 104
Point Pleasant, NJ 08742
USA

First issued in paperback 2021

Exclusive worldwide distribution by CRC Press, a Taylor & Francis Group

ISBN 13: 978-1-77463-235-2 (pbk)
ISBN 13: 978-1-926895-17-8 (hbk)

Library of Congress Control Number: 2012935667

Library and Archives Canada Cataloguing in Publication

Nanomedicine and drug delivery/edited by Mathew Sebastian, Neethu Ninan and A.K. Haghi.
(Recent advances in nanoscience and nanotechnology; v.1)

Includes bibliographical references and index.
ISBN 978-1-926895-17-8
1. Nanomedicine. 2. Drug delivery systems. 3. Nanotechnology.
I. Sebastian, Mathew II. Ninan, Neethu III. Haghi, A. K IV. Series:
Recent advances in nanoscience and nanotechnology; v.1

R857.N34N363 2012   610.28   C2011-908741-3

Advances in Nanoscience and Nanotechnology

Volume 1

NANOMEDICINE AND DRUG DELIVERY

Edited By

**Mathew Sebastian, MD, Neethu Ninan,
and A. K. Haghi, PhD**

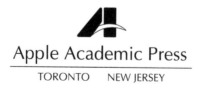

Apple Academic Press

TORONTO   NEW JERSEY

NANOMEDICINE AND DRUG DELIVERY

Contents

List of Contributors

Kirill A. Afonin
Center for Cancer Research Nanobiology Program, National Cancer Institute, NCI-Frederick, National Institutes of Health, Frederick, Maryland-21702, USA.

Zahoor Ahmad
Infectious diseases PK/PD Lab, Life Science Block, Indian Institute of Integrative Medicine, Sanat Nagar, Srinagar, Kashmir India.

M. A. Aleksandrova
N. K. Koltzov Institute of Development Biology of RAS, Russia-119334.

I. Banerjee
Department of Applied Physics, Birla Institute of Technology, Mesra, Ranchi-835215, India.
Department of Physics, University of Pune, Ganeshkhind, Pune-411007, India.

S. V. Bhoraskar
Department of Physics, University of Pune, Ganeshkhind, Pune-411007.

Eckart Bindewald
Basic Science Program, SAIC-Frederick, Inc, NCI-Frederick, Frederick-21702, USA.

Maria Bryszewska
Department of General Biophysics, University of Lodz, Pomorska, 141/143, Lodz, Poland.

Erin R. Calkins
Department of Chemistry and Biochemistry, University of California, Santa Barbara, CA 93106–9510, USA.

Clément Campillo
Laboratoire d'Electronique Moléculaire Organique et Hybride/UMR 5819 SPrAM (CEA-CNRS-UJF)/INAC/CEA-Grenoble, 38054 Grenoble Cedex 9 (France)

R. C. Carlisle
Department of Clinical Pharmacology, University of Oxford, Old Road Campus, Off Roosevelt Drive Headington, Oxford OX3 7DQ, UK.

Roberta Cavalli
Dipartimento di Scienza e Tecnologia del Farmaco, Università degli Studi di Torino, *via* P. Giuria 6, 10125 Torino, Italy.

R Narayana Charyulu
Vice Principal & HOD Department of Pharmaceutics NGSMIPS, Mangalore Karnataka, India.

R. K. Chilachyan
Gamaleya Scientific Research Institute of Epidemiology and Microbiology of RAMS, Russia-123098.

G. R. Dillip
Department of Physics, Sri Venkateswara University, Tirupati-517 502, India.

Volha Dzmitruk
Institute of Biophysics and Cell Engineering of NASB, Akademicheskaja, 27, Minsk, Belarus.

Pedziwiatr-Werbicka Elzbieta
Department of General Biophysics, University of Lodz, Pomorska, 141/143, Lodz, Poland.

Fabio Fenili
Dipartimento di Chimica Organica e Industriale, Università degli Studi di Milano, *via* Venezian 21, 20133 Milano, Italy and Consorzio Interuniversitario Nazionale per la Scienza e Tecnologia dei Materiali (IN-STM), *via* G. Giusti, 9–50121 Firenze, Italy.

Elena Ferrari
Dipartimento di Chimica Organica e Industriale, Università degli Studi di Milano, *via* Venezian 21, 20133 Milano, Italy and Consorzio Interuniversitario Nazionale per la Scienza e Tecnologia dei Materiali (IN-STM), *via* G. Giusti, 9–50121 Firenze, Italy.

Paolo Ferruti
Dipartimento di Chimica Organica e Industriale, Università degli Studi di Milano, *via* Venezian 21, 20133 Milano, Italy and Consorzio Interuniversitario Nazionale per la Scienza e Tecnologia dei Materiali (IN-STM), *via* G. Giusti, 9–50121 Firenze, Italy.

Cody Geary
Department of Chemistry and Biochemistry, University of California, Santa Barbara, CA 93106–9510, USA.

S. Goswami
Department of Polymer Engineering, Birla Institute of Technology, Mesra, Ranchi-835215, India.

Wade W. Grabow
Department of Chemistry and Biochemistry, University of California, Santa Barbara, CA 93106–9510, USA.

P. N. Gupta
Formulation and Drug Delivery Division, Indian Institute of Integrative Medicine (CSIR), Jammu-180001, India.

N. Gupta
Sagar Institute of Pharmaceutical Sciences, Sagar (M.P.) 470003, India.

Inessa Halets
Institute of Biophysics and Cell Engineering of NASB, Akademicheskaja, 27, Minsk, Belarus.

Luc Jaeger
Department of Chemistry and Biochemistry, University of California, Santa Barbara, CA 93106–9510, USA.
Biomolecular Science and Engineering Program, University of California, Santa Barbara, CA 93106, USA

Sanjay Jain
Principal & Professor Department of Pharmacognosy Smriti College of Pharmaceutical Education Indore, M. P. India.

R. K. Johri
Division of Pharmacology, Indian Institute of Integrative Medicine (CSIR), Jammu-180001, India.

Jagat R. Kanwar
Laboratory of Immunology and Molecular Biomedical Research (LIMBR), Centre for Biotechnology and Interdisciplinary Biosciences (BioDeakin), Institute for Technology Research and Innovation (ITRI), Deakin University, Waurn Ponds, Victoria-3217, Australia.

Rupinder K. Kanwar
Laboratory of Immunology and Molecular Biomedical Research (LIMBR), Centre for Biotechnology and Interdisciplinary Biosciences (BioDeakin), Institute for Technology Research and Innovation (ITRI), Deakin University, Waurn Ponds, Victoria-3217, Australia.

Wojciech Kasprzak
Basic Science Program, SAIC-Frederick, Inc, NCI-Frederick, Frederick-21702, USA.

K. Kiran
Department of Polymer Engineering, Birla Institute of Technology, Mesra, Ranchi-835215, India.

O.V. Kurskaya
Institute of Higher Nervous Activity and Neurophysiology of RAS, Russia-117485.

N. A. Loginova
Institute of Higher Nervous Activity and Neurophysiology of Russian Academy of Sciences, Russia.

E. V. Loseva
Institute of Higher Nervous Activity and Neurophysiology of RAS, Russia-117485.

S. K. Mahapatra
Department of Applied Physics, Birla Institute of Technology, Mesra, Ranchi-835215, India.

Ganesh Mahidhara
Laboratory of Immunology and Molecular Biomedical Research (LIMBR), Centre for Biotechnology and Interdisciplinary Biosciences (BioDeakin), Institute for Technology Research and Innovation (ITRI), Deakin University, Waurn Ponds, Victoria-3217, Australia.

K. Mallikarjuna
Department of Physics, Sri Venkateswara University, Tirupati-517 502, India.

Amedea Manfredi
Dipartimento di Chimica Organica e Industriale, Università degli Studi di Milano, *via* Venezian 21, 20133 Milano, Italy and Consorzio Interuniversitario Nazionale per la Scienza e Tecnologia dei Materiali (INSTM), *via* G. Giusti, 9–50121 Firenze, Italy.

M. V. Marey
Academician V. I. Kulakov Research **Center of Obstetrics, Gynecology**, and Perinatology, Russia-117997.

Apurba Krishna Mitra
Department of Physics, NIT Durgapur-713209, West Bengal, India.

G. Narasimha
Applied Microbiology Laboratory, Department of Virology, Sri Venkateswara University, Tirupati-517 502, India.

A. B. Panda
Department of Applied Physics, Birla Institute of Technology, Mesra, Ranchi-835215, India.

Rajesh Panday
Infectious diseases PK/PD Lab, Life Science Block, Indian Institute of Integrative Medicine, Sanat Nagar, Srinagar, Kashmir India.

Ashok R. Patel
Marie Curie International Incoming Fellow Vlaardingen-3134 XD, Netherlands.

M. Pechar
Institute of Macromolecular Chemistry, AS CR, Heyrovskeho sq. 2, Prague 6, 162 06, Czech Republic.

Brigitte Pépin-Donat
Laboratoire d'Electronique Mol*éculaire Organique et Hybride/UMR 5819* SPrAM (CEA-CNRS-UJF)/INAC/CEA-Grenoble-38054 Grenoble Cedex 9 (France).

O.V. Podgornyi
N. K. Koltzov Institute of Development Biology of RAS, Russia-119334.

R. Pola
Institute of Macromolecular Chemistry, AS CR, Heyrovskeho sq. 2, Prague 6, 162 06, Czech Republic.

R. A. Poltavtseva
N. K. Koltzov Institute of Development Biology of RAS, Russia-119334.

Francois Quemeneur
Laboratoire d'Electronique Moléculaire Organique et Hybride/UMR 5819 SPrAM (CEA-CNRS-UJF)/INAC/CEA-Grenoble, 38054 Grenoble Cedex 9 (France).

B. Deva Prasad Raju
Department of Physics, Sri Venkateswara University, Tirupati-517 502, India.

Elisabetta Ranucci
Dipartimento di Chimica Organica e Industriale, Università degli Studi di Milano, *via* Venezian 21, 20133 Milano, Italy and Consorzio Interuniversitario Nazionale per la Scienza e Tecnologia dei Materiali (IN-STM), *via* G. Giusti, 9–50121 Firenze, Italy.

Simon C. W. Richardson
School of Science, University of Greenwich at Medway, Central Avenue, Chatham Maritime, Kent ME4 4TB, UK.

Marguerite Rinaudo
Centre de Recherches sur les Macromolecules *Végétales (CERMAV-CNRS)* affiliated with Joseph Fourier University, BP53, 38041 Grenoble Cedex 9 (France).

K. Yu Sarkisova
Institute of Higher Nervous Activity and Neurophysiology of Russian Academy of Sciences, Russia.

L. W. Seymour
Department of Clinical Pharmacology, University of Oxford, Old Road Campus, Off Roosevelt Drive Headington, Oxford OX3 7DQ, UK.

Bruce A. Shapiro
Center for Cancer Research Nanobiology Program, National Cancer Institute, NCI-Frederick, National Institutes of Health, Frederick, Maryland-21702, USA.

P. P. Sharma
Department of Gynaecology and Obstetrics, Midnapur Medical College, West Medinipur-721101, West Bengal, India.

S. C. Sharma
Division of Pharmacology, Indian Institute of Integrative Medicine (CSIR), Jammu-180001, India.

Dzmitry Shcharbin
Institute of Biophysics and Cell Engineering of NASB, Akademicheskaja, 27, Minsk, Belarus.

G. D. Singh
Division of Pharmacology, Indian Institute of Integrative Medicine (CSIR), Jammu-180001, India.

S. Singh
Division of Pharmacology, Indian Institute of Integrative Medicine (CSIR), Jammu-180001, India.

B. Sreedhar
Indian Institute of Chemical Technology, Hyderabad-500 007, India.

Prathima Srinivas
Sri Venkateshwara College of Pharmacy, Affiliated to OsmaniaUniversity, Madhapur, Hyderabad, Andhra Pradesh India-500081.

B. V. SubbaReddy
Indian Institute of Chemical Technology, Hyderabad-500 007, India.

C. K. Sudhakar
Assistant Professor Department of Pharmaceutics, Smriti College of Pharmaceutical Education Indore, M. P. India.

G. T. Sukhikh
Academician V. I. Kulakov Research **Center of Obstetrics, Gynecology,** and Perinatology, Russia-117997.

Keka Talukdar
Department of Physics, NIT Durgapur-713209, West Bengal, India.

M. K. Tikoo
Division of Pharmacology, Indian Institute of Integrative Medicine (CSIR), Jammu-180001, India.

K. Ulbrich
Institute of Macromolecular Chemistry, AS CR, Heyrovskeho sq. 2, Prague 6, 162 06, Czech Republic.

Nitish Upadhyay
Research scholar Department of Pharmaceutics Smriti College of Pharmaceutical Education Indore, M. P. India.

Faye M. Walker
Department of Chemistry and Biochemistry, University of California, Santa Barbara, CA 93106–9510, USA.

R. A. Willemsen
Experimental Urology, Josephine Nefkens Institute, Erasmus MC, Dr. Molenwaterplein 50, 3015 GE Rotterdam, Netherlands.

Paul Zakrevsky
Department of Chemistry and Biochemistry, University of California, Santa Barbara, CA 93106–9510, USA.

List of Abbreviations

ALA	Aminolevulinic acid
AGIP	Amyloid growth inhibitor peptide
APC	Antigen-presenting cells
ATDs	Antitubercular drugs
BBB	Bloodbrain barrier
bGH	Bovine growth hormone
BSA	Bovine serum albumin
BSM	Bovine submaxillary mucin
BA	Butyl acrylate
CBD	Cannabidiol
CNS	Central nervous system
CTAR	Conditioned two-way avoidance reflex
CRH	Corticotropin-releasing hormone
CAR	Coxsackievirus and adenovirus receptor
CMC	Critical micelle concentration
COX-2	Cyclooxygenase-2
DA	Degrees of acetylation
DCs	Dendritic cells
DSC	Differential scanning calorimetry
DALYs	Disability-adjusted life years
DPI	Dry Powder Inhalers
DPPH	1,1-Diphenyl-2-picrylhydrazyl
DLS	Dynamic light scattering
EELS	Electron energy loss spectroscopy
EGF	Epidermal growth factor
EGCG	Epigallocatechin gallate
EGDMA	Ethylene glycol dimethacrylate
XDR-TB	Extensively drug resistant TB
FP	Flubriprofen
FDA	Food and drug administration
FTIR	Fourier transformed infrared
GAS	Gas anti solvent
G4-SNAP	Generation-4 polyamidoamine dendrimers
GUVs	Giant Unilamellar Vesicles
GBM	Glibenclamide

GFAP	Glio fibrillary acid protein
GLP	Glucagon-like peptide
GPCR	G-protein coupled receptor
GALT	Gut-associated lymphoid tissue
HBsAg	Hepatitis B surface antigen
HSV	Herpes simplex virus
HEA	2-Hydroxy ethyl acrylate
HRTEM	High resolution TEM
HAART	Highly active anti-retroviral therapy
HIV	Human Immunodeficiency Virus
HA	Hydroxyapatite
HH	Hypoxic hypoxia
IAR	IA receptors
ISCOM	Immune-stimulating complex matrix
INH	Incorporation of isoniazid
IDO	Indoleamine 2,3-dioxegenase
IA	Interferon-alpha
IF-γ	Interferon-gamma
IPN	Interpenetrating polymer network
JCPDS	Joint committee on powder diffraction standards
LUVs	Large unilamellar vesicles
LIF	Leukemia-inhibiting factor
LPS	Lipopolysaccharide
LCST	Low critical solution temperature
LDL	Low density lipoproteins
MRA	Magnetic resonance angiography
MMAD	Mass median aerodynamic diameter
MSC	Mesenchymal stromal cells
mRNA	Messenger RNA
MS	Metaprolol Succinate
MTX	Methotrexate
MBC	Methyl benzethonium chloride
MCC	Microcrystalline cellulose
MIC	Minimum inhibitory concentration
MD	Molecular dynamics
MC	Monte Carlo
MDR-TB	Multidrug resistant TB
NAC	N-Acetyl cysteine
NC	Nanocapsules

NP	Nanoparticles
NALT	Nasal lymphoid tissue
NSC	Neural stem cells
NETs	Neutrophil extracellular traps
ncRNA	Non-coding RNA
NDB	Nucleic acid database
O-MALT	Organized mucosal associated lymphoid tissue
PGRP	Peptidoglycan recognition protein
PMs	Physical mixtures
PNP	PoissonNernstPlanck
PHEA	Poly (2-hydroxyethyl acrylate)
PLL	Poly(L-lysine)
PLA	Poly lactic acid
PAA	Poly(amidoamine)
PAMAM	Poly(amidoamine)
PEO	Poly(ethylene oxide)
PEI	Poly(ethyleneimine)
PHPMA	Poly(N-(2-hydroxypropyl)methacrylamide)
PACA-NP	Polyalkylcyanoacrylate nanoparticles
PAAs	Polyamidoamines
PBA	Polybutyl acrylate
PBCA	Polybutylcyanoacrylate
PEG	Polyethyleneglycol
PIHCA-NP	Polyisohexylcyanoacrylate nanoparticles
PLGA	Polylactide *co*-glycolide
PLL	Poly-L-lysine
PCR	Polymerase chain reaction
PPI	Polypropyleneimine
PVA	Polyvinyl alcohol
PSMA	Prostate-specific membrane antigen
RESS	Rapid expansion from supercritical solution
ROS	Reactive oxygen species
RSV	Respiratory syncytial virus
RNA	Ribonucleic acid
SEM	Scanning Electron Microscope
SMEDDS	Self-micro emulsifying drug delivery systems
SUVs	Small unilamellar vesicles
SD	Solid dispersion
SLNs	Solid lipid nanoparticles

SDD	Spray dried dispersion
SEB	Staphylococcal enterotoxoid B
SC	Stratum corneum
SCOR	Structural classification of RNA
SLIT	Sublingual immunotherapy
SAP	Sweet arrow peptide
TT	Thiazolidine-2-thione
TIMP	Tissue inhibitor of metalloproteinase
TLR	Toll-like receptor
TCM	Traditional Chinese medicine
TEM	Transmission electron microscopy
THP	Trihexyphenidyl
TB	Tuberculosis
TNF	Tumor necrosis factor
UEA-1	Ulex europaeus agglutinin 1
WGA	Wheat germ agglutinin
WHO	World Health Organization
XRD	X-Ray diffraction

Preface

Nanomedicine is the speculative field in the vicinity of nanotechnology as it involves engineering and re-engineering of molecular assemblers that have the capability of re-ordering the matter either at the atomic level or at the molecular level. It can also be described as the control, construction, monitoring and repairing of human systems at the basic molecular level by making use of the state of the art nanostructures and nanodevices. It is believed to enhance the natural healing powers of the human body as well as increase its immunization capabilities and because of its wider applications, it is sub branched into various categories such as nanonephrology, a special field of nanomedicine that deals with the study of the protein structure of the kidneys. In the longer term, perhaps 10 to 20 years from today, the earliest molecular machine systems and nanorobots may join the medical armamentarium, finally giving physicians the most potent tools imaginable to conquer human disease, ill health, and aging. In general, miniaturization of our medical tool will provide accurate, controllable, versatile, reliable, cost-effective, and faster approaches to enhance the quality of human life, which gives an overview of this rapidly expanding and exciting field. Nanomedicine includes three progressively more powerful molecular technologies. The first category includes raw materials like nanoparticle coatings and nanocrystalline materials. The second category encompasses nanoscale-structured materials and devices like cyclic peptides, dendrimers, detoxification agents, fullerenes, functional drug carriers, MRI scanning (nanoparticles), nanobarcodes, nanoemulsions, nanofibers, nanoparticles, nanoshells, nanotubes, quantum dots and the third includes molecular machine systems and medical nanorobots.

The advantages of nanomedicine are two-fold. In the short term we are looking at advances in drug discovery and drug delivery, as well as the continued miniaturization of analytical/ diagnostic procedures. In the long term, we are looking at the ability to do *in vivo* diagnostics coupled with much more targeted, focused therapy. Now we just do general drug therapy: sometimes it works and sometimes it doesn't, and some medications produce significant side-effects. If the promise of nanomedicine holds true, we will be able to avoid those side-effects and have better response to therapy. Nanotechnology gives us the ability to do analytical procedures in the lab on a much smaller scale. We can look for drug targets on a cellular basis as opposed to a multicellular or tissue basis, as we do now. Advances in biosensors and molecular probes will allow for more detailed examination of cellular processes. This will help in identifying molecular targets for drug development. Nanomedicine is well under way in oncology. Once nanomachines are available, the ultimate dream of every healer, medicine man, and physician throughout recorded history will, at last, become a reality. Programmable and controllable microscale robots comprised of nanoscale parts fabricated to nanometer precision will allow medical doctors to execute curative and reconstructive procedures in the human body at the cellular and molecular levels. Nanomedical physicians of the early 21st century will still make good use of the body's natural healing powers and homeostatic mechanisms, because, all else equal, those interventions are best that intervene least. But the ability to direct events in a controlled fashion at the cellular level is the key that will unlock the indefinite extension of human health and the expansion of human abilities.

Recent advances in drug delivery deal with the development of synthetic nano-meter sized targeted delivery systems for therapeutic agents of increased complexity, and biologically active drug products. Therapeutic systems in this class are up to a million times larger than classical drugs like aspirin. Being larger there is more scope for diversity and complexity, which makes their description much more challenging and their delivery more difficult. Their increased complexity however, gives these systems the unique power to tackle more challenging diseases. Targeted delivery systems can have multiple functions, a key one being their ability to recognize specific molecules which can be located either in the membrane of target cells, or in specific compartments within the cell. A challenging objective of targeted drug delivery is the development of innovative multidisciplinary approaches for the design, synthesis and functionalization of novel nanocarriers for targeted delivery of drugs via oral, pulmonary and Blood Brain Barrier (BBB) crossing administration routes.

This book focuses on the recent advances in nanomedicine and drug delivery. This forward-looking resource outlines the extraordinary new tools that are becoming available in nanomedicine. The book presents an integrated set of perspectives that describe where we are now and where we should be headed to put nanomedicine devices in to applications as quickly as possible, including consideration of the possible dangers of nanomedicine. This book will consider the full range of nanomedical applications which employ molecular nanotechnology inside the human body, from the perspective of a future practitioner in an era of widely available nanomedicine, including: health benefits of phytochemicals and application of colloidal delivery systems; study of non-covalent attachment of recombinant targeting proteins to polymer-modified Adenoviral gene delivery vectors; role of nanoparticles as adjuvants for mucosal vaccine delivery; poly(amido-amine)s as delivery systems for biologically active substances; antimicrobial activity of silver nanoparticles; cancer treatment; dendrimers, capsules based on lipid vesicles for drug delivery and many other recent achievements. Written by some of the most innovative minds in medicine and engineering, this unique volume helps professionals understand cutting-edge and futuristic areas of research that can have tremendous payoff in terms of improving human health. Readers will find insightful discussions on nanostructured intelligent materials and devices that are considered technically feasible and that have a high potential to produce advances in medicine in the near future.

— **Mathew Sebastian, MD**

Chapter 1

Ethosomes as Non-invasive Loom for Transdermal Drug Delivery System

Sudhakar C. K, Nitish Upadhyay, Sanjay Jain, and R Narayana Charyulu

---

INTRODUCTION

The application of medicinal substances to the skin is a concept doubtless as old as humanity, the Papyrus records of ancient Egypt describes variety of such medication for external use. Galen described the use in Roman times of a forerunner of today's vanishing cream. Medications are applied in variety of form reflecting the ingenuity and scientific imagination of pharmacist through centuries. New modes of drug delivery have been developed to remedy the shortcomings of earlier vehicle or more recently to optimize drug delivery. The first official ointment appearing in the USP of 1820 consist of lard. Medications are applied to the skin in the form of ointments, creams, pastes, lotion, gels, and plasters (John et al., 1980).

For more than two decades, researchers have attempted to find a way to use the skin as a portal of entry for drugs in order to overcome problems associated with traditional modes of drug administration (Touitou, 2002). Delivery of drugs to the skin is an effective and targeted therapy for local dermatological disorders. The topical administration of drugs, in order to achieve optimal cutaneous and percutaneous drug delivery, has recently gained an importance because of various advantages such as ease of administration and delivery benefits. This route of drug delivery has gained popularity because it avoids first-pass effects, gastrointestinal irritation, and metabolic degradation associated with oral administration (Kikwai et al., 2005). The topical route of administration has been utilized either to produce local effects for treating skin disorders or to produce systemic drug effects. With topical dosage forms, great attention has been devoted to new formulation that ensures adequate localization of drug within the skin to enhance the local effect or increase the penetration through the stratum corneum and viable epidermis for systemic effects (Kumar et al., 2005). In search of a vehicle to deliver the medicament into the skin layers (cutaneous delivery), or through the skin and into the systemic circulation (percutaneous absorption), varied kinds of formulation systems and strategies have been evolved. Among the many, the lipid-based formulations have been in use for decades. However, of late, there has been a surge in their number with wide variation and flexibility in the interior designs and structures. The importance of lipids has especially increased after realizing the utility of phospholipids, the natural bio-friendly molecules, which in collaboration with water can form diverse types of supramolecular structures (Hadgraft 1996; Kumar, 2005; Schmid, 1994).

In treating skin disease, the primary purpose of applying drugs to the skin is to induce local effects at very close to the site of application. In the case of dermato-pharmacotherapy, the realization is to develop selective delivery system that enhances penetration of active ingredient, localizes the drug at site of action and reduce the percutaneous absorption. The main problem in dermatopharmcothearpy is the penetration of skin by most of drugs as with only a small portion of dose finally reaches the sites of action within the skin, producing limited local activity. Moreover, a few drugs which penetrate the skin easily are quickly removed by blood circulation, thus producing systemic effect rather than local effects. This has been a complicated task due to the highly effective barrier properties of the skin. In order to deliver drugs through the skin, most compounds require various degrees of permeation enhancement (Ranjit et al., 1996). Classic enhancement methods focused primarily on chemical enhancement or modulation of interactions between the drug and the vehicle. More recent research makes use of innovative vesicular carriers, electrically assisted delivery and various micro invasive methods, some incorporating technologies from other fields. The best avenue to improve drug penetration and/or localization is obviously to manipulate the vehicle or to utilize a drug carrier concept. Dermatological and cosmetic preparations frequently contain active principles, which can only act when they penetrate at least the outermost layer of the skin. However, the efficacy of topically applied actives is often suboptimal because the transport into the skin is slow due to the resistance of the outermost layer of the skin, the stratum corneum (Daniel, 2004).

The intact stratum corneum thus provides the main barrier; its "brick and mortar" structure is analogous to a wall (Figure 1). The corneocytes of hydrated keratin comprise of "bricks", embedded in "mortar", composed of multiple lipid bilayers of ceramides, fatty acids, cholesterol, and cholesterol esters. These bilayers form regions of semicrystalline, gel, and liquid crystals domains.

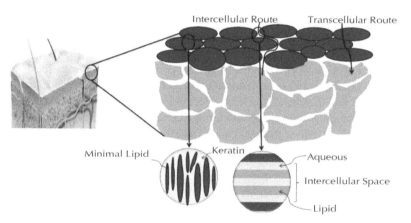

Figure 1. Simplified diagram of stratum corneum and two microroutes of drug penetration.

Most molecules penetrate through skin via this intercellular microroute and therefore many enhancing techniques aim to disrupt or bypass elegant molecular architecture.

(Daniel, 2004). Viable layers may metabolise a drug, or activate a prodrug. The dermal papillary layer is so rich in capillaries that most penetrants clear within minutes. Usually, deeper dermal regions do not significantly influence absorption, although they may bind for example, testosterone, inhibiting its systemic removal (Merdan et al., 1998). Vesicular systems are drug delivery system to deliver the drug dermally and transdermally (Daniel, 2004). Liposomes have the potential of overcoming the skin barrier, as these are bilayered lipid vesicles, consisting primarily of phospholipids and cholesterols (Hogaki et al., 2003).

The rationale for the use of lipid vesicles as topical drug carriers is 4-fold: (Hans et al., 1994)

(i) They may serve as "organic" solvent for the solubilization of poorly soluble drugs, for instance corticosteroids; as a result, higher local drug concentrations at the thermodynamic activity maximum can be applied,

(ii) They may serve as a local depot for the sustained release of dermally active compounds including antibiotics, corticosteroids or retinoic acid,

(iii) By virtue of penetration of individual phospholipid molecules or nonionic ether surfactants into the lipid layers of the stratum corneum and epidermis they may serve as penetration enhancer and facilitate dermal delivery leading to higher localized drug concentrations,

(iv) They may serve as rate-limiting membrane barrier for the modulation of systemic absorption, that is, they may serve as controlled transdermal delivery systems.

The vesicles have been well known for their importance in cellular communication and particle transportation for many years. Researchers have been understanding the properties of vesicle structures for use in better drug delivery within their cavities, that would allow to tag the vesicle for cell specificity. Vesicles would also allow to control the release rate of drug over an extended time, keeping the drug shielded from immune response or other removal systems and would be able to release just the right amount of drug and keep that concentration constant for longer periods of time. One of the major advances in vesicle research was the finding a vesicle derivative, known as an ethosomes (Barry, 2001; Jain et al., 2004; Touitou et al., 2000). Flexible liposomes are common vectors in transdermal drug delivery systems, with relatively good liquidity and deformability. Currently there are three types of flexible liposomes like transfersomes, ethosomes and niosomes. In recent years, ethosomes have become new liposome carriers with high deformability; high entrapment efficiency and a good transdermal permeation rate in the drug delivery system, and are suitable for transdermal administration (Fang et al., 2008; Jain et al., 2007).

Ethosomes are soft, phospholipid nanovesicles (tiny, bubble-like, lipid spheres), which, due to their structure, are able to overcome the natural dermal barrier, delivering drugs through the skin layers. The ethosome delivery system can be modulated not only for enhanced skin penetration but localizes the drug at the site of action, enables drugs to reach the deep skin layers (Merdan, 1998).The enhanced delivery of actives by means of ethosomes over liposomes can be attributed to an interaction between ethosomes and skin lipids (Figure 2). A possible mechanism for this interaction has been proposed. It is deliberation that the first part of the mechanism is due to the "ethanol effect", whereby intercalation of the ethanol into intercellular lipids enhances lipid fluidity and decreases the density of the lipid multilayer. This is followed by the "ethosome effect", which includes interlipid penetration and permeation by the opening of new pathways due to the malleability and fusion of ethosomes with skin lipids, resulting in the release of the drug in deep layers of the skin (Touitou et al., 2000). Ethosomes, phospholipid vesicles of short-chain alcohols, were shown to deliver model drug molecules, for example, testosterone, to a skin depth of 240 μ, compared with the delivery of testosterone to a depth of 20 μ by liposomes. Ethosomes also have a high entrapment capacity so that more drug can be delivered (David, 2001).

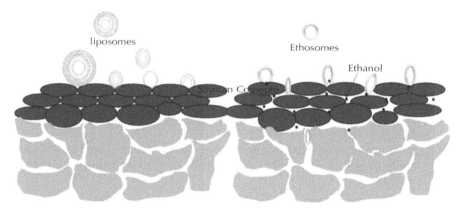

Figure 2. Comparative diagram of transport through liposomes and ethosomes vesicles. Ethosomes penetrate through the stratum corneum and the underlying viable skin into the blood circulation. Stratum corneum (SC) lipid disruption by ethanol and ethosomes deform itself to penetrates in the pores of stratum corneum to reach the blood stream.

Enhanced Transdermal Drug Delivery from Ethosomes

Mechanism of skin permeation of elastic liposome vesicle (ethosomes) is still unstated but anticipated mechanism is claimed by different authors

a) Lipid layers perturbation (SC lipid disruption)

b) Osmotic gradients

c) Elasticity of vesicles

Ethosomes represent the third generation of elastic lipid carriers, developed by Touitou et al. (1997, 2000a, 2000b, 2001). The ethosomal system is composed of phospholipid, ethanol, and water. Ethosomes have been reported to improve delivery of various drugs to skin (Figure 3). Although, the exact process of drug delivery by ethosomes remains a matter of speculation a combination of processes, most likely, contributes to the enhancing effect. As ethanol is a well known permeation enhancer, a synergistic mechanism was suggested among ethanol, vesicles, and skin lipids. Ethanol may provide the vesicles with soft flexible characteristics which allow them to more easily penetrate into deeper layers of the skin.

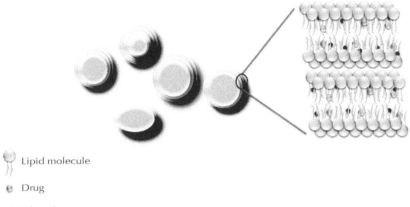

Lipid molecule

Drug

Ethanol

Figure 3. Ethosomal systems are sophisticated conceptually. Ethosomes could be unilamellar or multilamellar through to the core. Ethosomes contain soft phospholipid vesicles in the presence of high concentrations of ethanol. It was also proposed that phospholipid vesicles with ethanol have the ability to penetrate into the skin and influence the bilayer structure of the stratum corneum and that may lead to enhancement of drug penetration (Elsayed et al., 2006).

It is claimed that ethosomes significantly enhance drug delivery across the skin by two principle mechanisms: (a) a fluidizing effect of ethanol on phospholipid bilayers creating a "soft", deformable vesicle and (b) The SC lipid disruption by ethanol thereby permitting entry of ethosomes and their associated "payload" into the deeper skin layers (Dayan et al., 2000; Godin et al., 2004, 2005; Touitou et al., 2000). Ethosomes are variations of liposomes which incorporate ethanol to confer the property of ultradeformability. It is claimed that this allows significantly enhanced transport of associated active species into the deeper skin layers via a variety of (not unambiguously proven) mechanisms, including an action as true "carriers", SC lipid disruption, osmotic gradients, and so on (He et al., 2009).

Mechanism of Ethosome Permeation Proposed by Cevc
The mechanism proposed by Cevc, et al. (1992) is that the high deformability of these vesicles facilies their penetration through the intracellular lipid pathway of the SC. The driving force for the movement of the elastic liposomes (and their payload) is presumably generated by the hydration gradient across the skin, which varies from 15–20% water content in the SC up to 60% in the stratum granulosum (Figure 4). When the elastic liposomes are applied onto the skin and allowed to dry, the vesicles are attracted by the moisture in the epidermis and due to their flexibility they penetrate the skin. The osmotic gradient, caused by the differences in water concentration between the skin surfaces and interiors, has been proposed as the major driving forces for the penetration of vesicles. The osmotic gradient, for example, which is created by the difference in the total water concentrations between the skin surface and the skin interior, provides one possible source of such driving force. It is sufficiently strong to

push at least 0.5 mg of lipids per hr and cm² through the skin permeability barrier in the region of stratum corneum. The lipid concentration gradient, on the contrary, does not contribute much to the lipid penetration into dermis. Occlusion, therefore, is detrimental for the vesicle penetration into intact skin.

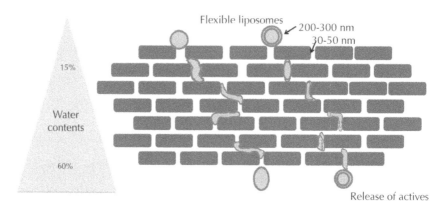

Figure 4. Penetration of the flexible liposomes through the intracellular lipid pathway of the stratum corneum (SC).

Mechanism of Ethosome Permeation Proposed by Touitou E

Ethosome is a novel vesicular carrier developed by Touitou et al., showing enhanced skin delivery. The ethosomal system is composed of phospholipid, ethanol, and water (Touitou et al., 2000a). Although, the exact process of drug delivery by ethosomes remains a matter of speculation (Dayan and Touitou, 2000), most likely, a combination of processes contribute to the enhancing effect (Touitou et al., 2000a). Ethanol is a well known permeation enhancer (Williams, 2003). A synergistic mechanism was suggested between ethanol, vesicles, and skin lipids (Touitou et al., 2000a, 2000b). Ethanol may provide the vesicles with soft flexible characteristics which allow them to more easily penetrate into deeper layers of the skin. It was also proposed that phospholipid vesicles with ethanol may penetrate into the skin and influence the bilayer structure of the stratum corneum (Kirjavainen et al., 1999) and this may lead to enhancement of drug penetration (Figure 5).

"Ethanol interacts with the lipid molecules in the polar head group region resulting in a reduction in the transition temperature of the lipids in the stratum corneum, increasing their fluidity and decreasing the density of the lipid multilayer. This is followed by the 'Ethosome effect', which includes lipid penetration and permeation by the opening of new pathways, due to the malleability and fusion of ethosome with skin lipids, resulting in the release of the drug into the deep layers of the skin. Ethanol may also provide vesicles with soft flexible characteristics, which allow them to penetrate more easily into the deeper layers of the skin."

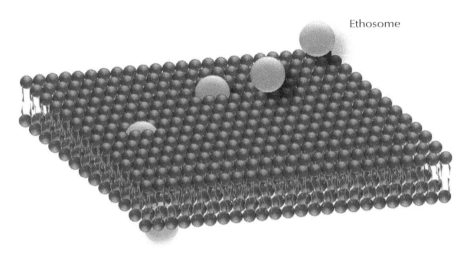

Ethosome

Figure 5. Lipid perturbation, along with elasticity of ethosome vesicles seems to be the main contributor for its improved skin permeation.

Factor Affecting the Penetration of the Vesicles

Factor affecting the penetration of the vesicles into skin elucidated by different authors. El Maghraby et al., suggested that the reasons for variable effects and explanations may arise from different vesicle compositions, alternative methods of preparation which result in vesicles having diverse characteristics with respect to size, lamelarity, charge, membrane fluidity and elasticity and drug entrapment efficiency, and the selection of skin membranes (man or animal, *in vivo* or *in vitro*). Other aspects of the experimental design (such as receptor solution composition) and the technique used in evaluation may have profound effects on the recorded action (El Maghraby et al., 2001, 2006; Verma et al., 2003). They support the existence of an important penetration enhancing effect. The intact vesicle permeation mechanism will have also an important role specially in improving skin deposition. Drug release from vesicles in the stratum corneum is an important step that affects transdermal flux (Honeywell-Nguyen and Bouwstra, 2003). These different interpretations reported in literature can be explained by the fact that vesicle–skin interactions are powerfully dependent on the physicochemical properties of the vesicular systems. Infact, it has been shown that vesicle–skin interactions are strongly affected by vesicle composition, and in particular by their phase state and elasticity. Liquid state vesicles have demonstrated higher capability to interact with human skin than gel-state vesicles (Bouwstra et al., 2003; Honeywell-Nguyen et al., 2002a, 2000b; Jacobs et al., 1988).

Stability and Scale up Process

Drug delivery from liposomes in transdermal formulation has been studied for many purposes but unstable nature and poor skin permeation limits their use for topical delivery. In order to increase the stability of liposomes, the concept of proliposomes was proposed (Deo et al., 1997). This approach was extended to niosomes, which exhibited superior stability as compared to liposomes (Vora et al., 1998). However, due to poor skin permeability, liposomes and niosomes could not be successfully used for systemic drug delivery and their use was limited for topical use (Lasch et al., 1991). To overcome problems of poor skin permeability (Cevc et al., 1996; Touitou et al., 2000a). Recently introduced new vesicular carrier systems ethosome, for non-invasive delivery of drugs into or across the skin. Ethosomes incorporated penetration enhancers (alcohols and polyols), to influence the properties of vesicles and stratum corneum (Cevc et al., 1997).

A number of methods have been used to prepare stable ethosomal formulations depending on the drug characteristics and on the drug delivery target (Touitou, 1996, 1998). The manufacturing processes are easily scaled-up. Relatively to manufacture, with no complicated technical investments required for the production of ethosomes. The presence of ethanol allows for efficient entrapment of hydrophilic, lipophilic, and amphiphilic molecules. This feature is illustrated by research in which three fluorescent probes of distinct physicochemical properties were encapsulated in ethosomes and liposomes, and their behavior was then examined by laser scanning confocal microscopy (Touitou, 2000a, 2000b). Ethosomes, invented by Touitou et al. (1996, 1998, 2000a), were so named to emphasize the presence of ethanol in a vesicular structure. Due to the interdigitation effect of alcohol on lipid bilayers, it was previously thought that the ethanol milieu is destructive to vesicular structures and that vesicles could not coexist with high concentrations of alcohol (Chin et al., 1997; Harris et al., 1987). In contrast to this belief, the existence of vesicles and the structure of ethosomes were evidenced by various methods including 31P-NMR, transmission electron microscopy (TEM), and scanning electron microscopy (SEM). Compared with other liposomes, the physical and chemical properties of ethosomes make these more effective for drug delivery through the stratum corneum into the blood circulation, which is very important in the design of a transdermal drug delivery system. It has been reported that there were no significant changes in average particle size, distribution, and structure of ethosomes over two years (Touitou and Godin, 2006).

One study has found that the size of liposomes significantly increased with time, while the average size of ethosomes basically remained constant over four weeks. It has also been found that ethosomes are well distributed when cholesterol is included in the formulation, and that they are prone to aggregation in the absence of cholesterol. It is thought that cholesterol stabilizes into a bilayer when ethosomes are maintained in a gel state, and that the high concentration of ethanol in ethosomes can ensure mobility of the vesicles, and that a moderate amount of cholesterol could ensure stability (Liu et al., 2011). It was possibly guaranteed the stability during long-term storage ethosome suspensions by freeze-dried. It was found that the freeze-dried ethosomes' cakes were compact, glassy characterized by low density and quick re-hydration. However, the storage time slightly influences the percentage of drug encapsulation within ethosomes showing a drug leakage after re-hydration around 10% (Cortesi et al., 2010).

Entrapment of (-)-epigallocatechin gallate (EGCG) into ethosome was carried out for improving its stability against decomposition. The stability of EGCG in solution and in ethosome exposed to UV or high temperature, results showed the EGCG stabilization effect through its entrapment in ethosome. Incorporation of tocopherol into ethosome retarded the decomposition of EGCG under UV (Hyo and Byung,

2007). Stability changes of ethosome membrane with temperature, lipid composition, and storage time were verified through the calcein release test. Calcein release was observed to be less than 5% at 45°C for 30 days, while most of calcein was released at 60°C. Incorporation of cholesterol into ethosome delayed calcein release at high temperature (Byung et al., 2004).

To increase the stability of ascorbyl palmitate ethosome, which is hydrated liquid crystalline vesicle, was used to entrap it in ethosome. Thermal stability of AP entrapped in ethosome was enhanced compared to that in standard solution (Sang and Byung, 2005). Data on SupraVir cream (Trima, Israel), a marketed ethosomal formulation of acyclovir, indicate that the formulation and the drug had long shelf-lives with no stability problems. Acyclovir in SupraVir cream has been shown by HPLC assay to be stable for at least 3 years at 25°C. Furthermore, skin permeation experiments showed that the cream after 3 years retains its initial penetration enhancing capacity (Touitou and Godin, 2006).

The determination of a zeta potential is predictive of the storage stability of colloidal dispersions. Lack of toxicity, good stability, and uncomplicated manufacturing make ethosomal carriers a valuable tool for novel and more efficient dermal and transdermal drug delivery system (Touitou and Godin, 2007).

Ethosomes versus Other Vesicular Carriers

At foremost glimpse, ethosomes appear to be remotely related to lipid bilayers vesicle, liposomes. However in functional terms, ethosome differ immensely from commonly used liposomes in that they are much more flexible and adaptable. The extremely high flexibility of their membrane permits ethosome to squeeze themselves even through pores much smaller than their own diameter. This is due to ethanol effect of the ethosome and is achieved by judiciously combining at least two components (phospholipids plus ethanol) with sufficiently different packing characteristics into a single bilayer. In Table 1, it is enumerated the comparsion of ethosome and other vescular carrier.

Kinetics of Ethosomes

These ethosomal systems showed improved performance both in terms of drugs concentration in the skin and flux or penetration through the skin. Although, ethanol is a proven penetration enhancers, there appear to be some synergy between the enhancing performances of ethanol, vesicles, and skin lipids. Phospholipid may interact with SC lipids of the intercellular layers enhancing their permeability (William, 2007). After having penetrated through the outermost skin layer, ethosomes reach the deeper skin layer, the so called dermis. From there, it reaches to systemic circulation via lymph and distributes throughout the body. If applied and exposed suitable conditions, ethosomes can thus reach all such body tissues that accessible to the subcutaneously injected liposomes. Ethosomes penetration through the skin is very efficient but it preceeded by lag time. Such time delay is due to the ethanol takes time for lipid perturbation and the vesicle penetrates the stratum corneum. The kinetic of therapeutic action is a function of velocity of transdermal carrier penetration and speed of drug distribution and action. The precise reach as well as kinetics of ethosomes penetration through the intact skin is affected by skin characteristics, applied dose and application condition and form (Gupta et al., 2004).

Ethosomes as Hauler of Restorative Agents

Ethosomes presents interesting features correlated with its ability to permeate intact through the human skin due to its high deformability. In fact, ethosomes are soft, malleable vesicles tailored for enhanced delivery of active agents. It has been shown that the physicochemical characteristics of ethosomes allow this vesicular carrier to transport active substances more efficaciously through the stratum corneum into the deeper layers of the skin than conventional liposomes.

This aspect is of great importance for the design of carriers to be applied topically both for topical and systemic drug administration. Furthermore, the ethosomal carrier is also able to provide an effective intracellular delivery of both hydrophilic and lipophilic molecules and also the penetration of an antibiotic peptide (i.e., bacitracin) within fibroblast cells was facilitated. A novel ethosomal carrier containing trihexyphenidyl (THP) HCl was investigated for the delivery of THP from ethosomes versus classic liposomes. As the THP concentration was increased from 0 to 3%, the size of vesicles decreased from 154 to 90 mm. That was most likely due to the surface activity of THP. When compared with standard liposomes, ethosomes had higher entrapment efficiency and a greater ability to deliver entrapped fluorescent probe to the deeper layers of skin (Dayan and Touitou, 2000). It was studied that ethosomes, phospholipid vesicles of short-chain alcohols, were shown to deliver model drug molecules, for example, testosterone, to a skin depth of 240 μ, compared with the delivery of testosterone to a depth of 20 μ by liposomes. Ethosomes also have a high entrapment capacity so that more amount of drug can be delivered (David et al., 2001). Cannabidiol (CBD) ethosomal formulation for transdermal delivery of cannabiol for the treatment of rheumatoid arthritis was prepared. Results of the skin deposition study showed significant accumulation of CBD in the skin, and underlying muscles after application of CBD-ethosomal formulation to the abdomen of mice. Plasma concentration study showed that a steady state level was reached in 24 hr, which was maintained through 72 hr (Lodzki et al., 2003). The dermal and intracellular delivery of bacitracin, a model poly peptide antibiotic, from ethosomes and demonstrated that the antibiotic peptide was delivered into deep skin layers through intercorneocyte lipid domain of stratum corneum. Efficient delivery of antibiotics of deep skin strata from ethosomal application could be highly beneficial in reducing possible side effect and other drawbacks associated with systems treatment (Godin and Touitou, 2004). Erythromycin ethosomes were designed and characterized for their antibacterial efficiency and evaluated *in vitro* and *in vivo*. The TEM, CLSM, DLS, DSC, and ultracentrifugation tests indicate that erythromycin ethosomes are small unilamellar soft vesicles encapsulating 78.6% erythromycin. Ethosomes are efficient carriers for erythromycin delivery to bacteria localized within the deep skin strata for eradication of staphylococcal infection (Godin et al., 2005a, 2000b). It was reported ethosomes for transcutaneous immunization, and antigen-loaded ethosomes for transcutaneous immunization against hepatitis B were prepared and characterized, which showed greater entrapment efficiency, optimal size range, and unilamellar, spherical shape in comparison to conventional liposomes.

Transcutaneous delivery potential of the antigen-loaded system using human cadaver skin demonstrated a much higher skin permeation of the antigen in comparison to conventional liposomes and soluble antigen preparation (Mishra et al., 2007).

Ethosomal carrier for of methotrexate (MTX) showed the feasibility for dermal and transdermal delivery of MTX, which provides better transdermal flux, higher entrapment efficiency, and possesses the ability of a self-penetration enhancer as compared to conventional liposomes (Dubey et al., 2006). The Ibuprofen applied transdermally from the ethosomal gel was present in plasma for a longer period of time as compared to the oral administration and showed a high relative bioavailability (Shumilov et al., 2010). The *in vitro* transdermal testing of the ligustrazine ethosome patches showed that the cumulative 24 hr amount of ligustrazine was up to 183 ± 18 µg/cm^2. The pharmacokinetic results revealed that the relative bioavailability was 209.45%. It can be conclude that transdermal drug delivery via ethosomes has potentially extensive applications in medicine as a result of its high efficiency, convenient administration, and limited toxicity (Liu et al., 2011). List of application of ethosome were listed in Table 2.

Table 1. Diversity between the Ethosome and various other vesicular carriers.

Characters	Liposome	Niosome	Transferosomes	Ethosomes
Vesicles	Bilayer Lipid vesicle	Non ionic surfactant vesicles	2nd generation elastic lipid vesicle carriers	3rd generation elastic lipid vesicle carriers
Composition	Phospholipids and Cholesterol	Cholesterol and Non-ionic surfactant	Phospholipids and Surfactant	Phospholipids and Ethanol
Characteristics	Microscopic Spheres (Vesicles)	Flexible liposome	Ultraflexible Liposome	Elastic Liposome
Flexibility	Rigid in nature	Rigid due to cholesterol. Moderate deformability	High deformability due to surfactant	High deformability and elasticity due to ethanol
Permeation Mechanism	Diffusion/Fusion/ Lipolysis	Adsorption and fusion of vesicles	Deformation of vesicle	Lipid Perturbation
Extent of Skin Penetration	Penetration rate is very less as the stiff shape and size does not allow to pass through stratum corneum	Penetration is more than conventional liposome	Can easily penetrate through paracellular space by flexible structure	Can easily penetrate through paracellular space by ethanol effect
Route of administration	Oral, Parenteral. Topical and transdermal	Oral ,Topical and Transdermal	Topical and Transdermal	Topical and Transdermal
Limitation	Cannot penetrates to deeper skin	Due to surfactant it may cause skin irritation. Leaking of entrapped drug	Due to surfactant it may cause skin irritation. and stable in gel form only	All drugs are not soluble in ethanol
Marketed products	Ambisome, DaunoXome, Doxil, Abelect	Lancome, Niosome™	Transfersomes® (Idea AG)	Nanominox, Cellutight EF, Noicellex, Decorin Cream

Phospholipid

Surfactant

Cholesterol

Ethanol

Table 2. Ethosomes as Hauler of restorative agents for topical/ skin delivery.

Formulations	Principle ingredients	Rationale of Ethosomal delivery	Application	Route of administration	Ref.
5-Aminolevulinic acid ethosomes	5-Aminolev-ulinic acid(ALA)	Significantly improved the delivery of ALA in the inflammatory skin	Anti-psoriasis	Topical	Yi-Ping et al., 2009
Ammonium glycyrrhizinate ethosomes	Ammonium glycyrrhiz-inate	Ethosomes reduced the erythema more rapidly with respect to drug solutions.	Anti-inflammatory	Topical	Paolino et al., 2005
Epigallocatechin gallate ethosomes	Epigallocat-echin gallate (EGCG)	Entrapment of (-)-epigallocatechin gallate (EGCG) into ethosome was carried out for improving its stability against decomposition.	Anti-infective	Skin	Hyo et al., 2007
Erythromycin ethosomes	Erythromy-cin	Ethosomal erythromycin was highly efficient in eradicating S. aureus-induced intradermal infections	Antibacterial	Skin	Godin and Touitou, 2005a,b
Isoeugenol ethosomes	Isoeugenol	Chemicals (allergen) in vesicular carrier systems can enhance the sensitizing capacity.	Allergens	Skin	Jakob et al., 2010
Matrine ethosomes	Matrine	Improves the percutaneous permeation	Anti-inflammatory	Topical	Zhaowu et al., 2009
Methotrexate ethosomes	Methotrexate	Ethosomes showed favorable skin permeation characteristics	Anti-psoriasis	Skin	Dubey et al., 2007
Minoxidil ethosomes	Minoxidil	Enhances the penetration and accumulation of Minoxidil in the skin by Pilocebaceous targeting	Hair growth promoter	Topical	Lopez-Pinto et al., 2005
Testosterone ethosomes	Testosterone	Testosterone ethosomes for enhanced transdermal delivery	Steroidal hormone	Skin	Touitou et al.,2000
Trihexyphenidyl HCl ethosomes	Trihexyphe-nidyl HCl (THP)	Increased drug entrapment efficiency, reduced side effect & constant systemic levels	Anti Parkinsonian	Skin	Dayan and Touitou, 2000

Table 2. *(Continued)*

Formulations	Principle ingredients	Rationale of Ethosomal delivery	Application	Route of administration	Ref.
Acyclovir ethosomes	Acyclovir Palmitate (ACV-C16)	Binary combination of the lipophilic pro-drug ACV-C16 and the ethosomes synergistically enhanced ACV absorption into the skin.	Antiviral	Skin	Zhou et al., 2010
Azelaic acid ethosomes	Azelaic acid	Release rate was higher from ethosomes than from liposomes	Anti-keratinizing	Topical	Esposito et al., 2004
Bacitracin ethosomes	Bacitracin	Ethosomal enhances intracellular delivery of bacitracin and reduced drug toxicity in the skin	polypeptide anti-biotic	Topical	Godin and Touitou, 2004
Colchicine ethosomes	Colchicine	Enhance skin accumulation, prolong release and improve the site specificity	Anti-gout	Skin	Singh et al., 2008
Finasteride ethosomes	Finasteride	Ethosomes are promising vesicular carriers for enhancing percutaneous absorption of finasteride.	5α-reductase inhibitor	Skin	Roa et al., 2008
Fluconazole ethosomes	Fluconazole	Enhances the skin permeation	Antifungal	Topical	Bhalaria et al., 2009
Ibuprofen ethosomes	Ibuprofen	Transdermal nanosystem, designed by using an ethosomal carrier	Antipyretic	Topical	Shumilov et al., 2010
Ligustrazine ethosomes	Ligustrazine	Ethosome patch enhances the permeation in the skin	Pulmonary vaso-dilator	Skin	Liu et al., 2011
Salbutamol ethosomes	Salbutamol	Enhanced drug delivery through skin with ethosomes	Anti-asthmatic	Skin	Bendas and Tadros, 2007
Sotalol ethosomes	Sotalol	Enhances the systemic absorption	Antiarrhythmic	Skin	Kirjavainen et al., 1999
Vitamin A Palmitate, Vitamin E, Vitamin C ethosomes	Vitamin A Vitamin E Vitamin C	Anti-oxidation of phospholipid was increase due to the synergistic interaction of all three together as compare to individual use	Vitamins	Topical	Koli et al., 2008

Ethosomes in the Service of Marketed Drug Delivery

Transdermal drug delivery generated major interest among large pharmaceutical companies in the 1980s and 1990s. Many topical preparations contain active ingredients which can only act when they penetrate at least the outermost layer of the skin, the stratum corneum. However, due to the resistance of the stratum corneum to the transport into the skin, the efficacy of topically applied actives is often far from required. Attempts to improve formulation of topical products are a continuing process and the development of micro- and nanovesicular systems as well as polymeric microparticles has led to marketing of topical drugs and cosmetics using these technologies. The ethosomes were found to be suitable for various applications within the pharmaceutical, biotechnology, veterinary, cosmetic, and nutraceuticals markets. List of marketed approved ethosomal formulation in Table 3.

Table 3. Marketed products based on Ethosomal formulation.

Products	Narrative	Mechanism
Body Shape (Maccabi-CARE)	Gel Executive solidification Cellulite reduction, stretching the skin flexible and based on a technology called Ethosome	Deeper diffusion into the skin
Cellutight EF (Hampden Health, USA)	Topical cellulite cream, contains a powerful combination of ingredient to increase metabolism and breakdown fats	Deeper penetration into the skin
Nanominox (Sinere, Germany)	Nanominox composed of 4% Minoxidil, Adenosine, Sophora Flavescens extract, Creatine Ethyl Ester, Cepharanthine, B12, Ethanol, distilled water, and uses ethosomes as the vehicle to deliver the active ingredients. Nanominox absorb for 10 minutes prior to washing your hair when other Minoxidil solutions, including those with nanosomes and/or liposomes, suggest 2-4 hr for adequate absorption.	Pilosebaceous Targeting and High penetration into deep layers of the skin.
Noicellex (NTT, Israel)	Topical anti-cellulite creams	Deeper diffusion into the skin
Osmotics Lipoduction Cellulite Cream (Osmotics, Israel)	Ethosomal cream is designed to help reduce cellulite and burn fat when applied to the skin.	Deeper penetration into the skin
SkinGenuity (Physonics, Nottingham,UK)	Using a unique blend of active anti-cellulite ingredients with the ingenious Ethosomes™ Delivery System to ensure good penetration, Skin Genuity drastically reduces those dimples. It also firms and softens your skin with natural antioxidants and moisturising agents to give you the peachy thighs and dimple-free derrière	High penetration into deep layers of the skin.
Supravir cream (Trima, Israel)	For the treatment of herpes virus , formulation of acyclovir drug has a long shelf life with no stability problems, stable for at least 3 year, at 25°C. skin permeation experiments showed that creams retained its initial penetration enhancing properties even after 3 years	Lipid Perturbation

The NTT, Novel Therapeutic Technology Inc., is biopharmaceutical company, having a portfolio of pharmaceutical formulations based on ethosomes technology, including formulations for the treatment of alopecia, deep skin infection, herpes, hormone deficiencies, inflammation, post-operative nausea, atopic dermatitis, and erectile dysfunction (Elsayed et al., 2007). Ethosomes are composed from safe and approved materials for pharmaceutical and cosmetic use and take the form of creams, gels, patches, spray and other semi solid forms, which have the advantage of high levels of patient compliance. Products using the technology are already on the market and company generating revenues.

CONCLUSION

Transdermal route is promising alternative to drug delivery for systemic effect. The rate of penetration of most drugs through the skin is controlled by the structure of the stratum corneum. The ability of the skin to impede the permeation of molecules means that, to date, only a small number of pharmaceutically active compounds have been suitable for conventional transdermal delivery. Liposomes have their limitations, however they are most effective for local skin delivery. Liposomes create a drug reservoir in the upper layer of the stratum corneum. If a compound needs to enter systemic circulation, ethosomes are more effective. In the skin, it increases permeability by disrupting the lipid bilayer of the stratum corneum. Lipid vesicles for enhancing drug skin permeation have been specially designed using various approaches. For this purpose, ethosomes, soft vesicles with fluid bilayers, and the elastic vesicles, have been invented. Although, each vesicle type has its own characteristics, their common feature is their ability to improve the delivery of drugs across the skin barrier. The high tolerability and efficiency of vesicular systems, such as ethosomes, open vast potential therapeutic uses. These carriers might offer advanced local and systemic new therapies with agents that are unable to efficiently penetrate the stratum corneum via passive diffusion. Concurrently, the ethanol concentration causes the lipid membrane to be more malleable than conventional vesicles but just as stable. This increased flexibility allows the ethosome to squeeze through smaller openings in the stratum corneum, namely the ones created when the skin came into contact with the ethanol in the ethosome. This efficient transport system has been demonstrated to be effective with macromolecules such as peptides, making ethosomes a promising candidate for future TDD products. Enhanced delivery of bioactive molecules through the skin and cellular membranes by means of an ethosomal carrier opens numerous challenges and opportunities for the research and future development of novel improved therapies. Ethosomal systems are sophisticated conceptually, but characterized by simplicity in their preparation, safety and efficiency–a rare combination that could expand their applications. The highly efficient delivery makes this system a promising candidate for the administration of bioactive compounds in gel, cream, and spray dosage forms.

KEYWORDS

- **Cannabidiol**
- **Dermatopharmacotherapy**
- **Ethosomes**
- **Methotrexate**
- **Scanning electron microscopy**
- **Stratum corneum**
- **Trihexyphenidyl**

Chapter 2

Colloidal Delivery Systems for Phytochemicals

Ashok R. Patel

INTRODUCTION

Over the last decade or so there has been a sea change in the thought process of common man. More and more people have started linking food intimately to optimal health. This recent popularity among the masses of having healthy food as a part of their routine diet has driven the food industry to invest heavily and aggressively into the research dealing with fortification of food products (with phytochemicals) leading to the growth of a specialized category of food products called "functional foods". On the other hand, the pharmaceutical sector is vigorously working on identification of potential novel actives from natural product based traditional medicine systems (Ayurveda and Traditional Chinese Medicine), which could be used for treating complicated health conditions (cancer, diabetes, HIV/AIDS etc.). This combined interest from both food and pharmaceutical sectors has led to increased exploratory research on phytochemicals. Phytochemicals are naturally occurring, biologically active chemical compounds in plants.

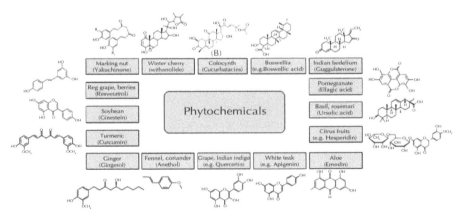

Figure 1. Examples of some of the phytochemicals with their sources.

The prefix "Phyto" is derived from a Greek word meaning "plant". Although there is no exact definition, "Phytochemicals" can be referred to as group of plant secondary metabolites that have little or no role in photosynthesis, respiration or growth and development but which may accumulate in surprisingly high concentrations (Cozier, et al., 2006). They differ from traditional vitamins as they are not essential nutrients and are often classified as non-nutritional. Also, there is a difference in the way human body perceives them. Whereas, there are specific mechanisms in the human body for accumulation and retention of vitamins, phytochemicals, in contrast, can be treated as non-nutrient xenobiotics (foreign substances) and metabolised to more excretable forms (Cozier, et al., 2009).

Phytochemicals includes a range of chemically unrelated compounds (e.g., carotenoids, flavonoids, phenolics, sulphoraphane, limonene, indoles, allium compounds etc.) having various biological properties (i.e., antioxidant, antiproliferative, antiinflammatory, etc., See Figure 1 and 2 for more examples), assumed to have evolved to allow plants to cope with environment challenges and harsh conditions like exposure to radiation and toxins, and defence against pests and infectious agents (Huffman, 2003; Tuteja et al., 2001).

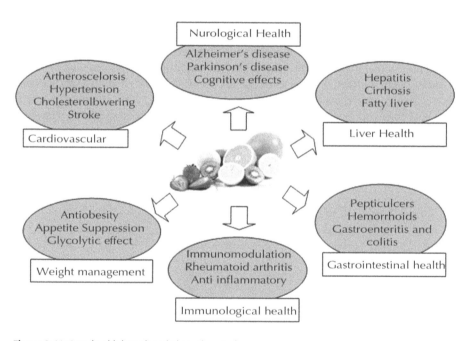

Figure 2. Various health benefits of phytochemicals.

PHYTOCHEMICALS AND SOME OF THEIR IMPORTANT HEALTH BENEFITS

Though, non-nutritional phytochemicals have been found to show a range of physiological effects and long term health benefits (Table 1). Some of their most important health benefits are emphasized with specific examples in the following section.

Table 1. List of some phytochemicals with their most commonly cited health benefits.

Compounds	Class	Health benefits	Ref.
Apocynin	Iridoid glycoside	Immune modulation	(Van et al., 2001)
Arjunolic acid	Triterpene	Lipid lowering	(Tiwari et al., 1990)
Artemisinin	Sesquiterpene lactone	Immune modulation	(Zhang et al., 1995)
Berberine	Alkaloid	Hypoglycemia	(Prabhakar et al., 2009)
Beta carotene	Carotenoid	Cardiovascular	(Riccioni, 2009)
Lycopene	Caretenoid	Cardiovascular	(Riccioni, 2009)
Astaxanthin	Caretenoid	Cardiovascular	(Riccioni, 2009)
Catechins	Polyphenols	Antihypertensive	(Negishi et al., 2004)
Diosgenin	Saponin	Hypolipidemic	(Sharma et al., 1996)
Evoline	Alkaloid	Nervine sedative	(Gupta et al., 2007)
Limonin and	Triterpenoids	Hypolipidemic	(Kurowska et al., 2000)
Limonoids Gingkolides	Diterpenoids	Neuroprotective effects	(Ahlemeyer et al., 2003)
Marsupin	Phenolics	Anti diabetic activity	(Manickam et al., 1997)
Withanolide	Steroidal lactone	Nervine sedative	(Kulkarni et al., 2008)
Reservatrol	Stilbene	Cardiovascular effects	(Bradamante et al., 2004)
Kadsurenone	Lignan	Antirheumatic	(Gurib-Fakim, 2006)
Swerchirin	Xanthone	Hypoglycemic activity	(Saxena et al., 1996)
Karanjin	Flavone	Hypoglycemic activity	(Mandal et al., 1986)
Shatavarin	Triterpenoid saponin	Immunostimulant	(Gautam et al., 2004)
Guggulsterone	Phytosterol	Cholesterol lowering	(Nityanand et al., 1989)

Cardiovascular Health

Despite the decline in rates of mortality due to heart diseases during the past two decades, cardiovascular diseases remain the most frequent cause of death. Hypertension is a common and most powerful contributor to all of the major cardiovascular diseases including coronary disease, stroke, peripheral artery disease, renal disease and heart failure. It affects up to 30% of the adult population in most countries. It is estimated that 7.6 million premature deaths (about 13.5% of the global total) and 92 million deaths and disability-adjusted life years (DALYS) (6.0% of the global total) are attributable to hypertensive conditions (Lawes et al., 2008). Epidemiological studies have shown an inverse relationship between intake of phenolics and flavonoids rich vegetables/fruits and chronic diseases such as cardiovascular diseases (Iriti et al., 2009; Soler et al., 2009; Yang, 2009).

Specific Examples

Chronic administration of flavanol quercetin (5 or 10 mgkg^{-1}day^{-1}) lowered blood pressure or prevented the development of hypertension in various experimental animal models (Duarte et al., 2001; Perez-Vizcaino et al., 2006). Results from *in vitro* and *in vivo* studies have also suggested curative and preventive effects of quercetin related flavanol on atherosclerosis (Pappas et al., 2009). Briefly, atherosclerosis is assumed to be initiated by the gradual incorporation of oxidized lipoproteins into blood vessel walls. Flavonols are believed to act via an inhibitory effect on low density lipoproteins (LDL) oxidation owing to their strong antioxidant properties (Catherine, 2007). Organosulfur compounds from garlic like allicin and S-allylcysteine have shown some promising results on blood pressure and cholesterol lowering in preclinical studies (Ali et al., 2000; Cruz et al., 2007; Sharifi et al., 2003).

Neurological Health

There has been a lot of convincing data on age related loss of neurological function due to the reduced ability of aged brain to counter oxidative insults (Markesbery, 1997). Accordingly, strong antioxidant properties of phytochemicals have been exploited to derive neuroprotective effects (Youdim et al., 2001).

Specific Examples

Polyphenolics from different sources (e.g., strawberry, spinach, blueberry, tea, red bell pepper, aged garlic extract, and herbal remedies) have been studied for their neuroprotective effects with some promising results. The antioxidant effects of quercetin have been associated with a reduced risk of neurodegenerative disorders in animal models (Anand et al., 1994; Shutenko et al., 1999). Benefical neuroprotective effects of curcumin, a polyphenol obtained from *Curcuma longa*, have been demonstrated successfully in different animal models (Peeyush et al., 2009; Yadav et al., 2009). Apart from neuroprotective effects, phytochemicals have also been studied for other pharmacological central nervous system (CNS) effects like tranquillizer, anticonvulsant, and depressant activity. For example, Jatamansone a sesquiterpene ketone found in *Nardostachys jatamansi*, Pongamol, a flavonoid found in *Pongamia pinnata* and Swertiamarin, a secoiridoid glycoside obtained from *Swertia chirata* have been found to show tranquillizer, anticonvulsant and CNS depressant effect respectively (Arora et al., 1962; Basu et al., 1994; Bhattacharya et al., 1976).

Liver Health

Chronic liver diseases represent a major health burden worldwide, with liver cirrhosis being among the leading cause of death in Western countries. Therapies developed along the principles of Western medicine are often limited in efficacy, carry the risk of adverse effects, and are often too costly, especially for the developing world. Therefore, treating liver diseases with plant-derived compounds which are accessible and do not require laborious pharmaceutical synthesis seems highly attractive. Many herbs belonging to alternative medicine systems have a long history of traditional use in revitalizing the liver and treating liver dysfunction and disease. Many of these herbs have been evaluated in clinical studies and are now being investigated phytochemically to understand their actions in a better way (Mukherjee et al., 2009).

Specific Examples

Extract of ayurvedic medicinal herb, *Sida acuta* have been found to show significant hepatoprotective activity in animals attributed to its phenolics constituent-ferulic acid (Sreedevi et al., 2009) Terpenes and flavanoid constituents of *Cleome droserifolia* have also proved to possess hepatoprotective activities (Abdel et al., 2009). Hepatotprotective effects of apigenin and kutkins in extracts of *Eclipta alba* and *Picrorhiza kurroa* have been demonstrated in *in vivo* studies (Saraswat et al., 1997; Saxena et al., 1993). Silymarin from *Silybum marianum*, listed in pharmacopoeial monographs for herbal drugs and herbal preparations is one of the main therapeutic used for its hepatoprotective effects (Stickel et al., 2007).

Gastrointestinal Health

Stomach ulcers are one of the main age-related ailments among general population. They were traditionally believed to be caused by non infectious mechanisms because the stomach is highly acidic and thus hostile environment for bacterial survival. However, *Helicobacter pylori* have recently been implicated as the primary cause of these diseases and are estimated to cause 60–90% of all gastric cancers (Malfertheiner et al., 2005). Adhesion of *H. Pyroli* to the cell lining of gastro intestinal tract is considered as an important parameter responsible for progression of stomach ulcers. Condensed phenols and flavonoids from cranberries have found to inhibit the adhesion of *H. pylori* to gastric mucosal constituents and gastric cell lines (Burger et al., 2000).

Specific Examples

Bergenin and neobergenin, isocoumarin phytochemicals, isolated from *Fluggea micrcarpa Blume* demonstrated significant protection against aspirin-induced peptic ulcer and pylorus-ligation in animal models. The mechanism of gastro-protective action was attributed to the increased prostaglandin production (Kumar et al., 1985). Luvangetin, a pyranocoumarin isolated from *Aegle marmelos Correa* has gastro-protective action similar to bergenin and neobergenin however mode of action is proposed to be different (Goel et al., 1997).

Immunological Health

The human defensive system is based on a highly organised and well coordinated immune response which performs complex and prompt molecular functions to maintain homeostasis. Immunomodulation, a collection of immunoregulatory cascades to bring about their specific stimulatory, suppressive or regulatory effect, has been utilized in clinical settings for cancer treatment, to combat specific infection and inflammation. Though, immunomodulation have mostly been achieved in past with the use of synthetic immuno drugs, of late many studies have been focussed on exploiting bioactive molecules as a source of immunodrugs.

Specific Examples

Recently, active constituents of *Glycyrrhiza glabra* (glycyrrhizic acid and its aglycone) were shown to exert a hepatoprotective effect via modulation of immune-mediated hepatocyte toxicity (Yoshikawa et al., 1997). Glycyrrhizic acid has also been reported to increase the resistance to *Candida albicans* and herpes simplex virus-1 infection in animal models (Sekizawa et al., 2001; Utsunomiya et al., 2000). Oxindole alkaloids from *Uncaria tomentosa* have shown positive influence on IL-1, IL-6 and IFN-γ production, suggesting immunoregulatory activity (Winkler et al., 2004).

Randomized clinical studies on a purified extract rich in pentacyclic alkaloids from same plants, also demonstrated benefit in patients with active rheumatoid arthritis (Mur et al., 2002).

Weight Management

Obesity have been increasingly considered by many as a lifestyle disorder and gaining newer findings of the genes and molecules involved in the development of obesity is creating new methods of obesity regulation.

Specific Examples

Ayurvedic herbs like Vrikshamla (*Garcinia*) have a long history of use as anti obesity agents. The actives like hydroxy citric acid present in Vrikshamla reduce the body's translation of carbohydrates to fats, helping burn calories. It also averts the loss of lean body mass (muscle) and augments the body's basal metabolic rate (Bagchi et al., 2006). Investigation suggests that this natural extract may also hold back the conversion of excess calories to body fat. Additionally, appetite is also suppressed by promoting synthesis of glycogen (Bagchi et al., 2006; Lewis et al., 1965). *Meshashringi/ Gymnema or Gurmara Gymnema*, whose Hindi name exactly means 'sugar destroyer', has been shown *in vitro* to have a glycolytic action and the capability to reduce the strength of a glucose solution (Yoshikawa et al., 1989). It has been used in Ayurveda for numerous centuries to regulate sugar metabolism. *Gymnema* increases the insulin production, possibly by repairing or regenerating pancreas cells, the site of insulin production. It also eliminates the taste of sugar, which effectively suppresses and reduces the effect the craving for sweets. The active constituent responsible for its activity has been identified as Gymnemic acids (Yoshikawa et al., 1989).

CHALLENGES RELATED TO FORMULATION AND DELIVERY OF PHYTOCHEMICALS

Although thousands of phytochemicals have been identified and many of their benefits have already been proven in animal models, their incorporation in food or pharmaceutical products has been sparse. Also, the diverse health potentials of Alternative medicine systems like Ayurveda and Traditional Chinese medicine (TCM) actives remain to be exploited completely by the food and pharmaceutical industries and their application in these filed is still in its infancy. One of the reasons for this underutilisation could be attributed to the array of problems associated with formulating and efficient delivery of these phytochemicals. Several formulation issues encountered are briefly outlined below (tabulated in scheme I for concise view).

Solubility

Many phytochemicals are poorly water soluble and hydrophobic in nature owing to their molecular structures. Low solubility can pose some serious problems with respect to formulation (difficulty in incorporating them into products) and *in vivo* performance (e.g., limited absorption, low bioavailability, and requirement of higher doses for producing desired effect). For example, Curcumin, a natural polyphenol isolated from turmeric (*Curcuma longa*) is a low molecular weight compound with a wide array of pharmacological activity, including antioxidant, anti inflammatory, neuroprotective etc. (Musthaba et al., 2009a). However, most of these effects have shown limited benefits in clinical settings. Limited aqueous solubility of curcumin was considered as one of the main factors responsible for such low bioavailability. When it comes to food products, hydrophobic actives are often delivered by using oil/lipid base for solubilisation. However, the introduction of low fat and fat free products has led to reopening of the problem of incorporating low solubility compounds in food products.

Chemical Reactivity and Degradation

Phytochemicals can be very unstable compounds once taken outside their natural environment in the plant and are thus susceptible to degradation and loss of bioactivity. Phytochemicals with reactive functional groups like allylic sulphides (allicin obtained from garlic), polyphenolics (e.g., Catechins, from green tea) etc., are reactive and more prone to have chemical incompatibility with common ingredients used in formulation. Apart from reactivity, some of the phytochemicals are also photolabile (e.g., curcumin and curcuminoids) and are thus susceptible to degradation when exposed to light. Tanins, a class of polyphenolic compounds show susceptibility of complex formation with proteins or other macromolecules and oxidation by trace metallic contaminants (Negishi et al., 2004). Formulation problems coupled with stability issues thus poses a great challenge for formulating effective systems of reactive phytochemicals.

Stability in Physiological Conditions

Orally ingested molecules have to go through the hostile journey of gastrointestinal tract with variation in pH, acidity, alkalinity and enzymatic attack to finally get absorbed and reach the systemic circulation. Due to their reactive nature, many phytochemicals show variable levels of instability in physiological conditions leading to degradation and loss of activity. For example Catechins, a polyphenolic plant metabolite abundant in tea derived from *Camellia sinensis,* shows susceptibility to chemical degradation in alkaline conditions resulting in an oral bioavailabilty of less than 5% (Musthaba et al., 2009a; Patel et al., 2011). Silymarin, a flavonol glycoside obtained from dried fruits of *Silybus marianum*, has a very poor oral bioavailability attribute to its degradation in gastrointestinal tract (Samaligy et al., 2006).

First Pass Metabolism and Pharmacokinetics

The first-pass metabolism (also known as first-pass effect or presystemic metabolism) is a phenomenon of drug metabolism whereby the concentration of drug is greatly reduced before it reaches the systemic circulation. It is the fraction of lost drug during the process of absorption which is generally related to the liver and gut wall metabolism. Many phytochemicals with their susceptibility to enzymatic attack undergo rapid first pass metabolism resulting in low bioavailability. Curcumin is heavily metabolised in the enterocytes of gut wall due to the attack by enzyme alcohol dehydrogenase and in hepatocytes of liver owing to the presence of various hepatic enzymes (Anand et al., 2007). Apart from first pass metabolism, poor pharmacokinetics of phytochemicals can be in form of poor absorption due to limited permeability (e.g., ellagic acid, a dietary antioxidant) (Sonaje et al., 2007) or rapid systemic clearance due to instability in plasma. For example camptothecin, a natural alkaloid extracted from *Camptotheca acuminate,* gets hydrolysed in physiological conditions (pH 7.4 at 37°C) and in blood resulting in reduction of its biological activity. The rapid hydrolysis in plasma occurs within only few minutes after 4. injection leading to prompt systemic clearance (Musthaba et al., 2009a).

Organoleptic Properties and Aesthetic Appeal

Organoleptic properties and appearance of products becomes very important for acceptance of food products by consumers. Unfortunately, phytochemicals are generally associated with undiserable organoleptic properties. For example, flavonoids, isoflavones, terpenes, and glucosinolates are almost always bitter, acrid, or astringent (e.g., Quercetin, present in fruit juices has extremely bitter taste). Most polyphenols generally give strong astringent taste due to their interaction with salivary proteins. Allicin, a polyphenolic compound extracted from garlic gives strong unacceptable odour (Drewnowski et al., 2000). Thus, it is quite a challenge to add these functional ingredients to food products without compromising the product functionality.

Based on the conventional definition, colloidal delivery systems can be categorised as one of the following dispersion systems:

- Solid-in-liquid dispersions such as colloidal particles formed from pure bioactive compound or embedded in polymeric, polymer conjugates and solid lipid carriers, or molecular complexes in colloidal form.
- Liquid-in-liquid dispersions such as colloidal emulsions from pure bioactive compounds and their melts or solutions in liquid carriers.
- Dispersions of self-assembled colloidal systems such as micelles (from surface active molecules and polymers), liposomes, liquid crystal phases (e.g., cubosome), and procolloidal systems (that forms colloidal structure after administration) (Boyd, 2008).

The selection of appropriate colloidal system depends a lot on the desired requirement. For example, solubilization of bioactive molecules can be achieved by simpler colloidal systems like micelles. However, if controlled release of bioactive molecules is desired, we have to find ways to encapsulate bioactive molecules using polymeric carriers (e.g., polymeric nanoparticles) or lipidic carriers (liposomes). Sophisticated requirements like targeting to specific site or decreasing metabolism requires use of advanced systems like immuno-conjugates, modified liposomes etc.

The following section summarizes application of various colloidal technologies for delivery of phytochemicals along with some cited examples. Since, delivery of phytochemicals in food product is relatively new field, the examples are pooled together for delivery systems of phytochemicals in general (also including pharmaceutical field).

- Low solubility

Formulation challenges:

- Big challenge in formulation of oral liquid products like beverages.

- Some phytochemicals show limited solubility in oil as well thus creating problem for development of oil based products.

- Low solubility could result in precipitation on storage thereby affecting the shelf life of the product.

Delivery challenges:

- Dissolution rate limited absorption.

- Low and variable oral bioavailability.

- **Chemical reactivity**

Formulation challenges

- Interaction with the component of formulation.

- Instability related to the pH of the product.

- Interaction with contaminants (metallic traces).

-Requirement of special packaging or storage condition for the products containing photolabile phytochemicals.

Delivery challenges

- Interference with absorption.

- Loss of bioactivity.

- Side effects due to reaction products.

- Instability in physiological conditions

- Degradation in GI tract.

- Low bioaccessability (amount of drug available for absorption).

- **Poor pharmacokinetics**

- Susceptibility to enzymatic metabolism.

- Low bioaccessibility and bioavailability.

- Variable clinical results.

- **Organoleptic properties**

- Difficult incorporation of phytochemicals in product formats (imparting undesired color and odor).

- Affecting the aesthetic appeal (consistency, appearance, and clarity).

- Unacceptability of product (bitterness and off-taste).

Scheme 1. Formulation and delivery challenges commonly encountered with incorporation of phytochemicals in food and pharmaceutical products.

Polymeric Nanoparticles and Polymer Conjugates

Nanoparticles (NP), are bioactive loaded colloidal particles prepared using natural polymers (e.g., chitosan, gelatin, albumin etc.) or synthetic biodegradable polymers such polylactide *co*-glycolide (PLGA) and poly lactide (PLA) as carrier stabilised using a surfactant or by other means(Gelperina et al., 2005; Patel et al., 2008b; Soppimath et al., 2001). Depending on the particle morphology, the bioactive molecules are embedded in the polymeric matrix or encapsulated in capsules with core-shell morphology (i.e., drug is encapsulated in the core surrounded by polymeric wall).

Features

As a delivery system, polymeric nanoparticles provide many advantages, such as solubility enhancement, improvement of absorption, protection of labile active against degradation, protection against enzymatic metabolism and enhancement of therapeutic efficiency. Furthermore, their distribution *in vivo* can be easily tuned by chemical or physical modification and thus, can be used for targeting to specific site. Hydrophobicity of polymeric nanoparticles makes them susceptible to opsonization resulting in decreased *in vivo* circulation time. To overcome this problem, nanoparticles have been derivatized using polyethylene glycol (PEG) resulting in extending the circulation times in blood after oral absorption (Owens et al., 2006).

Reported Applications

Catechins have known to have a low bioavailability (< 5%) and a short half life owing to strong systemic clearance. Chitosan nanoparticles were developed for oral delivery for improvement of its oral bioavailability (Zhang et. al., 2007). Polymeric nanoparticles with an average particle size of less than 50 nm were prepared in order to improve the solubility and stability of curcumin (Sahu et al., 2008a). Table 2 gives the list of polymeric nanoparticles of phytochemicals.

Polymer conjugation techniques include covalent modification of bioactive molecules in order to achieve desired advantages. Polymer conjugates have been successfully applied for the delivery of phytochemicals for example water soluble 4-poly ethylene glycol derivatives of podophyllotoxin and polymer bound campotheticin have been developed for effective antitumor activity (Caiolfa et al., 2000; Greenwald et al., 1999).

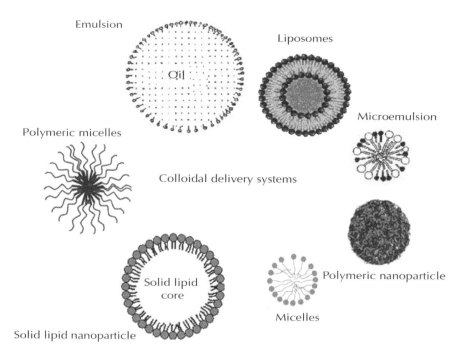

Figure 3. Schematic representation of some colloidal delivery systems (not in scale).

Table 2. Phytochemicals formulated in polymeric nanoparticles.

Bioactive	Carrier material	Ref.
Paclitaxel	D,L- polylactic acid	(Fu et al., 2006)
Triptolide	D,L- polylactic acid	(Liu et al., 2005)
Camptothecin	Hydrophobically modified chitosan	(Min et al., 2008)
Hypericin	Poly lactic acid and polylactic-*co*-glycolic acid	(Zeisser-Labouebe et al., 2006)
Berberine	Chitosan	(Lin et al., 2007)

Solid Lipid Nanoparticles

Solid lipid nanoparticles (SLN) refer to submicron size spheres prepared using lipids that remain solid at room temperature. The lipid component could comprise of one or more of following, fatty acids, fatty alcohols, mono-, di- or tri glycerides, and glyceride mixture or waxes (Mehnert et al., 2001; Wissing et al., 2004).

Features

The SLN as a delivery system presents many potential advantages: (a) protection of labile molecules against chemical degradation by minimising effect of light and oxygen; (b) controlled release of incorporated molecule due to the slower digestion rate; (c) possibility of drug targeting and (d) no issues with sterilization (Pardieke et al., 2009).

Reported Applications

The SLN have been explored for the delivery of phytochemicals (Table 3 gives the list of phytochemicals formulated as SLN). Quercetin, a natural flavonoid compound have been formulated as SLN in order increase its oral absorption and as per the results from animal studies, it was found that SLN showed more than 90% absorption of quercetin (Li et al., 2008). Triptolide was encapsulated in SLN to achieve controlled release and it was seen that incorporation of triptolide led to an increase in its anti-inflammatory activity and decreased toxicity (Mei et al., 2005). Curcuminoids loaded SLN were incorporated in cream in order to minimize its chemical and photo degradation, SLN formulation was found to be stable for up to 6 months (Tiyaboonchai et al., 2007).

Colloidal Particles

Preparing nanoparticles from bioactive compound itself is a very useful technique in oral delivery for enhancement of dissolution/solubilisation rate for poorly water soluble compounds and thus can be used as an effective technique for improvement of solubility limited low oral bioavailability. Formation of nanosized particles can be achieved either by top-down processes, based upon milling, or bottom up processes based upon molecular condensation (e.g., precipitation). The most common methods using the former principles includes (1) milling which includes mechanical reduction of size of molecules to sub-micron level using media mills. This technique has been commercialized by many pharmaceutical (e.g., Nanocrystal® which finds extensive application in pharmaceutical field) and chemical companies and (2) High pressure homogenisation where large drug crystals are subjected to high energy attrition leading to formation of drug particles in nanometer ranges (Liversidge et al., 2009). Other methods involve spontaneous precipitation and stabilisation of bioactive molecule by removing the solubilising solvent. Techniques like rapid expansion from supercritical solution (RESS) and gas antisolvent recrystallisation (GAS) uses supercritical fluid as a solvent whereas technique like (nano) precipitation and solvent evaporation uses organic solvent (Boyd, 2008; Patel et al., 2010a).

Features
Simple preparation method, no requirement of additional carrier material, enhanced dissolution rate due to increase in the surface area owing to the decreased particle size.

Reported Applications
Oleanolic acid, a naturally derived triterpene was formulated as nanosuspension using precipitation method without use of any other excipients in order to improve its oral bioavailaibility (Yajun et al., 2005). Curcumin was formulated as composite colloidal particles along with zein protein (using solvent evaporation) to enhance its water dispersibility and pH stability (Patel et al., 2010b).Whereas, formulations of Nab-paclitaxel and Phytosterols were prepared by similar method (solvent evaporation) using albumin and Tween 80 as stabilisers respectively (Laura et al., 2010; Stinchcombe, 2007).

Table 3. Phytochemicals formulated as SLN.

Bioactive	Main lipid material	Ref.
Glycyrrhizic acid	Lecithin	(Hou et al., 2008)
Podophyllotoxin	Soybean lecithin	(Chen et al., 2006)
Triptolide	Tristearin glyceride	(Mei et al., 2003)
Hydroxy camptothecin	Soyabean lecithin	(Xi. et al., 2007)
Silibinin	Bean lecithin	(Li et al., 2007)

Emulsions
Emulsions are the most common of the colloidal delivery systems used. Emulsion refers to a dispersion system that is composed of two immiscible liquids stabilised using surface active molecules (or particles). They can have very broad droplet size ranges. For clarity, we will refer to microscale emulsion (droplet size 1–20 μm) and nanoscale or submicron emulsions (<1 μm). The later ones are also known as miniemulsions and nanoemulsions. Another class of emulsions which form spontaneously, are historically called as microemulsions, (0.005–0.05 μm). Microemulsions are very close to micelles in their behaviour than the other emulsions classes.

Features
Microscale emulsions though used commonly as a delivery system in pharmaceuticals, suffers from disadvantages of being thermodynamically unstable and tendency to cream and coalesce over the time if other means for stabilisation are not used. Microemulsions on the other hand are thermodynamically stable and spontaneously formed. As a delivery system, microemulsions can offer numerous advantages, such as optical clarity, enhanced solubilisation and dissolution rate, increased absorption through the lymph and sustained release of the drug packed in the inner phase (Lu et al., 2005; Patel

et al., 2007). Nanoscale emulsions are kinetically very stable and also provide similar advantages like microemulsions but at lower surfactant concentration or without using surfactant but proteins.

Reported Applications
So far, phytochemicals have been formulated as emulsions for transdermal and topical use. For example, microemulsion based gel formulation of babchi oil (*Psoralea coryfolia*), containing bioactive molecule furocoumarin psoralen for topical use (Ali et al., 2008). Nanoemulsion of curcumin prepared using high pressure homogenization showed good anti-inflammatory activity in animal models (Wnag et al., 2008). Microemulsion of dietary isoflavoid and flavanoids (Genistein, Fisetin and Luteolin) was used to increase their bioavailability and was used topical for the treatment of ocular neovascularisation (Joussen et al., 2008). Table 4 gives a list of phytochemicals formulated as nanoscale emulsion.

Table 4. Phytochemicals formulated as emulsions.

Categories	Purpose	Bioactive	Ref.
Berberine nanoemulsion	Nanoemulsion for oral use	Berberine	(Sun et al., 2007)
Paclitaxel submicron emulsion	Injectable emulsion	Paclitaxel	(Constantides et al., 2000)
Triptolide microemulsion	For transdermal delivery	Triptolide	(Chen et al., 2004)
Silybin nanoemulsion	Liver targeted delivery	Silybin	(Song et al., 2005)
Docetaxel submicron emulsion	Injectable emulsion	Docetaxel	(Li et al., 2007)

Micelles

Micelles is easily one of the earliest known colloidal systems. It is ubiquitously present from simple surfactant micelles to complex digestive mixed micelles formed in GI tract by the body during digestion of lipophillic compounds. Micelles can be defined as a colloidal aggregate of amphiphilic molecules, which occurs at a well-defined concentration called the critical micelle concentration (CMC). In polar media such as water, the hydrophobic part of the amphiphiles forming the micelle tends to locate away from the polar phase while the polar parts of the molecule (head groups) tend to locate at the polar micelle solvent interface. Micelles formed in non-polar media, with polar phase oriented towards the core and non polar phase forming the interface are termed as reversed micelle. A micelle may take several forms, depending on the conditions and composition of the system, such as distorted spheres, disks, or rods. When a combination of surfactants is used, we can also form a mixed micellar system which can be used as drug delivery system (Patel et al., 2008a).

Features
Micellar systems have following attributes to be considered as effective delivery systems: (a) small size (typically < 10 nm); (b) thermodynamic stability (spontaneous formation above CMC) and (c) colloidal stability (Boyd, 2008). Also, these systems can be introduced into various product formats without any issues of instability or interactions with other formulation components. However, the limited solubilisation

capacity of micelles means that there is a requirement of high amount of surfactants or surface active agents. Also, these surfactant based systems (also including microemulsions and self-emulsifying systems) have a tendency to impart undesirable taste to the formulation limiting their applicability in oral products.

Reported Applications

Curcumin was solubilised using the natural structure of casein micelles resulting in enhanced solubility and stability in physiological conditions (Sahu et al., 2008b). Carotenoids were solubilised in phospholipid micelles to improve their cellular uptake (Sugawara et al., 2001).

Polymeric Micelles

Block co-polymers have been known to form self assembling structure called polymer micelles. Polymeric micelles have been developed as an alternative to low molecular surfactant-based systems as they offer greater versatility in terms of formation of micellar structure at lower critical micellar concentration, relative higher stability and greater flexibility of chemical modification (Torchillin, 2007). The polymeric micelles generally comprise of a relatively hydrophobic block such as poly-lactic acid, poly-caprolactone and poly-aspartic acid, with a hydrophilic PEG segment (Boyd, 2008). Miceller carrier loaded with curcumin was prepared using methoxy poly (ethylene glycol) as the hydrophilic part, palmitic acid as the hydrophobic part and encapsulated curcumin showed enhanced solubility and bioavailability (Sahu et al., 2008a). In another study, docataxel was formulated in polymeric micelles for efficient anti-tumor activity (Ji et al., 2008). Recently, immunomicelles were developed by covalently linking functional moieties to poly ethylene glycol and poly ethylene micelles for porphyrin to achieve increased solubilisation (Roby et al., 2006). However, this delivery system does not find many applications in food products because the polymers used are synthetic and non food grade.

Table 5. Modified liposomes as delivery systems for phytochemicals.

Categories-Description and Purpose	Bioactive	Ref.
Immunoliposomes-Liposomes conjugated with antibodies for site specific delivery	Docetaxel	(Wang et al., 2006)
Magnetic liposomes-Liposomes loaded with ferromagnetic material for targeting and triggered release	Paclitaxel	(Zhu et al., 2007)
PEGylated liposomes-Liposomes with PEGylation to make the surface more hydrophilic in order to circumvent uptake by reticuloendothelial system	Curcumin	(Hong et al., 2008)
Glucoronide modified-Surface modification using uronic acid derivative palmityl-d-glucuronide to achieve longer circulation time	Vincristine	(Tokudome et al., 1996)

Liposomes

Liposomes are arguably the most studied colloidal delivery system, in fact, they were first developed for drug delivery purposes as early as 1970s (Musthaba et al., 2009b).

Liposomes consist of vesicular self-assembled system comprising of one or more bi-layers, usually formed using a phospholipid, surrounding an aqueous core.

Features

They are biodegradable, biocompatible and can be used as carriers for both lipophilic and hydrophilic molecules. Encapsulation of bioactive molecules could help in im-proving the solubilisation, stabilisation, enhanced permeation and protection from physiological degradation. Moreover, release of the drug can be modulated based on the amount of cholesterol incorporated. It is also possible to target liposomes to spe-cific organs like liver by manipulating its surface characteristics (Table 5 gives a list of modified liposomes used as delivery systems for phytochemicals).

Reported Applications

Given, the advantages it has to offer and the fact that it's an established delivery sys-tem in pharmaceuticals, liposomes have been extensively researched as a delivery system for problematic phytochemicals. For example, liposomal delivery for buccal administration was developed for improving the oral bioavailaibility of Silymarin. *In vitro* permeation and absorption studies resulted in better permeation of formula-tion as compared to free silymarin (El-Samaligy et al., 2006). Ginsenoside, a steroid glycoside, and triterpene saponin, found exclusively in the plant genus *Panax (gin-seng)* wereencapsulated in liposomes prepared using film dispersion method, is one of the earliest studied liposomes of Traditional Chinese Medicine (TCM) (Ding et al., 1995). Antioxidant and chemoprotective properties of tea catechins encapsulated in liposomal formulations for transdermal applications were studied and it was found that encapsulated catechins showed better permeation as compared to unencapsulated catechins (Fang et al., 2006). There are many studies to prove the usefulness of lipo-somes as a delivery system of phytochemicals; however, their instability in acidic pH limits their use in food products.

Pro-colloidal Systems

These are the dispersions, solutions, liquid crystal like systems which undergo a phase-transition and form a new colloidal structure on dilution with aqueous phase. Self-microemulsifying drug delivery systems (SMEDDS) are currently the most stud-ied systems and finds its application in delivery of water insoluble but lipid soluble compounds. Researchers have explored SMEDDS as a delivery system for improve-ment of oral bioavailability of poorly soluble phytochemicals. For example silymarin was formulated as SMEDDS using Tween 80, ethyl alcohol and ethyl linoleate and *in vivo* results showed remarkable improvement in its oral bioavailability (Wu et al., 2006). Enhancement in oral bioavailability was also observed for *Pueraria lobata* isoflavone when formulated as SMEDDS using ethyl oleate, Tween 80 and Trancutol P (Cui et al., 2005).

CONCLUSION

Phytochemicals have been shown to have various health benefits. Alternate medi-cine systems like Ayurveda and TCM are also becoming popular and there has been a growth of awareness among consumers about the safety and beneficial effect of plant based products. All these factors together have led to increased large scale production of herbal drugs and nutraceuticals. As more and more phytochemicals are identified and more of their health benefits are confirmed in biological conditions, there will be an equivalent rise in the demand for their delivery. The delivery of phytochemicals is rather challenging as they pose an array of problems and formulators are faced with challenges of solving multiple delivery problems. And this is where the knowledge of colloidal systems could come into play. Colloidal delivery can address many of the delivery problems while preserving desired product functionalities such as appearance, taste and stability. This could be exploited to develop new products of phytochemicals. Colloidal systems like gels, foams, emulsions and suspensions have long been used in food products for aesthetic properties or for obtaining desired consistency; however, use of colloidal systems developed with an aim of delivering specific nutrient is still limited. The potential of colloidal delivery has been well recognized, as demonstrated by the drastic increase in the number of research papers aimed at delivery of nutrients using novel delivery techniques. However, it should be kept in mind that colloidal delivery systems in foods need to be developed using edible and food grade materials and at concentrations of actives that are proven safe and meet all regulatory requirements. To achieve this, a lot of efforts are needed to be focussed on identifying natural polymers and materials which could be used as a replacement of synthetic raw materials used in drug delivery. Some of the potential materials include animal proteins (gelatine, collagen, albumin, casein and whey protein) and plant proteins (zein, soy glycinin, wheat gliadin). It is still an infant frontier and successful application to delivering functional ingredients in the complex food systems will require a collaborative effort from colloid scientists, food technologists, formulation scientists and biologists. But looking at the recent trend, it can be easily stated that colloidal delivery systems are really a step forward towards effective and efficient delivery of phytochemicals for incorporation in both foods as well as pharmaceuticals products.

KEYWORDS

- **Central nervous system**
- **Flavonols**
- **Hypertension**
- **Immunomodulation**
- **Low density lipoproteins**
- **Phytochemicals**
- **Solid lipid nanoparticles**
- **Traditional Chinese medicine**

ACKNOWLEDGMENT

This research is financially supported by Marie Curie International Incoming Fellowship within the 7th European Community Framework Programme.

Chapter 3

Polymer-modified Gene Delivery Vectors Retargeted with Recombinant Proteins

R. Pola, M. Pechar, K. Ulbrich, R. C. Carlisle, R. A. Willemsen, and L. W. Seymour

---

INTRODUCTION

Viral gene therapy is a very promising approach for treatment of oncological diseases. The transduction efficacy of viruses is still several orders of magnitude higher than that of any non-viral vectors. However, clinical applications of the viral vectors have been so far compromised by the poor target cell selectivity, high immunogenicity and rapid clearance of the vectors from the body. It has been demonstrated that modification of adenoviruses with hydrophilic synthetic polymers based on poly(ethylene glycol) (Eto et al., 2008) or poly[N-(2-hydroxypropyl)methacrylamide] (PHPMA) (Fisher et al., 2007; Kreppel and Kochanek, 2008) significantly prolongs plasma circulation times and ablates the non-specific cell entry. At the same time, surface modification of the viral capsids with multivalent polymers enables retargeting of the vectors with receptor-specific ligands, such as growth factors (Morrison et al., 2008), tumor-specific peptides (Stevenson et al., 2007) or folates (Oh et al., 2006).

It has been repeatedly reported that attachment of a low-molecular-weight drug to a polymer carrier often leads to improved pharmacokinetics, lower non-specific toxicity and better therapeutic efficacy. Polymer therapeutics (Duncan and Vicent, 2010) can be also targeted using various ligands (peptides, growth factors, cytokines, antibodies and their fragments) to specific organs or tissues, for example. to tumors.

Antibodies and their fragments have the highest targeting specificity. Unfortunately, covalent attachment of the two macromolecules (protein and synthetic polymer) is often non-selective and leads to a complex mixture with compromised biological activity. Precisely defined structure is also highly desirable because well defined chemical entities get eventual regulatory approval for clinical applications much easier. Supra-molecular non-covalent self-assembly of the two macromolecules represents a possible solution of the general problem.

In this work, we introduce a new universal tool for specific, high affinity and non-destructive attachment of recombinant proteins to other macromolecules such as synthetic or natural polymers or proteins. The principle of the method is based on the strong and non-covalent interaction between acetylcholine receptors and α-bungarotoxin (BTX).

It has been reported (Katchalski-Katzir et al., 2003) that synthetic peptide with amino acid sequence GSGGSGGTGYRSWRYYESSLEPYPD (BTXbp) derived from the structure of acetylcholine receptor binds BTX with high affinity.

We linked BTXbp to a reactive HPMA-based hydrophilic copolymer containing reactive thiazolidine-2-thione (TT) groups. The resulting peptide-bearing copolymer (PHPMA-BTXbp) was used for surface modification of an adenoviral gene delivery vector. A recombinant anti-PSMA antibody scFv fragment containing the BTX binding region (BTX-scFv) was prepared and added to the polymer-modified BTXbp-bearing adenovirus (Ad-PHPMA-BTXbp) encoding luciferase as a reporter gene (Ad) as shown in Figure 1. The fusion protein BTX-scFv served as a targeting ligand redirecting the natural viral tropism to prostate-specific membrane antigen (PSMA) on prostate cancer cell lines.

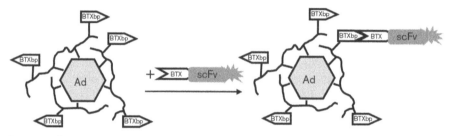

Figure 1. Schematic representation of a polymer-modified adenovirus targeted with a recombinant scFv antibody fragment attached via a bungarotoxin linker.

EXPERIMENTAL

Abbreviations

The AIBN, 2,2′-azobisisobutyronitrile; BTX, α-bungarotoxin; BTXbp, bungarotoxin binding peptide; DMSO, dimethyl sulfoxide; Dox, doxorubicin; HPMA, N-(2-hydroxypropyl) methacrylamide; Ma, methacryloyl; PSMA, prostate specific membrane antigen; scFv, single chain variable fragment; SEC, size-exclusion chromatography; TT, thiazolidine-2-thione. Standard single letter amino acid abbreviations are used.

Synthesis of the Peptide and Copolymers

Peptide BTXbp (GSGGSGGTGYRSWRYYESSLEPYPD, 2728 g mol^{-1}) was prepared by standard 9-fluorenylmethoxycarbonyl/tertiary butyl solid phase peptide synthesis on 2-chlorotrityl resin. The HPMA was prepared by reaction of methacryloyl chloride with 1-aminopropan-2-ol in dichloromethane (Ulbrich et al., 2000). The copolymer poly(HPMA-co-Ma-GG-TT) (polymer 1) was prepared by radical solution copolymerization of HPMA (90 mol%) and Ma-GG-TT (10 mol%) performed in DMSO at 50°C for 6 hr. The concentration of monomers in the copolymerization mixture was 15 wt% and that of AIBN initiator was 2 wt% (Šubr and Ulbrich, 2006).

The polymer-peptide conjugate (PHPMA-BTXbp) was prepared by reaction of the polymer 1 with the peptide in aqueous buffer at constant pH 7.4 for 2 hr at 25°C. The resulting polymer 2 was purified by gel filtration on Sephadex G-25 in water and lyophilized. Recombinant PSMA-specific BTX-scFv fusion protein was constructed, expressed in *E. Coli* and purified as described earlier (Willemsen et al., 2010).

Modification of the Adenoviruses with Polymers and Infection of the Cells

Polymer coating of Ad was performed by mixing Ad with PHPMA or PHPMA-BTXbp (polymer 1 or 2) in 10 mM HEPES buffer (1 hr, 10 mg/ml, pH 7.4). Recoveries were calculated using a Picogreen assay as previously reported for Ad-PHPMA using Oligreen (Carlisle et al., 2008). Mixing of 17 µl (10^9 copies) of polymer-coated Ad with 0.05 mg/ml solution of BTX-scFv in a total volume of 60 µl was then performed.

The LNCap and PC-3 carcinoma cells were obtained from ATCC; PSMA status was confirmed using an anti-PSMA antibody (AbCam) and flow cytometric analysis. The E1, E3 deleted Ad5 expressing CMV IE promoter driven luciferase was purchased from Hybrid Systems Ltd (Oxford, UK) and is denoted 'Ad' throughout.

Uptake studies were performed in suspension by incubating 200,000 cells with 10^7 copies of polymer-modified Ad sample for 90 min with constant agitation after purifying away unreached polymer using S400 columns 27-5140-01 (GE Healthcare). Cells were then spun (2000 g, 5 min), supernatant removed and a PBS wash performed. After re-suspension in 400 µl fresh media, half of the sample was analyzed for Ad genome content by QPCR as in (Carlisle et al., 2009) and half of the sample was re-plated and assayed at 24 hr for luciferase expression.

RESULTS AND DISCUSSION

Our initial attempts to bind the deprotected BTXbp to copolymer poly(HPMA-*co*-Ma-GG-TT) (polymer 1) in organic solvent always led to highly branched or even insoluble cross-linked product, probably due to acylation of the side chain of the two Arg and four Tyr residues in the amino acid sequence of BTXbp. As the pK_a value of the guanidino group of arginine is 12.5, it remains protonated under physiological conditions and is hardly available for the acylation at pH 7.4 used for the reaction. We also assumed that the eventual product of acylation of the phenolic group in tyrosine would be quickly hydrolyzed back as a result of general reactivity of phenyl esters with nucleophiles. Relative stability of the TT groups towards hydrolysis allowed us to bind most of the peptide to polymer in aqueous solution during 2 hr and still preserve half of TT groups for the subsequent modification of Ad (Scheme 1). The course of the binding reaction was monitored by HPLC. The resulting polymer 2 ($M_w = 65000$, $M_w/M_n = 2.7$) contained 16.7% w/w of BTXbp and 4.1% mol of TT.

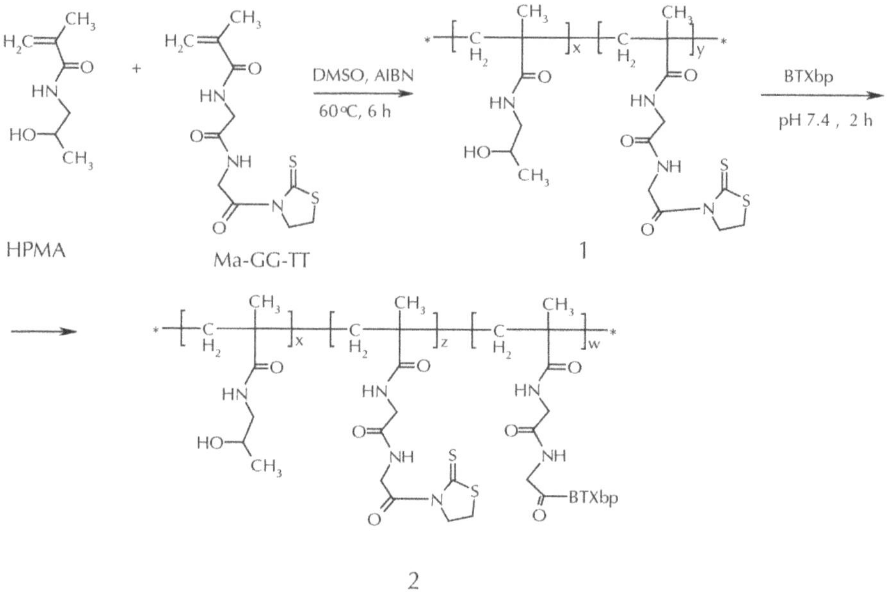

Scheme 1. Synthesis of the reactive copolymers

Successful systemic application of adenoviruses as gene delivery vectors is still associated with many serious hurdles such as immunogenicity, low target selectivity and short blood circulation times of the vectors. Surface modification of the viruses with hydrophilic synthetic polymers based for exampleon PEG or HPMA is a possible promising strategy overcoming at least to some extent the mentioned obstacles (Kreppel and Kochanek, 2008).

The first step in changing the undesirable natural Ad tropism is detargeting of the virus from its natural cell entry mechanism via coxsackie virus and adenovirus receptor (CAR). In this study, this was achieved by surface coating of Ad with multivalent highly hydrophilic HPMA-based copolymers 1 or 2. The ELISA studies confirmed that high efficiency of coating and protection of the capsid had been achieved. The finding was further confirmed by the fact that in cancer cell line infection studies, the polymer modification of Ad caused a knock-down in transgene expression of more than 100-fold. We assume that this decrease of infectivity is a result of polymer-shielding of the knob domain of Ad which is responsible for CAR receptor-mediated cell entry. Moreover, efficient coating of the adenovirus with hydrophilic HPMA copolymer protects it from interaction with anti-adenovirus antibodies. This result is in accordance with previously published data showing significant decrease of immunogenicity of proteins after their modification with HPMA copolymers and PEG (Rihova, 2002; Šubr et al., 2002).

The second important step is retargeting of the polymer-coated Ad to a specific cell receptor. Prostate-specific membrane antigen (PSMA) expressed on LNCaP cells was chosen in this work as a model target. To achieve PSMA targeting, a recombinant fusion protein BTX-scFv consisting of anti-PSMA antibody scFv fragment and BTX binding region was prepared. After the addition of BTX-scFv to Ad-PHPMA-BTXbp, the recombinant protein was non-covalently bound to the BTXbp sequences on the polymer-coated virus forming PSMA-targeted viral gene delivery vector (Ad-PHP-MA-BTXbp/BTX-scFv). This resulted in partial restoration of the luciferase transgene expression. Notably, no such restoration of luciferase expression was observed when BTX-scFv ligand was added to Ad-PHPMA with no BTXbp attachment handle. The results of a control experiment with PSMA-negative PC-3 cells showed no response to the addition of the targeting ligand, demonstrating the impressive selectivity and specificity of the system (Figure 2).

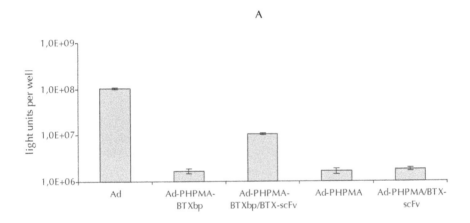

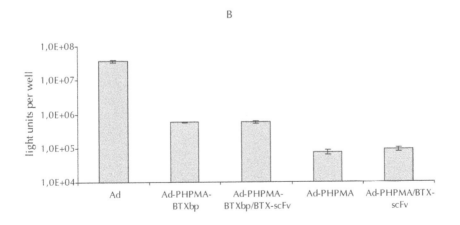

Figure 2. Luciferase expression in PSMA-positive LNCaP cells and PSMA-negative PC-3 cells after incubation with unmodified or polymer-modified Ad. Ad, polymer coated Ad or polymer-coated, retargeted Ad were prepared as described in the methods and used to infect LNCaP (panel A) or PC-3 cells (panel B). Luciferase reporter gene expression was assayed at 24 hr (see methods). N = 4, standard deviation shown, ** = p < 0.005.

CONCLUSION

We have successfully linked a recombinant PSMA-specific antibody scFv fragment to a polymer-modified Ad using a strong, non-covalent interaction between BTX and BTXbp. The retargeted Ad achieved significantly higher reporter gene expression in the PSMA receptor-positive cell line compared with the receptor negative cells. The presented data demonstrate the impressive activity and flexibility of the novel PHP-MA-BTXbp/BTX-scFv linker system that can provide a universal tool for achieving receptor-specific adenovirus gene transfer.

KEYWORDS

- **Bungarotoxin**
- **Poly(ethylene glycol)**
- **Prostate-specific membrane antigen**
- **Viral gene therapy**

ACKNOWLEDGMENT

The work was supported by Grant Agency of the Czech Republic, grant 203/08/0543 and by Ministry of Education of the Czech Republic, grant No. IM4635608802.

Chapter 4

Study of Drug Transport Properties of Acrylic Based Iron (III) Oxide Filled IPN

S. Goswami, K. Kiran, A. B. Panda, P. P. Sharma, S. K. Mahapatra, S. V. Bhoraskar, and I. Banerjee

INTRODUCTION

Synthetic polymer hydrogels are gaining interest for the control release of the drugs because of their good biocompatibility and water permeation properties. Interpenetrating polymer network (IPN) type hydrogel has proved to be more promising nowadays on account of its interlocked morphology along with hydrophilicity to hold as well as release the drug in required rate. The IPN is defined as a special class of polymer alloys, in which the possibility of phase separation has been arrested to a great extent by suitably engineering the morphologies of the participating components. In IPNs, one polymer is synthesized or cross-linked in the immediate presence of the other and they are at least partially interlaced on a molecular scale but not covalently bonded to each other and cannot be separated unless chemical bonds are broken. Also an IPN can be made suitable as carrier of drug delivery system, for periodic administration as required in chronic infection via oral or systemic routes when it is made biocompatible. Various studies have established that the local application of antibiotics provides high concentration of drug at the site of infection with a low systemic toxicity (Kaul et al., 2005; Nelson, 1987). Different local drug delivery systems with antibiotics have been attempted; however the most widely studied material has been an antibiotic-acrylic composite. Hydrophilic acrylics, for example poly acrylic acid, polyacrylamide, poly(2-hydroxyethyl acrylate), poly(hydroxylethyl methacrylate) and so on, are used for biocompatibility and/or biodegradability (Frutos et al., 2002; Majid et al., 1985; Nelson et al., 1993). The weight ratio of hydrophilic and hydrophobic components taken in the polymer blend, controls a range of properties for example, porosity, biocompatibility, toughness, % drug loading and release, swelling characteristics and cross-linking density etc. These are by far the leading factors governing the diffusional transport properties of the drugs into the matrix. Ferrer et al. showed formation of nanodomains (30–100 nm) in hydrophilic-hydrophobic IPN based on poly(2-hydroxyethyl acrylate) and poly(ethyl acrylate) and suggested their suitability for cell adhesion on that basis (Ferrer et al., 2007).

The transport properties of the drugs into the carrier matrix can further be enhanced by embedment of nanoparticles in the IPN matrix. Especially, targeted delivery of drugs by magnetically active drug carriers (polymers) using an externally applied magnetic field is very common. Super paramagnetic particles are widely used for such deliveries as they can be active even under much smaller magnetic field ~ 2–8 (Bean and Livingston, 1959; Neuberger et al., 2005; Vays and Khar, 2004). Literature reveals that in presence of magnetic field, the magnetic carriers demonstrated 16-fold increase in the maximum drug loading, 6-fold increase in drug release and 6-fold increase in the drug targeting efficiency to rat tail target segments (Widder et al., 1978).

The main aim of the present study is to see the difussional transport properties of a semi –II IPN, based on hydrophilic poly(2-hydroxyethyl acrylate) (PHEA) and hydrophobic polybutyl acrylate(PBA) and to find out its efficiency as multi drug carrier for targeted delivery. Elastomeric PBA was used to give the IPN enough toughness in combination to the hydrophilic nature of PHEA required for the biocompatibility and drug dissolution. The diffusion kinetics studies for metaprolol succinate (MS) and Aspirin (SA) have been done. The *in vitro* drug release studies have been conducted in presence of *E. coli*. Embedment of magnetic nanoparticles in the IPN-gel was carried out and the effect on drug transport phenomenon was checked.

MATERIALS AND METHODS

Butyl acrylate (BA) from CDH (New Delhi, India) was purified by washing first with 2% aqueous potassium hydroxide solution, then by thorough and repeated washings with distilled water (to make alkali free, as tested by litmus paper) and dried over anhydrous calcium chloride and finally vacuum distilled. The 2-hydroxy ethyl acrylate (HEA) from Aldrich Chemical Company (Germany) was used without further purification. Benzoyl peroxide (Bz_2O_2) from Loba Chemie Pvt Ltd. (Mumbai, India) was purified by repeated crystallisation from chloroform. Ethylene glycol dimethacrylate (EGDMA) (Aldrich Chemical Company, Germany), without any modification was used as the cross-linker and co-monomer.

The powders of iron oxide particles of sizes 20 nm were prepared by DC thermal arc-plasma method using iron block of commercial grade. The details of the experimental set-up of DC thermal arc plasma method are given in earlier report (Ferrer et al., 2007; Goswami et al., 2011). Also magnetic property of the particles was reported there.

Metaprolol succinate, as a model drug, was kindly provided by Dr. Reddy's laboratories, Bengaluru, India and Aspirin (2-acetoxy benzoic acid), was taken from CDH, New Delhi.

Poly butyl acrylate polymer was first formed, under constant stirring and inert atmosphere, in presence of 2% Bz_2O_2 initiator at 80°C, along with the nanoparticles of iron (III) oxide pre-mixed with it. The Fe_3O_4 nanoparticle embedded PBA mass was swollen in a mixture of 2-hydroxyethyl acrylate monomer, the initiator and 2% EGDMA crosslinker for 24 hr at room temperature and then allowed to heat again at 80°C till the white crosslinked gel was formed. Uniform mixing of iron oxide particles with the PBA polymer was assured from magnetic response of the NP-IPN sample taken randomly from the mass. The IPNs were prepared by taking the two acrylates in 50:50 blend ratio (w/w). The samples, designated as "NP-IPN" were purified by distillation from ethanol for 24 hr (Ferrer et al., 2007) to remove the unreacted monomers and finally vacuum dried to constant weight at 50°C. These dried samples were used for characterization. For comparison of properties, IPNs without iron (III) oxide particles, designated as "IPN-gel", were also prepared and purified in the same way.

THEORY/CALCULATION

Biocompatibility of Iron (III) Oxide Nanoparticles

Growth of *E. coli* in the presence of *arc* generated Fe_3O_4 nanoparticles in nutrient broth medium was studied to test their biocompatibility. *E. coli* bacteria were grown in 50 ml of nutrient broth at 37°C for 48 hr maintaining a pH of 7–7.2 with synthesized nano particles dispersed in the broth medium. The pre-weighed 25 µg of iron oxide powder was immersed in bacterial suspension and were kept in shaker incubator to set the whole of the bacterial suspension under uniform contact to the nanoparticles during growth. The optical density (absorbance at 660 nm) was then taken using UV-VIS Spectrophotometer, Perkin Elmer, USA at 1 hr intervals each for determining the cell counts to study the bacterial growth curve. A growth curve of mother culture had also been obtained in similar manner for comparison. The optical density at 660 nm has been calibrated to be equivalent to 107 cells/ml in our case through serial dilution viable count method. Number of cells per ml against time was then plotted for obtaining the bacterial growth curve.

Characterisation of IPNs

Polymer films of both the types of IPNs were characterized by FTIR spectroscopy (SHIMADZU IR Prestige-21, Japan) in ATR mode within the wavelength range 400–4000 cm⁻¹. Crosslink density of the IPNs, with or without the iron (III) oxide particles were determined by using Flory-Rehner equation (Gupta and Hung, 1989; Madhukumar et al., 1994) as follows:

$$\gamma = \frac{[V_p + \chi V_p^2 + \ln(1 - Vp)]}{[d_r V_s (V_p^{1/3} - V_p / 2)]} \qquad (1)$$

where, V_p = volume fraction of polymer in the swollen mass, V_s = molar volume of solvent, d_s = density of solvent, d_r = density of polymer, χ, polymer-solvent interaction parameter according to Bristow and Watson (Adegbite and Olorode,2002; Goswami et al., 2005; Shantha and Harding, 2003) is given by

$$\chi = \beta + \left(\frac{V_s}{RT}\right) \times (\delta_s - \delta_p)^2 \qquad (2)$$

where β = lattice constant (0.34); R, universal gas constant (cal/K/mol); T, absolute temperature (K), δ_p and δ_s are solubility parameter of IPN and solvent respectively γ=crosslink density of the polymer sample; M_c^{-1} = molecular weight of polymer chain in between two successive crosslinks. The parameter V_p was found out by using equation,

$$V_p = 1/1 + Q, \qquad (3)$$

Where,
$$Q = \frac{m - m_0}{m} \times \frac{d_r}{d_s}$$
(4),

m_0, m are mass of dry and swollen polymer in gm respectively. The IPN samples were dipped in a series of solvents having solubility parameter in the range (18–22 MPa$^{1/2}$) up to equilibrium swelling in each. The % swelling (Q) was then calculated and with the help of equation 1, degree of cross-linking was determined (Goswami et al., 2005; Gupta and Hung, 1989).

The cross-linked networked structure of the prepared IPNs was assessed by swelling behaviour of the circular samples of 1 cm diameter, as prepared by pressing the gel like mass in between two glass slides under vacuum drying. The dried and pre-weighed samples were immersed in water for 24 hr at 37°C during which period the polymer attained equilibrium swelling. Then the swollen samples were carefully taken out at 1 hr interval, wiped with a filter paper for the removal of free water on the surface, and then weighed. The degree of swelling was calculated using the following equation:

$$SR(\%) = \left[\frac{(w_t - w_d)}{w_d} \right] \times 100$$
(5)

where w_d and w_t are the weights of dry and wet samples at time t respectively. All measurements were triplicated for each sample.

For characterization of the response to different pH environments, the circular samples of IPNs, as mentioned in swelling experiment, were allowed to reach equilibrium swelling in three different pH solution namely 4, 6, and 9 at 37°C. The pH values were selected to allow comparison of swelling behavior in human G.I. conditions. Equilibrium swelling studies were conducted gravimetrically using the equation 5.

In vitro Drug Release Study in Presence of E. coli

The drug loading was carried out by swelling the known amount of IPN samples, in circular disc form of 1 cm diameter, in drug solution at 37°C. After immersing the samples in the drug solution for 24 hr, it was taken out, dried and reweighed. The increase in dry weight of the hydrogel was taken as the amount of drug loaded. The 2mg/ml solution of Metaprolol Succinate (MS) and Aspirin (SA) were used for drug loading in IPN samples.

In vitro release of the drugs loaded in IPN and NP-IPN was tested in presence of E. coli (NCIM 2809) bacteria. Proper cleaning of the equipments and IPNs was done with distilled water and autoclaved at 121.5°C, 15 psi for 30 min. The E. coli bacteria were grown in 50 ml of nutrient broth at 37°C for 48 hr maintaining a pH of 7–7.2 with drug loaded with IPN and NP-IPN samples (Brice et al., 2005).

Drug Release Through the IPN

The UV-VIS spectrophotometer was used to measure the absorbance at a fixed wavelength of 274 nm for MS and 296 nm for SA. The absorbance was tested at least twice on every sample to ensure stable and accurate results. All tests occurred at ambient temperature of 30°C. The MS and SA drug solutions of 0.056, 0.028, 0.014, 0.007, and 0.0035 mg/ml concentration were prepared by dilution of the 0.112 mg/ml stock prepared in a volumetric flask. The absorbance of these solutions was tested. A calibration curve for each of the drug sample were generated with concentrations ranging from 0.112 mg/ml to 0.0035 mg/ml. Using the correlation-regression analysis, a linear equation was applied to each set of calibration data. From these equations, the drug concentration in a given solution (e.g., the medium during release study) was calculated from its UV absorbance level.

The drug loading for this study was done following the same procedure as mentioned above. Drug release experiments were carried out in diffusion cell having two chambers side- to- side separated by a semi-permeable membrane. In one of the chambers the dried drug loaded IPN discs in solution (at pH 9) were taken and in the other, only solution was taken. This arrangement was done keeping in mind a comparison with the diffusion of drug through the mucous membrane inside the GI tract of human body.

The experimental set up is shown here in Figure 1. The entire diffusion cell was placed into an incubator at 37°C (JEIO TECH, SI-300R, Korea) for 30 min prior to the commencement of the experiment to ensure complete wetting of the drug loaded sample in the solution. The experiment started with the stirring of the cells at a constant 100 rpm, by the incubator. This ensured complete homogeneity of the released drug in solution within the diffusion cell. The top of the cell was sealed with a glass stopper to avoid the evaporation of water.

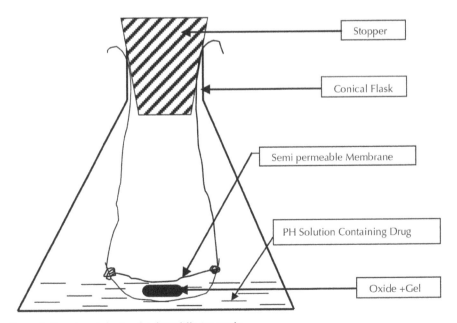

Figure 1. Experimental setup for drug diffusion study.

During the diffusion experiment, samples of 4 ml were withdrawn from the cell at specific time points. The time points were at 5, 15, 30, 60, 120, and 240 min. Each of the withdrawn samples was tested spectrophotometrically and the concentration of the specific drug was calculated. A series of time-release curves were developed based on the data collected from above experiments to describe the release behavior of the IPN materials. The fractional drug release (M_t/M_∞) of each IPN polymer sample was estimated using an optimization approach. Partition coefficient of drug between the IPN and solution was calculated using the modified method of Sato and Kim (Sato and Kim, 1984).

$$K_d = \frac{[V_0(C_0 - C_s)]}{V_m C_s} \tag{6}$$

where, V_0 is the volume of solution, V_m the volume of polymer film, C_0 the initial solute concentration and C_s the solute concentration in the solution at the equilibrium. The initial solute concentrations in the experiment were similar to those in the diffusion tests. The Cs was measured spectrophotometrically. The V_m was measured gravimetrically from the density of dry IPNs.

RESULTS AND DISCUSSION

Biocompatibility of Iron(III) Oxide

Figure 2a shows the undistorted growth curve of E. coli cells in presence of iron oxide nano particles hence confirming the biocompatibility of the nanoparticles. The iron oxide has caused prolonged stagnant phase of the E. coli in comparison to that in mother culture (MC). Iron acts as electron acceptor for bacteria that can couple organic matter oxidation to Fe (III) reduction in the absence of oxygen (Madhukumar et al., 1994).

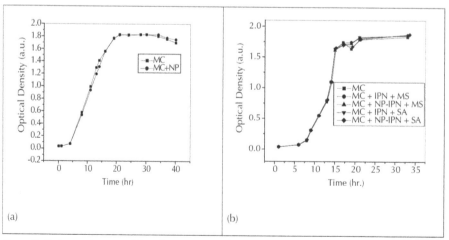

Figure 2. Cell growth curve of E. coli in presence of (a) pure Iron oxide nanoparticles in MC and (b) drug loaded IPN gel and NP-IPN

Iron-reducing bacteria are thus able to gain energy from the reduction of sol-uble or solid iron species (Ferrer et al., 2007). Also it is well established that iron act both as nutrient and as electron acceptor, on the growth and cultivability of bacteria like *E. coli,* which is a good source of penicillin amidase (Brice et al., 2005). In view of this, further the same growth study of the *E. coli* cells was per-formed in presence of drug loaded IPNs presented in Figure 2b. The graph also confirms the biocompatibility of the drug loaded IPNs and its suitability as drug delivery system.

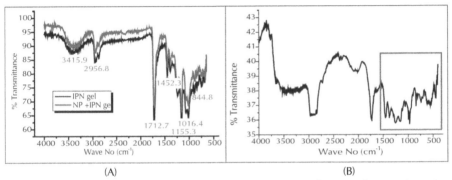

(A)   (B)

Figure 3. (a). FTIR spectra of IPN- gel and NP–IPN (b) FTIR spectra of NP-IPN showing absorption in the range 500–1500 cm^{-1}

Properties of IPNs

The FTIR spectra of IPN-gel and NP-IPN (Figure 3) shows characteristic transmit-tance peaks corresponding to O-H, C-H and C=O stretching with no change in peak intensities. This indicates the absence of direct chemical bonding of the nanoparticles with the acrylate components.

It could be inferred that acrylate polymerization in presence of the nanoparticles, might has taken place without any alteration in reaction mechanism. However, the embedment of iron (III) oxide particles in the gel is clear from the above results (peak in the range 440–650 cm^{-1}).

Decrease (approx.16.9%) in cross-link density is found (Figure 4) due to em-bedment of nanoparticles in NP-IPN compared to that of IPN-gel. Free radical polymerization and cross-linking of acrylics depends upon the ease of formation and mobility of the long chain radical through an increasingly viscous medium. Presence of clustered foreign particles (Goswami et al., 2011), for example, iron (III) oxide, in the medium may have restricted the mobility of the chain radicals thereby reducing the probability of the curing reaction. Higher the cross-link den-sity, lower is the penetration of solvent molecules in the network; hence is the observation here. Extent of swelling in distilled water is plotted here for both IPN-gel and NP-IPN.

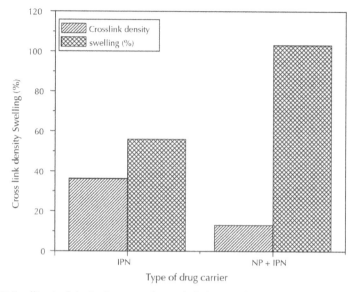

Figure 4. % Swelling in deionised water and cross-link density of the IPN-gel and NP-IPN

The swelling characteristic of IPN-gel with respect to that of the NP-IPN in different pH medium is demonstrated in Figure 5. Equilibrium swelling of the IPN-gel and NP-IPN has been found to be more significant in alkaline pH than in acidic pH. The NP-IPN has shown increased swelling compared to that of the IPN-gel. This may be due to preferred degree of ionization of the NP-IPN through the iron (III) oxide particles in the alkaline medium (Liu et al., 2003).

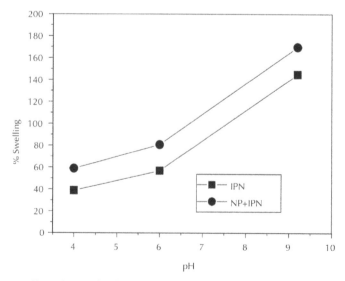

Figure 5. % Swelling of IPN-gel and NP-IPN in different pH medium after 3 weeks.

Study of Drug Loading and Release

Drug loading data as observed in Figure 6 shows enhancement of loading in NP-IPN compared to that in IPN-gel. This may be due to the higher porosity caused by lower degree of cross-linking in the former matrix. Percentage loading varies according to the nature of drug for example SA shows higher degree of loading in NP-IPN compared to that of MS whereas with IPN-gel, the trend is opposite. The amount of drug, which can be loaded into the polymeric material, depends on three parameters, namely, the drug solubility in the initial solution, the solvent volume fraction of the cross-linked hydrogel and the drug partition coefficient between the polymer and the solution (Varshosaz and Koopaie, 2002). The network cannot accommodate the entire volume of liquid if the crosslink density is too high and the solvent expels from the gel by contraction. It is evident from the partition coefficient values of SA and MS (Table 1) that NP-IPN gels can accommodate more solution compared to that of IPN-gel mesh. Solubility of SA (3.1 mg/ml) being lower than that of MS (276 mg/ml) (Ravishankar et al., 2011; Sumathi and Alok, 2002) is expected to be transferred to the IPN hydrogel pores more easily. In view of this, preferable loading of SA on IPN gel over MS in the present study could be inferred.

Table 1. Loading percentage (according to dry weight of the IPN-gel) and partition coefficient of MS and SA between IPN and solution (pH:9).

Samples	C_s (mg/ml)		C_0 (mg/ml)		Partition coefficient K_d		Loading% SA	MS
	SA	MS	SA	MS				
IPN-gel	1.77	1.87	2	2	0.028	0.015	4.7	2.14
NP-IPN	1.5	1.4	2	2	0.049	0.067	7.5	4.0

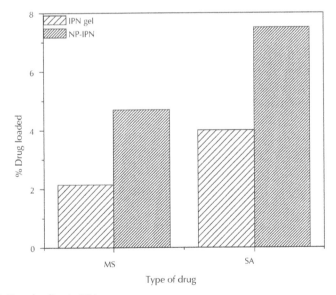

Figure 6. % Drug loading in IPNs.

Drug release study for the IPNs loaded with the different drugs reveals (Figure 7) that initial abrupt rise in the extent of drug release within 5 min is followed by steady release in next 20 min. Moreover, slower release from NP-IPN than that from IPN-gel particularly with SA is remarkable. Release rate of MS from NP-IPN was found to be independent of time beyond 20 min in contrast to the irregular release of the drug from IPN-gel.

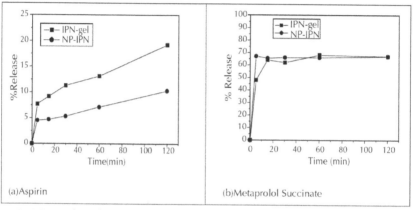

(a)Aspirin   (b)Metaprolol Succinate

Figure 7. % Drug release from IPNs with time.

In order to study drug transport mechanism from the different molecularly designed hydrogels, Ritger–Peppas (Zhou and Wang, 2001) diffusion equation was considered to fit the experimental data.

$$\frac{M_t}{M_\infty} = k_1 t^n$$

(7)

where M_t/M_∞ is the fractional drug release, k_1 is a kinetic constant, t is the release time and n is the diffusional exponent that can be related to the drug transport mechanism. The M_t/M_∞ values were calculated from the experimental curve in Figure 7 and log (M_t/M_∞) values were plotted against log(t) to find out the value of n from the slope of the line.

Table 2. Drug release kinetics parameters from log (M_t/M_∞) vs. log(t).

Sample	t (min)	-log (M_t/M_∞)		n	
		SA	MS	SA	MS
IPN-gel	5	1.1140	0.2516	0.48	0.16
	10	1.0375	0.1225		
	15	0.9469	0.1386		
	30	0.8823	0.1003		
	60	0.7158	0.1064		
	120	0.5053	0.1237		

Table 2. *(Continued)*

Sample	t (min)	-log (M_t/M_∞)		n	
		SA	MS	SA	MS
NP-IPN	5	1.3450	0.1153	0.52	0.05
	10	1.3293	0.1303		
	15	1.2726	0.1225		
	30	1.1468	0.1225		
	60	0.9871	0.1159		
	120	0.7073	0.0962		

The value of the diffusion exponent 'n' is found to be ~ 0.5 for SA which suggests the diffusion to be Fickian type. However, the diffusion behavior is deviated from the law in case of MS.

CONCLUSION

Super paramagnetic Fe_3O_4 nanoparticles were physically embedded in the bulk of acrylic IPNs. The effect of nanoparticles on the IPN properties in terms of cross-link density, swelling characteristics, drug transport phenomenon and biocompatibility was studied. The NP-IPNs showed lower degree of cross-linking but enhancement in swelling compared to IPN-gel. This is due to restricted mobility of growing polymer chains and unavailability of them for curing reaction, in the iron oxide embedded polymer matrix. *In vitro* biocompatibility test of the metal oxide nanoparticles and IPNs was successfully observed with *E. coli*. The presence of iron (III) oxide in NP-IPN, helped both as a nutrient and as an electron acceptor for *E. coli* cells, leading to bacterial cultivability and delayed death compared to that in IPN-gel. The NP-IPNs showed higher percentage of drug loading compared to that of IPN-gels which may be due to greater porosity in the later, on account of the lower degree of cross-linking. However, drug release study gives clear indication about the possibility of the NP-IPNs use as controlled release delivery system. In case of Aspirin, the transport of drug seems to be purely Fickian diffusion in contrast to that of Metaprolol succinate.

KEYWORDS

- **Interpenetrating polymer network**
- **Metaprolol succinate**
- **Mother culture**
- **Polybutyl acrylate**
- **Synthetic polymer hydrogels**

ACKNOWLEDGMENT

This research work is supported financially by Department of Science and Technology, Govt. of India, under a project in FAST Track scheme received by S. Goswami. The authors would like to thank Ms. Tishna Bal, Department of Pharmaceutical Sciences, for her kind presentation of the model drug for this work.

Chapter 5

Poly(Amido-amine)s as Carriers for Intracellular Delivery of Drugs and Proteins

Fabio Fenili, Elena Ferrari, Amedea Manfredi, Roberta Cavalli, Simon C. W. Richardson, Elisabetta Ranucci, and Paolo Ferruti

---

INTRODUCTION

Structure and Preparation

Polyamidoamines (PAAs) are synthetic polymers carrying amide- (a) and *tert*-amine (b) groups regularly arranged along the polymer chain according to the sequences …a…a…b…b… or …a…a…b…. They are prepared by Michael polyaddition of primary or secondary amines to bisacrylamides (Scheme 1) (Danusso and Ferruti, 1970; Ferruti, 1996; Ferruti et al., 1985).

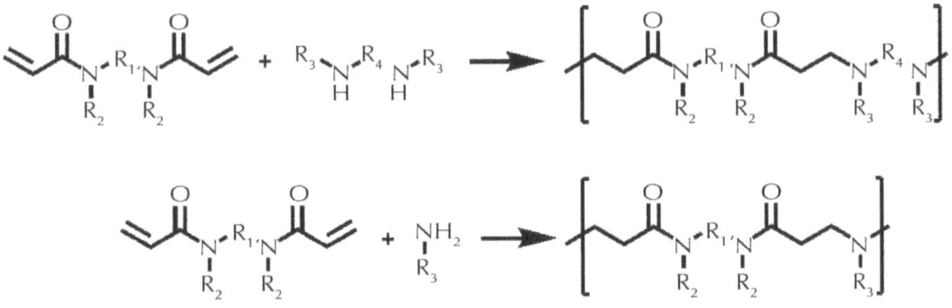

Scheme 1. Synthesis of linear PAAs. R_1, R_2, R_3 and R_4 can be any alkyl residues eventually containing carboxyl, amide, ester, ether groups.

The PAAs are endowed with a combination of properties that make them appealing for practical applications, particularly in the biotechnological field.

The preparation process of PAAs is simple, easily scaleable and environmentally friendly. It takes place in water or alcohols, at room temperature and without added catalysts (Ferruti et al., 1994; Manfredi et al., 2007). The number-average and weight-average molecular weights of the PAAs usually range between 5,000–40,000 and 10,000–80,000 respectively. The PAAs are water-soluble and nearly all of them are soluble in dilute acids. Narrow polydispersity fractions can be obtained by fractionation techniques, as for instance ultrafiltration through membranes of definite cut-off. By employing suitably functionalized monomers, additional functions, such as hydroxyl-, carboxyl-, allyl- and *tert*-amine groups may be distributed as pendants along the polymer chain. Other chemical groups such as thiols and primary or secondary amines can be introduced if first protected and then de-protected by standard procedures (Ferruti et al., 2002). Peptide moieties can be easily inserted for targeting purposes either as pendants or as integral portions of the polymer chain. The PAA-protein conjugates can be also synthesized. Other targeting moieties, such as sugar moieties, can be inserted by simply adding amino-sugars to the polymerization recipe (Casali et al., 2001). This imparts to PAAs a remarkable structural versatility, which is probably unique in stepwise polymers (leaving perhaps apart thermosetting resins) and is only surpassed by polyvinyl polymers.

Chemical Properties

Acid-Base Properties

All PAAs contain *tert*-amine groups in their main chain (Ferruti et al., 2000; Pattrick et al., 2001). In the absence of additional acid or basic substituents, they are low to medium strength polymeric bases with pK_{a1} and (when present) pK_{a2} values in the order of 7.5–8.5 and 3.5–6.5, respectively. They may experience sharp increase in their ionizations state, and become membrane-active, if as a consequence of cell internalization they localize in lysosomes, where the pH drops to 5.5 or whereabouts. Carboxylated PAAs are amphoteric, and by selecting the starting monomers their acid-base properties can be tuned in order to obtain PAAs prevailingly negatively or positively charged, and according to the body's district in which they reside, capable to pass from a negative to a positive species upon cell internalization (Ranucci et al., 2009). The acid-base properties of a typical amphoteric PAA named ISA 23 and its ionization state as a function of pH is shown in Figure 1.

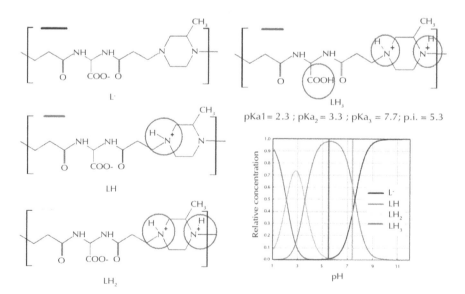

Figure 1. Relative amounts of the differently charged units of a typical amphoteric PAA as a function of pH.

For comparison purposes, the protonation profiles of three typical PAAs, including ISA 23, is shown in Figure 2.

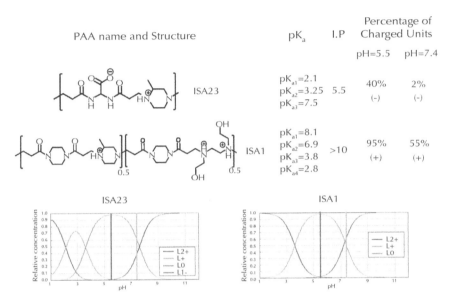

Figure 2. Comparison between the protonation profiles of ISA23 and ISA 1. Each set of curves represents the relative abundance of the differently charged units of the PAA as a function of pH.

Degradability

The PAAs are degradable in aqueous media. The degradation of several PAAs has been extensively studied by means of viscometric and chromatographic techniques (Franchini and Ferruti, 2005; Ranucci et al., 1994. It was found that the degradation rate is affected by the structure of both the amide and the amine moieties and increases by increasing temperature and pH. The mechanism of PAAs degradation is purely hydrolytic as no vinyl groups, such as those that would have derived from a β-elimination, that is, retro-Michael reaction, are present in degraded samples (Bignotti et al., 1994). The *tert*-amine groups in β position to the amide groups along the polymer chain catalyze the degradation reaction, but tritosomal enzymes do not affect it (Ranucci et al., 1991). In a biomedical context, the degradability of PAAs is important, since it allows renal clearance once the polymer has completed its function. The cytotoxicity of the low molecular weight degradation products was determined and found to be similar, or lower, then that of the native polymers.

Biological Properties

Toxicity

Cationic PAAs are usually two or more orders or magnitude less cytotoxic (IC_{50} in the range 0.5–3 mg/mL) than other commonly used polycations such as poly-L-lysine (PLL) and poly(ethyleneimine) (PEI). Amphoteric PAAs are even more biocompatible. The cytotoxicity of ISA23, and ISA1 is reported in Table 1 together with those of PLL and PEI.

Table 1. Cytotoxicity and net average charge at pH 7.4 of PAAs.

Sample	Average (%) of charge per unit (pH 7.4)	IC_{50}
ISA23	40 (-)	>5 mg/ml
ISA1	55 (+)	3 mg/ ml
PEI	>95 (+)	0.005 mg/ml
PLL	>95 (+)	0.01 mg/ml

Cell Uptake and Intracellular Trafficking

Uptake and intracellular trafficking of fluorescent labeled-PAA conjugates were performed in B16F10 cells *in vitro* using endocytosed and immunological markers to define specific intracellular compartments. Cells internalize PAAs *via* the endocytic pathway. In intracellular compartments, where the pH is first lowered to 6.5 (endosomes) then to 5.0 (lysosomes), they become prevailingly cationic and display endosomolytic properties (Lavignac et al., 2004; Richardson et al., 1999, 2010). Fluorescence microscopy revealed co-localization of ISA1 and ISA23 with Lysotracker (marker for lysosome and late endocytic structures). The ISA1 also co-localized with the Early Endosomal Antigen 1 (EEA-1) that accumulates in early endocytic structures (Richardson et al., 2010).

Body Distribution

The PAAs ISA23 and ISA1, re-named ISA22 and ISA4 after labeling with radioactive probes, were parenterally administered to mice. It was found that the purely cationic ISA4 had a different body distribution then the amphoteric ISA22 (Table 2). While the liver rapidly captured the former, the latter exhibited a "stealth-like" behavior, that is, circulates for prolonged time in the bloodstream (Richardson et al., 1999). Moreover, ISA22 administered to tumor-bearing mice showed a clear tendency to localize in the tumor mass (Table 3).

Table 2. Body distribution of ^{125}I-labelled PAAs after intravenous injection in rat.

Body district	Distribution (%)			
	ISA22		ISA4	
	after 1 hr	after 5 hr	after 1 hr	after 5 hr
Blood	≈70	≈20	≈1.5	≈0
Kidney	≈2	≈1	≈7	≈4
Liver	10	8	83	85
Lungs	≈2	≈4	≈4	≈3
Urine	≈13	≈65	≈0	≈15

Table 3. Distribution into tumoral tissues thanks to EPR effect of ^{125}I-Labelled ISA 22 after intravenous administration to mice with B16F10 cell Lines.

Tissue	Distribution (%)	
	After 1 hr	After 5 hr
Blood	≈10.7	≈4.5
Liver	≈2.1	≈2
Kidneys	≈2.2	≈1.8
Tumor	≈1.8	≈2.2

NEW GENERATION PAAS

PAA-SSPy as Intracytoplsmic Vehicle of Immunotoxines

Therapeutically relevant proteins such as antibodies, cytokines, growth factors, and enzymes are playing an increasing role in the treatment of viral, malignant, and autoimmune diseases. The development and successful application of therapeutic proteins, however, is often hindered by several difficulties, as for instance insufficient stability and shelf-life, costly production, immunogenic and allergic potential, as well as poor bioavailability and sensitivity towards proteases. To overcome these problems, a possible approach is to modify proteins by covalently conjugating them with water-soluble polymers, thus increasing their plasma residence, reducing protein immunogenicity and increasing their therapeutic index. Numerous polymer–protein conjugates with improved stability and pharmacokinetic properties have been developed by different authors, for example, by anchoring enzymes or biologically relevant proteins to polyethylene glycol components (PEGylation) (Duncan, 2003, 2006). Increasing attention has been devoted to the nature of the chemical linkage between the polymer backbone and the protein. In this work reductively cleavable disulphide bonds have been used. Disulfide bonds are stable in bloodstream but undergo reduction inside the cells, therefore can be regarded as "smart" stimuli-responsive linkages in polymer therapeutic design for intravenous administration (Arpicco et al., 1997).

Two PAAs bearing pendant 2-ethenyldithiopyridine (ISA1-SSPy and ISA23-SSPy) (Figure 3) were used to investigate their ability to mediate intracellular delivery of the type I ribosome-inactivating gelonin.

The strategy adopted consists of a three step synthesis. In the first step, a cystamine cross-linked PAA was synthesized generating a hydrophilic tri-dimensional network. In the second step, the hydrogel obtained was de-reticulated by direct disulfide exchange reaction with dipyridyl disulfide. Finally, the linear and soluble PAA-SSPy thus obtained was conjugated via thiol-disulfide exchange reaction to a thiol-containing gelonin, a ribosome inactivating protein (Scheme 2).

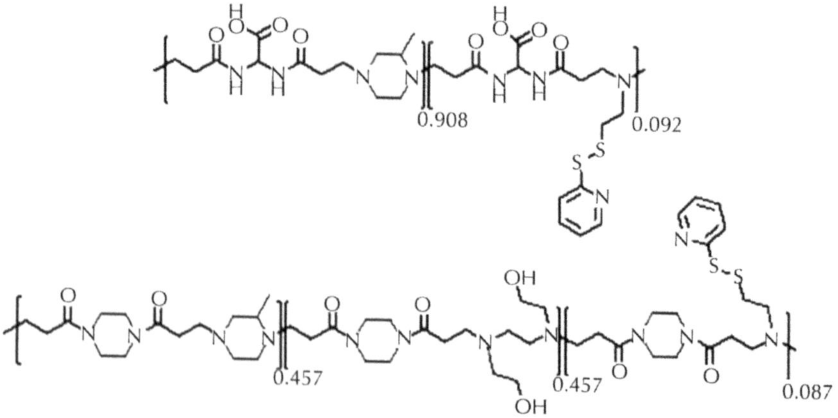

Figure 3. Structures of ISA23-SSPy (top) and ISA1-SSPy (bottom).

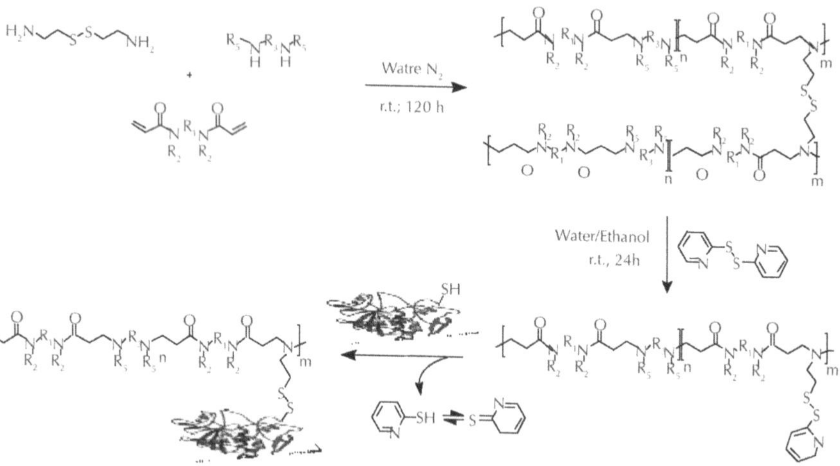

Scheme 2. Synthetic pathway leading to PAA-gelonin conjugates.

Two different recombinant protein, encoding gelonin with an N-terminal 6xHistidine (H or His) and V5 epitope tag (6H-V5 Gelonin) and gelonin encorporating a C-terminal HA and 6xHis tag flanking a cysteine residue (Gelonin HA-Cys-6H) were prepared introducing the required tag on a gelonin plasmid by polymerase chain reaction (PCR), isolated and purified from *E. coli*.

In vitro experiments were performed on B16F10 cells using non-toxic concentration of gelonin (1, 4 and 14 µg/ml) and polymeric samples up to 2 mg/ml. The ISA1-SSPy promoted the intracytoplasmic delivery of gelonin more efficiently than the parent non-functionalized ISA1 with IC_{50} values of 100 µg/ml.

The results obtained for ISA1-SSPy-HA-Cys-6H, designed to have a covalent bound between the polymeric vector and the toxin, and ISA1-SSPy-6H-V5 Gelonin were the same, suggesting a non-specific conjugation to the thiol-groups in the Gelonin HA-Cys-6H.

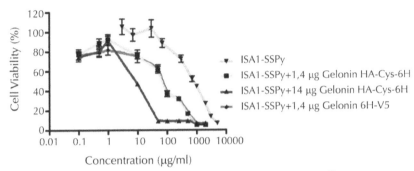

Figure 4. Cytotoxicity of ISA1-SSPy-Gelonin conjugates against B16F10 cells.

This findings could be attributed both to the ability of ISA1-SSPy to react with protein disulfide groups and to the interactions between the ethenyl-dithiopyridine pendants and the hydrophobic domains of the protein, giving stable complexes. The ISA23-SSPy was unable to mediate toxin delivery.

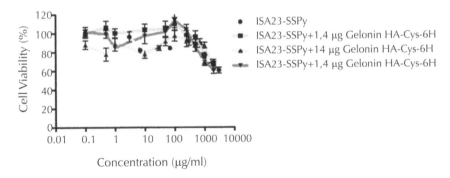

Figure 5. Cytotoxicity of ISA23-SSPy-Gelonin conjugates against B16F10 cells.

PAA-cholesterol Nanoparticles

Poor drug solubility is one of the most limiting problem in new drugs application. Hydrophilic-hydrophobic compounds, among which block co-polymer or polymer conjugates, are regarded as promising structure in view of their use in drug delivery. In fact, in aqueous environment these molecules self assemble into nano- or micro-particles in which the lipophilic part tends to segregate into domains, capable of remarkable payloads of hydrophobic molecules and increasing their solubility by orders of magnitude. Among amphiphilic polymers, increasing attention has been recently paid to cholesterol conjugates with hydrophilic polymers. Cholesterol is one of the most common membrane sterols and plays a relevant role in the metabolism of living organisms, in particular in self-association of molecules in biological environments (Devalapally et al., 2007).

Novel cholesterol-poly(amido-amine) (PAA) nanoparticles, based on ISA1 and ISA23 polymers, have been synthesized, in which cholesterol is bound to the PAA backbone through a thiol-disulphide exchange reaction between thiocholesterol and the PAA-SSPy precursors previously described (Figure 6) (Ranucci et al., 2008) .

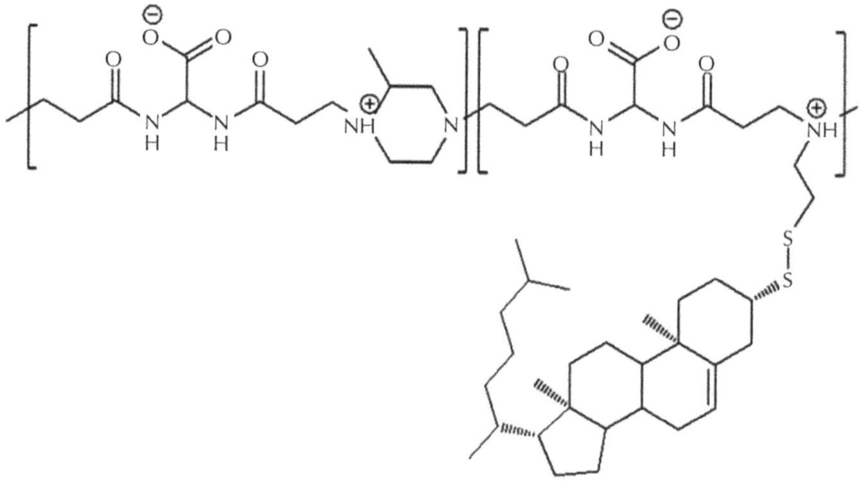

Figure 6. Structure of ISA23-cholesterol conjugates.

The PAA-cholesterol conjugates synthesized presented a strong tendency to form nanoparticles with a narrow mono-modal diameter distribution centered around 50 nm, as shown by TEM images and Light Scattering analyses.

These nanoparticles are susceptible to be specifically designed for intracellular delivery, thanks to the ability of PAAs to promote intracellular trafficking coupled to the strong reducing intracellular environment.

Table 4. DLS analyses of self-assembling PAA-cholesterol nanoparticles.

Samples	Cholesterol % (w/w)	Average diameter (nm)	Polydispersity Index
ISA1-SSChol1	8	243 ± 16	0.20
ISA1-SSChol2	15	264 ± 21	0.18
ISA23-SSChol1	8	124 ± 6	0.11
ISA23-SSChol2	15	131 ± 7	0.13

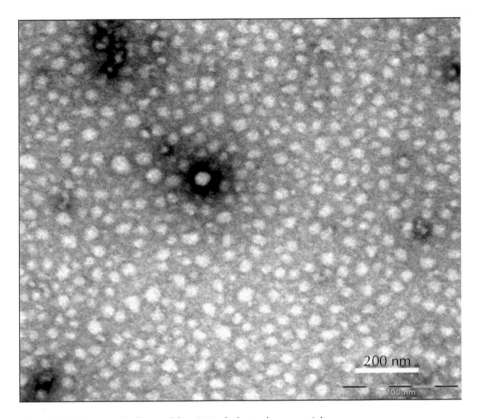

Figure 7. TEM image of self-assembling PAA-cholesterol nanoparticles.

The cytotoxicity of PAA-cholesterol conjugates was assessed by *in vitro* cytotoxicity assays performed against 3T3/BALB-c Clone A31 cell lines. All samples were found being non-toxic, with IC_{50} value of 2–3 mg/ml (Table 5).

Table 5. Cytotoxicity of PAA-cholesterol conjugates against 3T3/BALB-c Clone A31 cells.

Sample	IC_{50}
ISA23-SSChol	>3 mg/mL
ISA1-SSChol	>2 mg/ mL

The PAA-cholesterol nanoparticles containing lyphophylic drugs were formulated using two different techniques.

Using the electrospraying method, that is a method of liquid atomization consisting in the dispersion of a PAA-cholesterol solution into small charged droplets by an electric field, nanoperticles containing 9% of doxorubicin and 5% of tamoxifen on a weight-to-weight basis were prepared with dimension ranging from 200 to 300 nm (Figure 8).

Doxorubicin loaded (9%) PAA-cholesterol nanoparticles

Tamoxifin loaded (5%) PAA-cholesterol nanoparticles

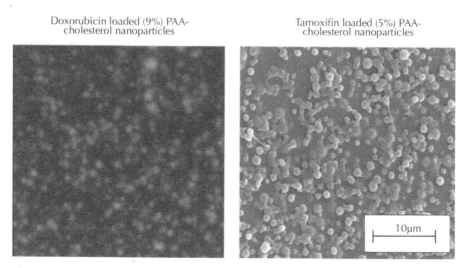

Figure 8. TEM image of doxorubicin (right) and tomoxifen (left) ISA23-cholesterol nanoparticles.

Doxorubicin-loaded ISA23-cholesterol nanoparticles were internalized into Vero cells and mainly localized in the perinuclear region.

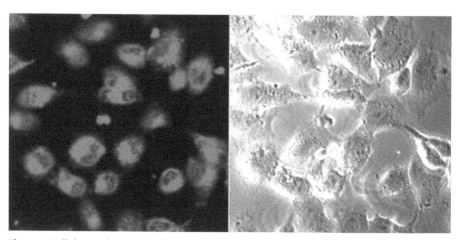

Figure 9. Cellular uptake of doxorubicin-loaded and fluorescent PAA-cholesterol nanoparticles with confocal laser scanning microscopy.

The second method consisted in the formulation of PAA-cholesterol nanoparticles by solvent injection from a water-ethanol mixture.

Table 6. DLS and Z-potential analyses of PAA-cholesterol nanoparticles obtained using the solvent-injection method.

Samples	Average diameter (nm)	Polydispersity Index	Z-Potential (mV)
ISA23-SSChol	80 ± 10	0.26	-14.86 ± 0.99

These nanoparticles showed no hemolytic activity tested on *in vitro* red blood cells.

PAA-β-cyclodextrin Nanoparticles

The β-cyclodextrin is widely used in the pharmaceutical field thanks to its ability to form host-guest complexes with lypophilic drugs. Since these complexes are themselves rather insoluble in water, many β-cyclodextrin derivatives have been prepared in order to improve the solubility but just few can be taken into consideration thanks to their smart synthetic process (Szejtli, 2004). To this purpose, β-CD-polymer conjugates have a great potential as drug solubilisers since the polymer could stabilise the β-CD-drug complex via secondary interactions with the host molecule.

β-CD-PAA copolymers can be obtained either as hyperbranched soluble products or crosslinked materials. We found that, in alkaline conditions, β-CD behaves as a multifunctional monomer since about 5 hydroxyl groups per molecule undergo Michael-type addition to bisacrylamides.

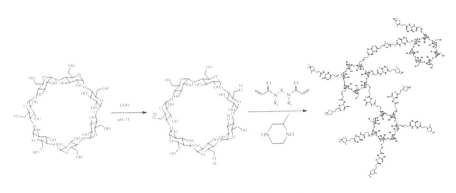

Scheme 3. Synthetic pathway leading to PAA-β-cyclodextrin conjugates.

During stepwise polymerization reactions involving multifunctional monomers, the reacting mixture may turn into a gel. Following the Flory-Stockmayer equation the conversion degree at which the gelling takes place can be determined (Equation 1). If p_c is equal to 1 the critical functional ratio r_c can be determined (Equation 2), that is the functional ratio above which the system is able to crosslink and below which hyperbranched but still soluble polymers are obtained (Flory, 1953).

Equation 1.
$$pc = \frac{1}{\{r[1+\rho(f-2)]\}^{1/2}}$$

Equation 2. $$rc = \frac{1}{1+\rho(f-2)}$$

Biological evaluations carried out on PAA-β-CD conjugates, including *in vitro* MCF-7 cell viability tests and *in vivo* haemolytic activity (human RBC), have confirmed the biocompatibility of the polymer.

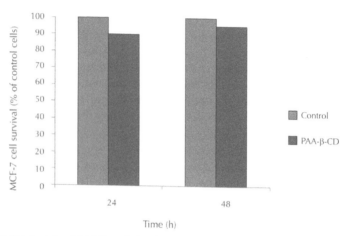

Figure 10. Cytotoxicity of PAA-β-cyclodextrin conjugates against MCF-7 cells.

The PAA-β-cyclodextrin micro- and nanogels were prepared by high-pressure homogeneization of a hydrogel suspension in water. These nanoparticles have been loaded with Paclitaxel obtaining water dispersable complexes on nanometric scale, with a loading of drug equal to 5% on a weight-to-weight basis. The dispersion can be freeze-dried and re-dispersed in water with no alteration.

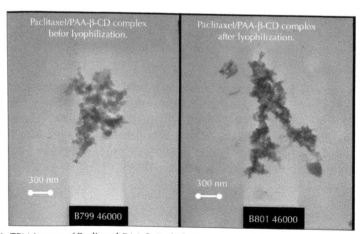

Figure 11. TEM images of Paclitaxel-PAA-β-Cyclodextrin nanoparticles.

Paclitaxel even complexed by the polymeric system, maintains its efficiency in the inhibition of cancer cell growth (*In vitro* MCF-7 cell cultures).

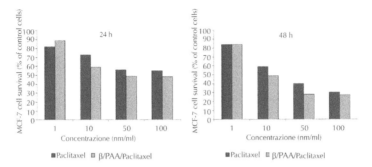

Figure 12. Study of the inhibition of MCF-7 cell growth by paclitaxel-loaded PAA-β-CD nanoparticles.

Further experiments on β-CD-PAA nanoparticles formulations with progesterone and dexamethasone are ongoing.

CONCLUSION

The PAAs constitute a family of ionic polymers that are easily synthesized and can be designed to be biocompatible and degradable in the body fluids. Those of second generation warrant potential, inter alia, as stimuli-responsive delivery system for proteins and drugs and for the synthesis and formulation of nanoparticles for different biomedical applications.

In more general terms, PAAs are highly versatile functional polymers and biotechnological applications do not exhaust their potential for practical exploitation. To give some examples, PAAs have been designed to act as excellent sequestering agents for heavy metal ions and are presently being investigated for fine purification of drinking water from traces of nasty micro-pollutants such as Chromium, Arsenic, Cadmium, Nickel, Lead and others; copolymers of cyclodextrins have been prepared as hydrogels that are potentially capable of purifying water by a single treatment from both inorganic and organic pollutants; hybrid products with natural organic polymers such as chitosan, cellulose, dextran and others as well as with silica and silicon-based materials have been prepared. It is our opinion that the unique combination of chemical and biotechnologically relevant properties of PAAs is still waiting to be fully exploited.

KEYWORDS

- **Cytotoxicity**
- **Poly(amido-amine)**
- **Poly(ethyleneimine)**
- **Polyamidoamines**
- **Poly-L-lysine**
- **Poor drug solubility**

Chapter 6

Nanoparticles as Adjuvant(S) for Mucosal Vaccine Delivery

PN Gupta, GD Singh, SC Sharma, S Singh, MK Tikoo, N Gupta, and RK Johri

---

MUCOSAL IMMUNE SYSTEM

The first productive interaction between most infectious agents and the host is with mucosal surfaces, specially, the nasal, oropharyngeal, respiratory, genitourinary, and gastrointestinal mucosa. Conventional vaccine strategies that involve parenteral immunization with inactivated viruses, bacteria or subunits of relevant virulence determinants of those pathogens do not prevent initial interactions. Infact, traditional vaccine strategies do not prevent infection but instead resolve infection before disease ensues. Moreover, many bacterial toxins bind to and interact with mucosal epithelial cells, in which case significant damage to the host may ensue before serum antibodies can play a role in protection. The mucosal surfaces of the gastrointestinal and respiratory tracts represent the main portals of entry for most human pathogens. Sexual contact is another mucosal mode of transmission of infection. Direct inoculation of pathogens into the bloodstream is other important route of infection. Most external mucosal surfaces are replete with organized follicles and scattered antigen-reactive or sensitized lymphoid elements, including B cells, T lymphocytes, T-cell subsets, plasma cells, and a variety of other cellular elements involved in the induction and maintenance of immune response. The mucosal surfaces encompass a critical component of the mammalian immunologic repertoire.

Numerous studies have indicated that induction of systemic immunity through parenteral immunization can effectively clear systemic infections, but it usually fails to protect the mucosal surfaces. Mucosal vaccine administration with an appropriate adjuvant, on the other hand, can induce immune responses at both systemic and mucosal sites and as a result, may prevent not only infectious diseases but also colonization at mucosal surfaces (Davis, 2001). The mucosal immune system differs in several ways from the systemic immune system. Mucosal immunization frequently results in the stimulation of both mucosal and systemic immune responses, while systemic immunization typically only induces systemic responses without activating the mucosal immune system. Induction of mucosal response leads to production of secretory IgA (sIgA) antibodies, which are not usually produced by systemic immunization (Nugent et al., 1998). The production of sIgA on the mucosal surfaces is the result of local exposure of antigens to the mucosal-associated lymphoid tissues, especially those in the upper respiratory tract (nasal associated lymphoid tissue, or NALT), and the gastrointestinal tract (gut-associated lymphoid tissue, or GALT). In most cases, infectious agents enter the body at mucosal surfaces and therefore the protective immunity at these surfaces can be effectively induced by mucosal immunization through oral, nasal, rectal or vaginal routes (Neutra and Kozlowski, 2006). The common features of all inductive mucosal sites include epithelial surface containing M cells (Figure 1) overlying organized lymphoid follicles. These cells are also envisaged as "gateway of mucosal immune system".

MUCOSAL IMMUNIZATION: AN EDGE OVER PARENTERAL VACCINATION

Vaccine delivery via mucosal route has several advantages over parenteral vaccination. (I) The most important reason for using a mucosal route of vaccination instead of a parenteral route is that the vast majority of infections occurs at or takes their departure from mucosal surfaces and in these infections topical application of vaccines is usually required to induce a protective immune response. The parenteral immunization induces poor mucosal immunity; however, mucosal immunization can induce both mucosal and systemic immunity (Holmgren et al., 2003). (II) The immunization at one mucosal site can induce specific responses at distant sites because of the expression of mucosa-specific homing receptors (site-specific integrins) by mucosally primed lymphocytes and complementary mucosal-tissue specific receptors (addressins) on the vascular endothelial cells (Holmgren and Czerkinsky, 2005). This interconnected network is important because protective immunity (for instance against sexually transmitted diseases) could be induced in segregated mucosal sites in a practical way such as by oral or intranasal immunization and without hampering cultural or religious barriers. (III) Mucosal vaccines are potentially useful to overcome the known barrier of parenteral vaccination caused by either pre-existing systemic immunity from previous vaccination or in young children from maternal antibodies or selective immuno-suppression such as that caused by HIV infection. For example, mucosal antibody response to oral cholera vaccination was observed in AIDS patients even after they had completely lost their ability to respond to injectable vaccines of tetanus toxoid (Eriksson et al., 1998). (IV) In addition to serum IgG and mucosal IgA antibodies, mucosal immunization can stimulate cell mediated responses including helper CD4+ T cells and CD8+ cytotoxic T lymphocytes, the latter being important to eliminate intracellular pathogens (Magistris, 2006). (V) The mucosal vaccine delivery is crucial for protective efficacy against non-invasive infections at mucosal surfaces that are normally impermeable to serum antibodies' transduction, or passive passage across an epithelium for example GIT infection with *V. cholerae* (Holmgren and Czerkinsky, 2005). (VI) The mucosal vaccine delivery is particularly important for pathogens that can infect the host through both systemic and mucosal route because induction of both sIgA and systemic IgG confer protection at both site. This mode of vaccine delivery could be explored for combating pathogens acquired through non-mucosal routes such as blood or skin. (VII) Mucosal vaccination is also beneficial to induce peripheral systemic tolerance especially against those T cell mediated immune reaction that are associated with development of delayed type hypersensitivity reactions. This strategy is important to avoid delayed type hypersensitivity reactions and other allergic reactions to many ingested food proteins and other allegens (Holmgren et al., 2003). Mucosal tolerance is a specific systemic hyporesponsiveness that arises after mucosal administration of an antigen. The tolerance is mediated by a combination of suppressor T-cells, inhibitory cytokines and factors which inhibit the inflammatory process. Oral tolerance can be used for the treatment of atopic diseases in human (Ogra et al., 2001).

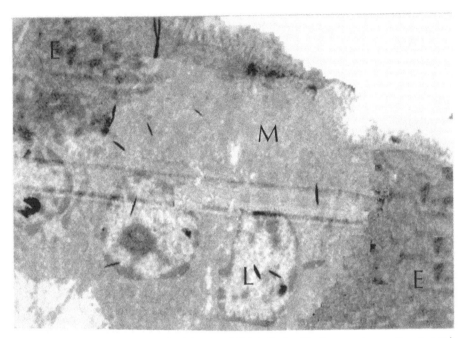

Figure 1. Electron photomicrograph of the M-cell (M) in ileal epithelium overlying a Payer's patch of BALB/c mouse. The M cell is flanked by enterocytes (E). Lymphoid cells (L) constitute the central hollow of the M cells.

But one major limitation with mucosal immunization is a striking balance between achieving an effective therapeutic response with a particular dose, whilst preventing the induction of tolerance. Therefore, it is important to understand the mechanisms involved in controlling these responses. The key cells that determine the success or demise of a vaccine are antigen-presenting cells (APC), for example, dendritic cells (DC) and T lymphocytes, including sub-populations of T-helper cells, T-cytotoxic cells, and regulatory T cells (Holmgren and Czerkinsky, 2005). Immune interactions at the local level will have a profound effect on the type of immune response generated (e.g., first nuclear factor of activated T cell proteins is involved in both the generation of Th1 or Th2 cells and the maintenance of T-cell tolerance), so a clear understanding of local immune responses at the site of antigen uptake is essential (Macian, 2005).

On the other hand, extreme mucosal administration of vaccines also offers a number of practical advantages. Mucosal vaccination, being non-invasive in nature, does not require the use of needles. This would carry less risk of transmitting type of infections still associated with needle re-use (Levine , 2003; Ryan et al., 2001) Additionally, mucosal vaccination is relatively easy and does not require expensive trained personnel. The production of mucosal vaccines may be cost effective in comparison to injectable vaccines that require high standards of purity, in addition to sterility. Moreover, oral vaccines can also be expected to have much greater acceptability than injectable vaccines by causing no sore arm etc. Further it can enhance vaccine safety and adverse effects by avoiding direct contact between potentially toxic vaccine component and systemic circulation. Finally, mucosal vaccines allow for the easy administration of multiple vaccines (Chen, 2000). There are various approaches for the vaccine delivery by the mucosal route, each having its own merits and demerits (Table 1).

Table 1. Comparison of parenteral and mucosal administration of vaccines.

Vaccination	Parenteral	Nasal	Oral
Vaccine administration	Injection neccessiates medically trained personnel	Delivery device demands full co-operation of the vaccinee	Easy; self-administration via simple ingestion
Risks	Infection (HIV, Hepatits B)	Inaccurate dosing	Inaccurate dosing
Formulation	Mostly with alum	Need of mucosal adjuvant	Requires potent mucosal adjuvant
Required antigen dose	Low	Efficient transfer across nasal epithelium necessitates medium dose	Hostile GIT environment necessitates comparatively higher dose
Immune response	Potent systemic antibody and T cell responses	Mucosal and systemic antibody and T cell responses, can induce tolerance	Mucosal antibody and modest systemic antibody responses, can induce tolerance
Protective Efficacy	Many viral, bacterial and parasitic disease models in animals and humans	Many animal models of viral and bacterial diseases	Small number of animal models of viral and bacterial diseases
Clinical use	Extensive	Limited number of clinical trials	Limited clinical trials of subunit but extensive use for attenuated vaccines
Safety	No major problems with subunit vaccines; mild to serious side effects with killed or attenuated vaccines	Largely unknown, evidence of antigen transfer to neuronal tissue via olfactory bulb in mice	Considered to be the safest route of vaccine delivery

POLYMERS FOR THE MUCOSAL ADMINISTRATION OF VACCINES

There are various options for the delivery of mucosal vaccines (Table 2). The polymer-based delivery systems for mucosal vaccine delivery are of considerable potential. To date, there are only a limited number of licensed mucosal oral vaccines available, including polio vaccine and a live typhoid vaccine Ty21a (Vivotif; Berna Biotech Ltd, Berne, Switzerland and Swiss Serum and Vaccine Institute, Berne, Switzerland). However, several additional oral vaccines are in late stages of development, including improved vaccines against *V. cholerae* and *Salmonella typhi*, and a rotavirus vaccine (Dietrich et al., 2003; Holmgren and Czerkinsky, 2005). These vaccines were mainly developed as live attenuated organisms. However, not all pathogens can be success-fully modified to allow the development of live mucosal-oral vaccines. Additionally there is inherent risk associated with live attenuated vaccines. The nonpathogenic at-tenuated organism may revert to virulent form. Therefore, development of new vac-cine delivery systems is warranted, which can be applied to a wide range of different pathogens, and can be administered mucosally.

The concept of a polymeric carrier system involves delivery of drugs/antigens to a specific target site where it is to be released from the carrier. The utilization of this ap-proach towards the development of mucosal vaccine delivery system was specifically dictated by the need to protect proteins and antigens against degradation in the hostile GIT and a desire to increase their uptake by the immune system. The encapsulation of proteins and antigens in polymeric matrices in the form of nanoparticles is a promising approach (Andrianov and Payne, 1998). Polymers have been one of the most popular choices as materials for such encapsulation since the tremendous potential of synthetic polymer chemistry allows fine-tuning of physicochemical properties of polymeric de-livery systems.

A number of different polymers have been evaluated for the development of mu-cosal vaccines (Table 3). The considerations of toxicity, irritancy, allergenicity, and biodegradability are of primary concern. The advantages of using natural polymers include their low cost, biocompatibility and aqueous solubility. However, the natural polymers may also be limited in their use due to the presence of extraneous contami-nants, variability from lot to lot and low hydrophobicity. In contrast, synthetic poly-mers are more reproducible and can be prepared with desired degradation rate, mo-lecular weight and co-polymer composition. Nevertheless, synthetic polymers may be disadvantageous due to their limited solubility; they are often soluble only in organic solvents and consequently may not release biologically active antigen.

Several approaches involving polymeric coatings or encapsulation are currently being evaluated for the development of mucosal delivery of vaccines. These approach-es include, PLG nanoparticles (Gupta et al., 2006; Jaganathan and Vyas, 2006), enteric coating polymers (Dea-Ayuela et al., 2006) alginate microcapsules (Tafaghodi et al., 2006), starch microcapsules (Sturesson and Degling, 2000), gelatin capsules (Litwin et al., 1996) and polymethacrylates (Haining et al., 2004). The objectives with all of these strategies are to improve upon one or more of the following parameters, to reduce gastric and intestinal degradation of the antigen, to enhance antigen absorp-tion, to extend residence time in the gut, to promote uptake of the antigen by the gut-associated lymphoid tissue (GALT) and to reduce the dose of antigen needed to induce a significant immune response.

NANOPARTICLE DEVELOPMENT FOR MUCOSAL VACCINE DELIVERY

The polymer characteristics profoundly affect nanoparticles' structure. The polymer should have desirable mechanical strength necessary to maintain integrity of the deliv-ery system during the in-process manipulations. The polymer should confer protection of the encapsulated antigens from the harsh environment that the nanoparticles will encounter in the GIT. Polymeric nanoparticles can enhance the immune response to mucosally administered antigens by several means. The encapsulation of an antigen in nanoparticles converts any antigen to particulate form which is much more efficient at inducing an immune response than the same antigens in the soluble state. Particulate antigens were the more effective immunogens because they were translocated more efficiently into the cells of the Peyer's patches (Andrianov and Payne, 1998).

Table 2. Various option for the vaccine delivery by mucosal route.

Option for mucosal vaccine delivery	Comments	Ref.
Live bacterial vector, (E. Coli.)	The capability of some microorganism to colonize and infect intestinal mucosa and the potential for including genes for unrelated microorganism encoding relevant antigens represent an attractive means for design of novel mucosal vaccines.	Banerjee et al., 2002;
Live viral vector (Vaccinia virus, Canary pox virus)	Live recombinant vector vaccines have the advantage that they can stimulate both humoral and cell mediated immune responses and have potential for immunization alone or in combination with a subunit vaccine.	Smythies et al., 2005
Virosomes	Viral surface glycoproteins possess high affinity for receptors on mucosal surfaces, thus providing a mechanism for efficient attachment of antigen to mucosal surfaces.	Durrer et al., 2003
Liposomes	Liposome vaccine may enhance uptake and processing by enclosing the antigen in the lipid vesicles. Although they are not completely resistant to lipases and bile salts found in the small intestine, cholesterol-containing liposomes can provide at least partial resistance. Polymerized liposomes are considered to be a good candidate for the oral immunization.	Clark et al., 2002
Nanoparticles and microparticles	Particles can be taken up by the M cells of the Peyer's patches. Nanoparticles/microparticles have advantage over microbial system in which immune response to the live vector can dominate.	Gupta et al., 2006
Cochleates	Induce a strong and prolonged immune response manifested by the presence of mucosal and systemic antibody and cytotoxic T cells.	Perez et al., 2006
Cholera toxin B subunit conjugates	Proteins coupled to CTB acquire its mucosal immunogenic properties due to the high affinity of CTB for cell surface G_{M1} ganglioside and its avid uptake by M cells on intestinal Peyer's patches.	Singh et al., 2004
Immune-stimulating complex matrix (ISCOM)	ISCOMs are cage like structures into which antigen can be incorporated resulting in enhanced immune response after their administration. ISCOMs are resistant to solubilization by the bile salts like, deoxycholate, cholate and taurocholate.	Aguila et al., 2006

Table 2. *(Continued)*

Option for mucosal vaccine delivery	Comments	Ref.
DNA delivery to mucosal surface	Direct mucosal administration of DNA plasmid expression vector encoding a protein antigen is more efficient than recombinant viral vector for gene transfer to muscle tissue.	Jain et al., 2005
Transgenic plants	This technology represents an important step for the production of inexpensive edible immunogen suitable for immunization of large population.	Thanavala et al., 2005

The enhanced immune response by the nanoparticles is a result of enhanced uptake of the antigen. Specialized epithelial cells, called M cells, mainly take up particles and the pathogen expressing invasion genes. A noble method for bacterial uptake in the mucosal tissue is mediated by dendritic cells (DCs) which open the tight junctions between the cells, send dendrites outside the epithelium and directly sample bacteria. Additionally particles or antigen may also penetrate through the para-cellular route (Rescigno et al., 2001). It appears that the Peyer's patches are the predominant sites for particle uptake in the GIT. The mucosal sites include the organized mucosal associated lymphoid tissue (O-MALT), which are the specialized antigen sampling sites of the mucosal immune system. The antigen sampling function of the O-MALT is performed predominantly by the membranous epithelial M cells, which are located in the Peyer's patches. The M cells translocate antigen from the gut lumen to the underlying aggregates of lymphoid follicles that constitute the patches. This is an environment rich in immunocompetent cells important in the induction of the immune response. Nanoparticles can also improve the immune response by a controlled release of antigen from the polymeric devices. Antigen release can be manipulated to maximize the induction of the immune response by controlling the release rate through proper polymer fabrication. Ideally the antigen release should mimic a classical prime and boost immunization scheme. Additionally some polymers can act as adjuvant *per se*. This can be exemplified by synthetic polyphosphazene, which has remarkable adjuvant effects when mixed with antigen and injected as a solution into experimental animals (Payne et al., 1998). This polymer in its ionized state can also be cross-linked with divalent cations to form microparticles that can enhance the immune response after mucosal immunization. Thus, in nutshell, polymers modulate various profiles of antigens to evoke heightened immune responses.

Table 3. Classification of some commonly used polymer in drug delivery.

I.   **Synthetic degradable polymers**
   (a) Polyorthoesters
   (b) Polyanhydrides
   (c) Polyamides
   (d) Polyalkylcyanoacrylates
   (e) Polyesters
       (i) Lactides/glycolides
       (ii) Polycaprolactones

(f) Polyphosphazenes
(g) Pseudo-polyamino acids
II. Synthetic non-degradable polymers
    (a) Silicone elastomers
    (b) Poly [ethylene-co-(vinyl acetate)]
    (c) Acrylic polymers
    (d) Polyethylene oxide
    (e) Polyethylene glycol
III. Natural polymers
    (a) Proteins: Albumin, globulin, gelatin, collagen, casein
    (b) Polysaccharides: Starch, cellulose, chitosan, dextran, alginic acid
IV. Genetically engineered polymers
    (a) Elastin-like polymers $[VPGXG]_n$ (X= any amino acid except proline)
    (b) Typical silk-like polymers $[(GAGAGS)_9 GAAVTGRGDSPASAAGY]_n]$
    (c) Silk elastin-like block copolymers $[(GAGAGS)_m(GVGXP)_n]_o$ (X=any amino acid except proline)
    (d) [Poly(alanylglycine)]–$(AG)_m X_n$ (X=any amino acid)

FACTORS AFFECTING UPTAKE OF NANOPARTICLES

The M cell appears to be the primary route of entry into the host for several enteric viral pathogens. The mechanism for the uptake of synthetic and biodegradable nanoparticles by M cells appears similar to that observed for bacteria. Nanoparticle uptake initially involves contact with the microvillus projections on the M cell surface followed by rapid phagocytosis through the extension of apical membrane processes. Various factors affecting the uptake of particles are summarized in Table 4.

Table 4. Various factors affecting uptake of nanoparticles/microparticles.

Particle size
Particle hydrophobicity
Dose of particle (Antigen dose)
Administration vehicle
Polymer composition
  ➤ Crystalinity
  ➤ Glass transition temperature
  ➤ Copolymer ratio
Effect of additives
Particle surface charge (Zeta potential)
Animal species used for evaluation
Age of the animal
Fed state of the animal
Mucosal layer characteristics
Use of targeting agent on the particles
Method for the quantitation for the extent of uptake

Particle Size

In general, nanoparticles are absorbed to a greater degree than microparticles. The smaller particles are distributed more easily to distant sites, and remain detectable for longer periods of time. These conclusions are consistent for microparticles made of different polymers and different size ranges. Jani et al. (1992) studied the comparative uptake of 50 nm, 500 nm and 1μm polystryrene particles and found that 50 nm particles are absorbed and distributed quicker than 500 nm and 1 μm particles. Florence suggested that decrease in particle diameter may result in increased uptake below 1 μm and particles above 3 μm are taken up by the Peyer's patches but remained there (Florence, 2005).

Hydrophobicity

Hydrophobicity of the particles influences profoundly their uptake behavior. Jung et al. reported that uptake of nanoparticles prepared from hydrophobic polymer was higher than from particles with more hydrophilic surfaces (Jung et al., 2000). They further added that hydrophobic polystyrene nanoparticles interact to M cells with more affinity than absorptive epithelia whereas less hydrophobic PLGA nanoparticles interact with both cell types. Other investigators have shown that decreasing surface hydrophobicity, by the adsorption of poloxamers 235, 238, 407, or poloxamines 901, 904, and 908, may decrease the uptake of polystyrene microparticles into cells of the immune system, thereby avoiding elimination (Moghimi et al., 1994). The charge on the particles also determines its uptake by the intestinal epithelia. Although the charged particles are taken up, their uptake is less compared to non-ionic hydrophobic particles (Florence, 2005). The negatively charged and neutral particles exhibited greater affinity to Peyer's patches in comparison to positively charged particles (Shakweh et al., 2005). This finding was in accordance with previous report that a combination of both, negative charge and increased hydrophobicity of the particles improve the gastrointestinal uptake (Jung et al., 2000).

Effect of Dose and Vehicle on Uptake

The extent of particle uptake is also influenced by the dosing. It was observed that polystyrene particles were identified in Peyer's patches with difficulty after 1 day of feeding, but were readily identified following chronic feeding. Le Ray et al. (1994), have shown that changing the vehicle in which the particles were administered could enhance the extent of uptake of polystyrene particles in mice. Further, volume and tonicity of the administered vehicle also have an effect on the extent of uptake (Eyles et al., 1995).

Glass Transition Temperature and Crystalinity of the Polymer

Glass transition temperature (Tg) and crystalinity of the polymer are two important bulk properties of the polymer affecting the release of incorporated components. Without proper release characteristics, drugs or vaccines incorporated into microparticles may be released either prematurely or to insignificant levels before elimination. The Tg is the temperature at which a transition occurs from the glassy state to the rubbery state resulting in increase in the molecular motion and free volume of the amorphous polymer, which in turn increases the drug release from the polymer. Above *Tg,* the polymer acquires sufficient thermal energy for isomeric rotational motion or for significant torsional oscillation to occur in most of the bonds in the main chain. This leads to an increase in the free volume of the amorphous polymer, and thus in turn, the release of incorporated bioactives (Norris et al., 1998).

Migliaresi et al. observed an increase in the degree of crystallinity of polylactic acid with the degradation of the polymer (Migliaresi et al., 1994). This could be related to the faster degradation of the amorphous phase of the semi-crystalline polymer, resulting in loss of amorphous material and concomitant increase in crystallinity. A decrease in crystallinity increases the drug release because the diffusion coefficient and solubility of the drug in polymer are inversely proportional to at least the first power of the amorphous content. The structural features, which influence the crystallinity of the polymer, are similar to those, which affect the glass transition temperature. Bioactive (drug/vaccine) may release from nanoparticles by several mechanisms including surface and bulk erosion, disintegration, microparticle hydration, drug diffusion and desorption. These bioactive release mechanisms are in turn controlled by bulk properties such as the molecular weight of the polymer (affecting crystallinity and glass transition temperature), the copolymer composition, polymer matrix density and the extent and nature of the cross linking. By adjusting the blend ratio of poly (DL-lactic-co-glycolic acid) (PLGA)/polyethyleneglycol (PEG), the release profile of entrapped dextran and rabbit gamma immunoglobulin (IgG) microparticles can be varied (Cleek et al., 1997).

Effect of Additives

Various additives are involved in the fabrication of nanoparticles. Polyvinyl alcohol (PVA) is the most commonly used emulsifier in the formulation of lactide and poly (D, L-lactide-co-glycolide) nanoparticles. A fraction of PVA remains associated with the nanoparticles despite repeated washing because PVA forms an interconnected network with the polymer at the interface. The residual PVA affect different pharmaceutical properties of the particles such as particle size, zeta potential, polydispersity index, surface hydrophobicity, protein loading and also slightly influenced the *in vitro* release of encapsulated protein. Importantly, nanoparticles with higher amount of residual PVA had relatively lower cellular uptake despite their smaller particle size (Sahoo et al., 2002). The lower cellular uptake of nanoparticles with higher amount of residual PVA is attributed to the higher hydrophilicity of the nanoparticle surface. Trehalose is a well-documented protein stabilizer. An increase in the release of HBsAg was observed with treahalose stabilized PLGA nanoparticles/microparticles when compared with PLGA nanoparticles/microparticles without trehalose (Gupta et al., 2006; Jaganathan et al., 2004). Since the protein stabilizer (trehalose) reduced denaturation at the aqueous-organic interface, the payload of HBsAg was increased and this was reflected in augmented cumulative percent release. Moreover, sugars (e.g., trehalose, sucrose) have appreciable solubility in aqueous media. They dissolve rapidly from the matrix leaving a porous matrix, which in turn releases antigen/bioactive relatively faster.

Effect of Species, Animal Age, and Food Ingestion on Uptake

The species variation can affect extent of uptake of the particles. The uptake of polystyrene particles in rabbit was at least an order of magnitude greater than mice because of the greater abundance of the M cells in the Peyer's patches (Pappo and Ermak 1989). Le Fevre et al. showed greater uptake of polystyrene particles in older mice (Le Fevre et al., 1989). Other investigator reported that age of the animal did not affect the extent of polystyrene particle uptake in rats (Simon et al., 1994). The extent of uptake in the mice was enhanced by the presence of food, which may delay the intestinal transit of the particles (Simon et al., 1994).

Intestinal Mucus Layer Characteristics

The uptake of the nanoparticles is preceded by their passage through two barriers *i.e.* the mucus gel layer and the mucosa. Intestinal mucus is a high molecular weight glycoprotein secretion, which covers the mucosa with a continuous adherent blanket. The mucus layer protects the gastrointestinal mucosa from potentially harmful bacteria, pathogens, or chemicals (Strous and Dekker, 1992). Several investigators have reported diminished diffusion of small and large compounds such as bovine serum albumin (BSA), lysozyme, tertiary amines, quaternary ammonium compounds (Desai et al., 1992). Mucus acts as a barrier by entrapping microparticles, causing agglomeration, which results in an increase in net size and by decreasing the diffusion coefficient through the mucus thereby restricting diffusion to the mucosa layer. Since the high number of sulfate, sialic acid and sugar moieties in the carbohydrate side chains of the mucin molecule imparts a highly negative charge to mucin (Strous and Dekker, 1992), it may be expected that electrostatic interactions between positively charged drugs and particles would cause binding within the mucin layer. Several mechanisms have been documented in literature (O'Hagan, 1996) for the uptake of the nanoparticles (Table 5).

Table 5. Site-specific mechanism for the uptake of the nanoparticles/microparticles.

Uptake Site	Mechanism	Particle size
Intestinal epithelial cells on villus tip	Paracellular transport	100-200 nm
Villus tips	Persorption	5-150µm
Intestinal macrophages	Phagocytosis	1 µm
Enterocytes/M-cells	Endocytosis	<200 nm
Peyer's patches	Transparacellular	<10 µm

TARGETING OF DELIVERY SYSTEM(S) FOR MUCOSAL IMMUNIZATION

Targeting to the specific site of the gastrointestinal tract is an effective means for the enhancing the uptake of the particulate systems. Depending on the pharmaceutical application, different targets within the gastrointestinal tract can be exploited (Figure 2) including mucus glycoproteins (mucins), epithelial cells, M-cells, Peyer's patches or gut-associated lymphoid tissue (GALT), and abnormal glycoproteins secreted by cancerous cells (local tumours). Brayden et al. (2005) reviewed various novel M-cell surface receptors that could be used to target orally delivered antigens. Gene expression technology has provided evidence that co-culture model has many characteristics of Peyer's patches. It has been demonstrated that epithelial genes that were unregulated in co-culture corresponds to genes expressed selectively in mouse FAE (Lo et al., 2004). These include claudin 4, laminin β3, tetraspanTM4SF3 and a matrix metalloproteinase. Claudin 4 appears to have dual location at tight junctions (M cell-enterocyte). As an M cell and enterocyte cytoplasmic receptor, it is involved in the trafficking of pathogens across M cells to lymphocyte or dendritic cells. Peptidoglycan recognition protein (PGRP)-S and PGRP-L are other potential targets co-localized with UEA-positive cells in microdissected mouse PP and in the FAE respectively (Lo et al., 2003). Other targeting agents like lectins, invasins, antibodies etc. can be used as means of enhancing targeting and thus in turn particle uptake. Various ligands for the targeted immunization are summarized in Table 6.

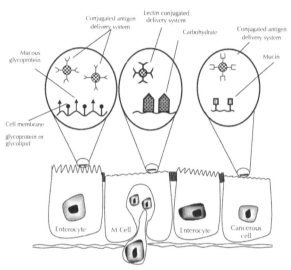

Figure 2. Various options for the targeted delivery. Mucus glycoprotein, M-cells and abnormal glycoprotein secreted by the cancerous cells can serve as receptor for binding with various ligands conjugated to drug/vaccine delivery system.

Table 6. Various ligands for targeted mucosal immunization.

Targeting Ligand	Targeting site	Conjugated material	Ref.
Ulex europaeus 1	Mouse Peyer's patch M cells	FITC, HRP Polystyrene microparticles Liposomes	Clark et al., 1995; Foster et al., 1998
mAb 5B11	Brush border of both M cells	Polystyrene latex microparticles	Kabok et al., 1994
Lycopersicon esculentum	Rat intestine	Polystyrene microparticles	Carreno-Gomez et al., 1999
Secretory IgA	Mouse Peyer's patch M	Liposomes	Zhou et al., 1995
Triticum vulgaris	Mouse intestine	Liposomes	Chen et al., 1996
Bandeiraea simplicifolia I isolectin B 4	Hamster NALT M cells	Biotin, HRP	Giannasca et al., 1987
Invasin-C192	Intestinal M cells	Polystyrene nanoparticles	Hussain and Florence, 1998
O-palmitoly mannan	Peyer's patch	Niosomes	Jain and Vyas, 2006
Cholera toxin B subunit	M cells of Peyer's patches	Bilosomes	Singh et al., 2004

Abbreviations: NALT, nasal-associated lymphoid tissue; FITC, fluorescein isothiocyanate; HRP, horseradish peroxidase mAb; monoclonal antibodies

Lectin Mediated Targeting

Lectins are proteins or glycoproteins capable of specific recognition of and reversible binding to carbohydrate determinants of complex glycoconjugates, without altering the covalent structure of any of the recognized glycosyl ligands. Lectin receptors are expressed on various cells such as endothelial cells, hepatocytes, macrophages, monocytes and lymphocytes. They are efficient in recognizing the complex oligosaccharide epitopes, which are also present on the cell surface or could be exogenous glycoconjugate ligands' mimics of endogenous carbohydrate epitopes (Vyas et al., 2001). Lectins are potential tools for the targeting of particulate vaccines to the M cell of the Peyer's patches, which are the sampling site of the mucosal immune system. Nanoparticles/microparticles may also be targeted to mouse Peyer's patch M cells by coating with the lectin UEA1 for the development of effective mucosally targeted vaccines. In studies reported by Foster et al. (1998), polystyrene microparticles (0.5 mm diameter) were covalently coated with the lectin UEA1 and administered to mice both by injection into ligated gut loops of anaesthetized animals and by oral gavage. In contrast to other proteins, lectin UEA1 coating selectively targeted the microparticles to mouse Peyer's patch M cells, and M cell adherent microparticles were rapidly endocytosed. Although the lectins specific for the human intestinal M cells await identification, human M cells preferentially display the sialyl Lewis A antigen (Giannasca et al., 1999) and this could be envisaged for targeting vaccines to the mucosal immune system. Future studies should determine whether lectins may similarly be used to target vaccine candidate in PLA/PLGA based delivery construct to intestinal M cells, and whether such targeting enhances the immune response to antigens delivered by these carrier systems. Our research group has developed biodegradable polymer based stabilized microparticles and nanoparticles for the mucosal vaccination (Jaganathan and Vyas, 2006) and also envisaged lectin for the targeted mucosal immunization (Gupta et al., 2006). Additionally we have also explored cholera toxin B subunit conjugated bilosomes (Singh et al., 2004) and mannosylated niosomes (Jain and Vyas 2006) as potential carrier-adjuvants for the targeted oral mucosal immunization.

Recently, we have developed hepatitis B surface antigen (HBsAg) encapsulated liposomes coupled with *Ulex europaeus agglutinin 1* (UEA-1) for increased transmucosal uptake by M-cells of the Peyer's patches (Gupta and Vyas, 2011). The liposomes were characterized for shape, size, polydispersity and encapsulation efficiency. Bovine submaxillary mucin (BSM) was used as a biological model for the *in vitro* determination of lectin activity and specificity. Dual staining technique was used to investigate targeting of lectinized liposomes to the M-cells (Figure 3). The serum anti-HBsAg IgG titre obtained after three consecutive days of oral immunizations with HBsAg encapsulated lectinized liposomes and boosting after third week, was comparable with the titre recorded after single intramuscular prime and third week boosting with alum-HBsAg (Figure 4). Moreover, lectinized liposomes induced higher sIgA level in mucosal secretions and cytokines level in the spleen homogenates (Figure 5). The results showed that the developed surface modified liposomes could be a potential module for the development of effective mucosal vaccines.

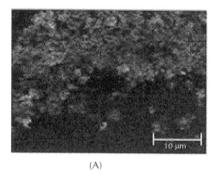
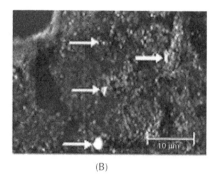

(A)   (B)

Figure 3. Confocal laser scanning microscopy images showing targeting of the liposomes to the M-cells of the Peyer's patches in mice by dual staining. M-cells were primarily stained with TRITC-UEA-1. Control liposomes (FITC-BSA coated) showed little or no binding to M-cells (A). Lectinized liposomes (shown by arrow) were associated predominantly with M-cells (B).

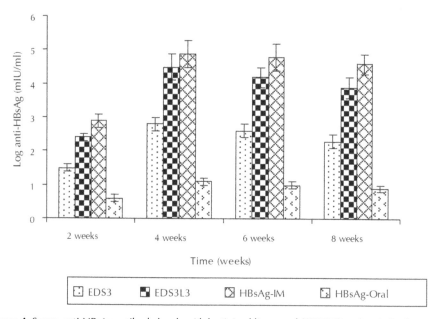

Figure 4. Serum anti-HBsAg antibody levels with lectinized liposomal (EDS3L3) and optimized non-lectinized liposomes (EDS3). The animals were immunized orally with the preparation equivalent to the 10 μg HBsAg for three consecutive days and booster dose was given after third week of first immunization. Single intramuscular immunization with booster dose after third week was given with the alum-HBsAg to serve as standard and HBsAg without liposomes was administered orally followed by a booster dose after third week for the comparison. After 4 weeks there was significant difference (P<0.001) among EDS3L3, EDS3, HBsAg-Oral or HBsAg-IM, however, the difference between EDS3L3 and HBsAg-IM was not significant (P>0.05).

Invasin Mediated Uptake

Invasins are virulent factor usually associated with the bacterial cell wall, and have the capacity to stimulate cytokine synthesis and to interact with mammalian cells by distinct mechanisms (Henderson et al., 1996). Young et al. (1992) demonstrated the potential of invasins for the internalization process. For this purpose, microparticles were coated with *Yersinia enterocolitica* invasin and the resulting conjugates put in contact with human laryngeal epithelial cells (Hep-2 cells). The presence or absence of internalised conjugates was monitored by TEM and light microscopy. It was clear that conjugates not only bound, but also were internalised by the Hep-2 cells. In contrast, control conjugates were rarely associated with these cells. *Salmonella typhimurium* selectively bind to, invade and destroy murine M cells and have been studied as live oral vaccine delivery vehicles. The M cell targeting by *S. typhimurium* is mediated by a specific adhesion (Jepson and Clark, 1998). Reovirus type 1 is another ligand, which selectively adhere to, and are endocytosed by intestinal M cells. It was demonstrated that proteolytic processing of native reovirus type 1 is required for adhesion to murin M cells and this is dependent on retention of modified σ1 and/or product of μ1 outer capsid protein. It has been suggested that σ1 protein is having potential for the targeted delivery (Clark et al., 2000).

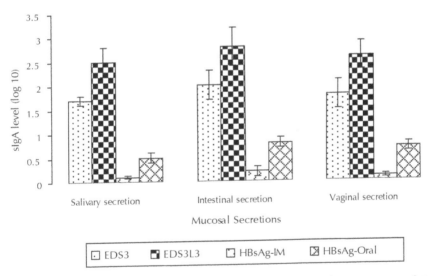

Figure 5. sIgA level in mucosal secretions after oral immunization with HBsAg encapsulating lectinized liposomes (EDS3L3) and optimized non-lectinized liposomes (EDS3). The animals were immunized orally with the preparation equivalent to the 10μg HBsAg for three consecutive days and booster dose was given after third week of first immunization. Single intramuscular immunization with booster dose after third week was given with the alum-HBsAg to serve as standard and HBsAg without liposomes was administered orally followed by a booster dose after third week for the comparison. The salivary, intestinal and vaginal secretions were collected after eight week of first immunization. The differences in the antibody level was significant (P<0.05) among EDS3L3, EDS3, HBsAg-Oral or HBsAg-IM.

Antibody Directed Targeting

The use of antibodies and monoclonal antibodies has been proposed for specific targeting within the gastrointestinal tract. It was observed that binding of the 5B11 monoclonal antibody, with specificity for rabbit M cells, to polystyrene particles, enhanced uptake by rabbit M-cells 3- to 3.5-times when compared to controls (Durrer et al., 1994). The ability of different conjugates, obtained by coating latex microparticles with albumin (BSA), bovine growth hormone (bGH), human IgG (hIgG), secretory IgA (hIgA), and bGH complexed with an IgG antibody raised against bGH (bGH-Ab), to be taken up by M cells were studied. It was found that the selectivity in binding to and entry into M-cells was improved by the use of IgG or bGH-Ab. Moreover, the appearance of conjugates in rat mesenteric lymph showed a similar selectivity to that found for binding and entry into M-cells. Ferritin-loaded liposomes conjugated to IgA were investigated for mucosal immunization via the rectum (Durrer et al., 1994). It was observed that the presence of IgA on the liposome surface increased the uptake of conjugates by PP, and the local rectal /colon immune response to ferritin, about five fold over uncoated liposomes.

NANOPARTICLES FOR VARIOUS MUCOSAL ROUTES

Although different mucosal surfaces are intimately networked with each other through the common mucosal immune system and homing of antigen-reactive cells from the organized lymphoid follicles, nevertheless there is significant degree of compartmentalization within the system. It has been shown previously that immunization of the inductive sites in the GALT and BALT is associated with the development of IgA antibody response and distribution of specific antigen reactive plasma cells in the lamina propria of respiratory, intestinal, and genital mucosa and in the nasopharynx and mammary glands (Kozlowski et al., 1997). However, differences exist in the magnitude of immune reactivity at different sites.

Oral Delivery of Vaccines

Particulate antigens are more effective for oral immunization than soluble antigens. The ability of particulate antigens to induce enhanced immune responses following oral immunization is mainly a consequence of their greater uptake into intestinal Peyer's patches. The microencapsulation step was undertaken to provide better protection for the antigen during intestinal transit and to target the antigen to the Peyer's patches. Poly (butyl-2-cyanoacrylate) microparticles induced enhanced antibody responses in comparison to oral immunization with soluble OVA. Moreover, smaller particles (100 nm) appeared to be more effective than larger ones (3 μm) for the induction of salivary IgA responses. The enhanced efficacy of the smaller particles may be attributed to their greater uptake into the Peyer's patches (O'Hagan, 1996).

The induction of enhanced serum, salivary and intestinal antibody responses following oral immunization in mice with 100 μg of staphylococcal enterotoxoid B (SEB) entrapped in PLG microparticles has been observed. The immunogenicity of OVA encapsulated microparticles has been shown to depend both on the dose of antigen administered and on the total number of particles per dose (Uchida et al., 1994). Particle size has a significant effect on the immunogenicity of PLG microparticles with entrapped OVA. It has been demonstrated that 4 μm microparticles were optimal for the induction of serum immune responses, but that 7 μm particles were optimal for mucosal IgA responses (Uchida et al., 1994). Despite the possibility of antigen denaturation during microencapsulation, PLG entrapped antigens have induced protective immunity following both systemic and mucosal immunization. In addition to protection of the respiratory tract following oral immunization, PLG microparticles could confer protective immunity against intestinal pathogens for example, *Vibrio cholerae, Helicobacter pylori* etc. (Del Giudice et al., 2001; Holmgren and Czerkinsky, 2005).

Nasal Vaccine Delivery

The nasal vaccine delivery can elicit either immune response or tolerance. The balance between active immunity and tolerance is influenced by the nature of the antigen and its interaction with the mucosal inductive site (Partidos, 2000). Factors such as the dose, the use of an adjuvant, frequency of administration and genetic background of the host are contributing factors. Thus, an understanding of the mechanisms that lead to a mucosal immune response is crucial in developing effective nasal vaccines. Intranasal immunization elicits both humoral and cellular immune responses. The antigen is sampled and passed to underlying lymphoid cells in the submucosa where antigen processing and presentation take place. As a result the activation of T-cells occurs, which help B-cells to develop into IgA plasma cells (Partidos, 2000; Wu and Russell, 1997). The interaction between an antigen and the nasal mucosa and the NALT will depend on a variety of factors but the physical nature of the antigen (solution or particulate), the dose and frequency of contact influenced profoundly the immune response.

Small soluble antigens are able to penetrate the nasal epithelium and interact with dendritic cells, macrophages and lymphocytes. Drainage is then to the superficial cervical lymph node which then drains to the posterior lymph nodes. Contrary to this, antigen in the form of nanoparticles is largely taken up by M-cells in the NALT. The NALT drains preferentially to the cervical lymph nodes. The antigen so taken up can elicit a local (and also a distant) mucosal response or lead to tolerance (Sminia and Kraal, 1999). Yanagitu et al. (1999) reported the antibacterial activity of mucosal Th1 and Th2 immune responses in mice responsible for the inhibitions of bacterial attachment to epithelial cells. They concluded that nasal vaccination was an effective immunization regime for the induction of antigen specific Th1 and Th2 cell driven IgA immune responses that possess an ability to inhibit bacterial attachment to epithelial cells and subsequent inflammatory cytokine production. Further, Wu and Russel (1997) confirmed that intranasal vaccination is more effective than intragastric immunization at generating earlier and stronger mucosal immune responses. Additionally, nasal lymphoid tissue (NALT) and its draining lymph nodes may retain long-term memory.

Rectal Delivery of Vaccine

The rectum in humans and mouse is well populated with lymphoid tissue, with well-defined lymphoid aggregates and typical M cells. These tissues offer a promising site for vaccine delivery, which may be convenient to exploit, particularly in young children. Immunization via the rectal route would avoid exposing vaccines to hostile environment that is the low pH and abundant proteolytic enzymes present in the upper gastrointestinal tract. The rectal route may be successfully exploited for vaccine delivery using particulate delivery systems (Zhou et al., 1995). At the same time, there are serious limitations associated with the potential exploitation of the rectal route of immunization. The vaccine may be expelled before it has time to be effective and this may be difficult to control in young children. Additionally, there may be considerable cultural resistance to the acceptance of formulations delivered by the rectal route. Due to these limitations rectal immunization has not been studied as intensely as other mucosal sites. However, studies carried out with poliovirus, SIV, influenza virus, and *S. enterica* have demonstrated that intrarectal administration of antigens is highly effective in inducing specific antibody responses in the intestine and other sites in the common mucosal system (Bergmeier et al., 1992).

Vaginal Vaccine Delivery

The vagina is envisaged as a component of the common mucosal immune system and oral and intranasal immunization in mice with microparticles induces a vaginal antibody response. The presence of aggregated lymphoid follicles or M cells in the vaginal epithelium is not reported so far yet, intravaginal immunization in humans induced local antibody responses. However, intravaginal immunization strategy in small animal models is not much successsful, despite the use of novel delivery systems (starch microparticles) and adjuvants (O'Hagan et al., 1993). Additionally, the local immune response in the vagina is under influence of hormonal control, with major changes in local antibodies at different stages of the cycle. Recently it has been shown that the intranasal route of immunization was more effective than the intravaginal route for the induction of immune responses in the vagina (Tommaso et al., 1996). As a result, the vaginal route of immunization seems unlikely to be successfully exploited for the development of novel vaccines. Moreover, the genital tract is a less potential site for the mucosal immunization because it displays several distinct features not shared by typical mucosal tissues and external secretions (Mestecky et al., 2005).

Sublingual Delivery of Vaccines

Vaccine delivery by sublingual route is an attractive alternative to conventional parenteral delivery. This non-invasive mode of vaccines administration is a potential approach for allergen vaccination (Olaguibel et al., 2005). Sublingual immunotherapy (SLIT) has been investigated as a non-invasive alternate in order to treat type I allergies (Van Overtvelt et al., 2006). Small molecules can cross the squamous epithelia, the basement membrane and the lamina propria at various sites within the mouth and thus are transported to the systemic circulation via the deep facial and brachio-cephalic veins. Sites do vary in the mouth in terms of keratinization of the outermost epithelium, in thickness and in other features, which render some tissues more suitable than others for the intentional delivery of drugs by this route. Various innate properties of drugs, lipid solubility, ionization and molecular size contribute to the ease at which they may diffuse across the oral membranes.

The possibility of delivering proteins by the mouth, to which immune response is required is worthy of consideration. Penetration enhancers and bio/mucoadhesives have been investigated for their suitability. Additionally, various devices such as patches, wafers and tablets have also been studied as physical aids to retain the applied drug on the required tissue (Wheeler and Sharif, 1996). Allergens cause local inflammation in the mouth in sensitive people and thus it is likely that these allergenic proteins are hitting targets such as IgE-coated mast cells. Moreover, allergens could be used as a model for immunization with other antigens. Thus it is assumed that allergens can desensitize patients when given sublingually. It is not proven, however, that these proteins do in fact cross the sublingual epithelium to stimulate local or systemic immunological tissues. It is possible that ingress occurs where the junctional epithelia are attached to the tooth surface, where there is a constant inflammation and where various cell types involved in the immune response are usually present. The delivery of allergen-specific immunotherapy by the oral route is termed as SLIT and it has reported to be effective and safer than subcutaneous administration. Sublingual-mucosal Langerhans cells can capture the allergen and transport it to local lymph nodes, which may lead to induction of T lymphocytes that suppress the allergic responses. However, the contact of allergen with the antigen presenting cells in the oral mucosal is crucial and is a key determinant (Akdis et al., 2006).

Pulmonary and Ocular Vaccine Delivery

Pulmonary and ocular vaccine delivery constitutes another mode of vaccine delivery via mucosal route. The vaccine delivery to the alveoli can be achieved by pulmonary route through aerosolized vaccine administration. The pulmonary vaccine delivery to the bronchus-associated lymphoid tissue has been reported for the immunization of human against measles using a live attenuated virus (Dilraj et al., 2000). Herpes simplex virus (HSV) commonly infect eye and ocular mucosal immunity to HSV has been raised by ocular immunization for the treatment of infection with HSV. Vaccines against HSV administered as drops to the eyes have shown effective ocular-mucosal immunity (Nesburn et al., 1998).

Mixed Mucosal Routes

An emerging concept is immunization by mixed mucosal routes or a combination of mucosal and parenteral routes of vaccine administration. Based on experiments carried out with *Shigella, N. gonorrheae, S. pneumoniae, V. cholerae, S. enterica* and poliovirus, it has been concluded that mucosal immune responses can be enhanced by parenteral priming followed by oral booster immunization. Enhancement of mucosal immune response can be achieved by parenteral or mucosal priming with infectious agents, although the mechanism underlying the enhancement of mucosal immune response following either route of priming is still undefined. Other investigations have also supported the beneficial effects of oral priming on parenteral booster immunizations with cholera, *S. enterica* influenza, and other vaccines (Coffin and Offit, 1998).

CONCLUSION

Recent discoveries in both mucosal vaccine delivery and mucosal adjuvant research have significantly improved the effectiveness of mucosal immunization in animal models. The mucosal immune system is a complex system that generate large amount of s-IgA as well as cell mediated immunity at mucosal surfaces to prevent pathogen infiltration and inflammation. The mucosal immune system should be most efficient in providing protection against pathogens and generating longer lasting protection using attenuated pathogen for vaccine. The only mucosal vaccines approved for humans are attenuated pathogens. Future mucosal vaccines will also involve vaccines strategies other than attenuated pathogens. New delivery strategies such as immunization of live recombinant vectors, DNA plasmids, and transgenic plants to deliver antigens present promises to improve the efficiency of mucosal antigen delivery. Further, DNA vaccines and subunit vaccines such as bacterial adhesion in combination with potent mucosal adjuvants (such as QS21; a saponin, unmethylated CpG motifs or cytokines such as IL-12) or mucosal delivery systems based on nanoparticles will have the potential to be the next generation of vaccines. Mucosal delivery of vaccines offers a number of significant advantages over systemic delivery. One potential approach to the mucosal delivery of vaccines is the encapsulation or entrapment of antigens into polymer based nanoparticles or microparticles. Polymeric delivery systems can be manipulated to enhance the efficacy of mucosally administered vaccines in a number of ways; they can protect antigens from degradation, concentrate them in one area of the mucosal tissue for better absorption, extend their residence time in the body, or target them to sites of antigen uptake (e.g., Peyer's patches in the gut).

Immunization does not always stimulate immunity because of the insufficient elicitation of immune responses. Such limitations have spurred the development of new adjuvant and antigen-delivery systems. Adjuvant plays an important role in enhancing the efficacy of vaccines. Recombinant proteins or synthetic peptides are safer than crude inactivated microorganism, but less immunogenic. This limitation can be overcome by using specific adjuvant. The adjuvant selection depends on several criteria, like the target species, the antigens, the type of desired immune response, the route of administration, or the duration of immunity. So far, biodegradable polymers particularly of PLGA have been used, considerably because of their well-known degradation properties. An area requiring additional efforts is analytical characterization of protein-encapsulated nanoparticles. Advanced methods for protein characterization is in demand to approach the problem of protein stabilization in polymer based delivery systems. Development of *in vitro–in vivo* correlation for protein release from protein nanoparticles is another issue. More intensive interactions between immunologists and drug delivery specialists are required to understand protein release and its presentation to the immune system. All the approaches involving encapsulation of antigens into nanoparticles are likely to suffer from the same significant drawback; the extent of uptake of the particles across the gut appears to be limited. Whether or not the extent of uptake in humans is sufficient to allow the development of an effective oral vaccine is currently unknown. However, it is clear that in rodents, the extent of uptake of nanoparticles can be enhanced using targeting ligands.

Numerous studies suggest that the efficiency of particle absorption can be improved through modification of particle surfaces with targeting molecules such as antibodies or lectins etc. Albeit the results are promising, it is not known if any of the strategies will be effective in humans because it is currently unclear whether particulates are taken up in human GIT. Additionally the uptake mechanisms and absorption efficiencies are not known. Thus current knowledge obtained from animal models may or may not be extendible to human beings. Continued research to understand the inter-connection and sub-compartmentalization of the common mucosal system will certainly guide the rational selection for routes of mucosal administration. An efficient delivery vehicle, combined with an effective adjuvant given through an optimal route of administration, will ultimately allow for the development of a successful needle-free (mucosal) vaccine in humans.

KEYWORDS

- **Antigen-presenting cells**
- **Dendritic cells**
- **Gut-associated lymphoid tissue**
- **Nasal associated lymphoid tissue**
- **Organized mucosal associated lymphoid tissue**

Chapter 7

Biosynthesis of Silver Nanoparticles, Characterization and Their Antimicrobial Activity

K. Mallikarjuna, G. Narasimha, B. V. Subba Reddy, B. Sreedhar, G. R. Dillip, and B. Deva Prasad Raju

INTRODUCTION

There has been an increasing interest in the development of a clean synthetic procedure often known as "green chemistry" for nanoproducts which are targeted as potential applications in the fields of catalysis in chemical reactions, drug delivery in medical field, biolabelling, microelectronic, information storage, and optoelectronic devices (Crooks et al., 2001; Bhumakar et al., 2007; Dai and Bruening, 2002; Gittins et al., 2000; Hayat, 1989; Murray et al., 2001). The broad spectrum of silver nanoparticles was produced by different physical and chemical methods. For environmental concerns, there is a need to develop benign nanoparticles using non-toxic chemicals in the synthesis protocols in order to avoid adverse effects in medical applications. At present, several groups of researchers concentrate on biomimetic approaches such as plant or plant leaf extracts, microorganisms and yeast to synthesize the metal nanoparticles called as "green chemical or phytochemical" approach (Sinha et al., 2009). One of the synthesis procedure such as leaf extracts of *geranium, lemon grass, neem and several others* has been reported (Dubey et al., 2010; Rajesh et al., 2009; Shankar et al., 2003, 2004a, 2004b; Song et al., 2009;). The *Piper betle* is a traditional medicinal plant of India, The betel leaf is used in a number of traditional remedies for the treatment of stomach ailments, infections, and as a general tonic. It is often chewed in combination with the betel nut *(Areca catechu)*, as a stimulatory. Some evidence suggests that betel leaves have immune boosting properties as well as anti-cancer properties. It is also well known for its phenolic content, and also for its antibacterial and antioxidant activities as well. So far, there have been no reports on the synthesis of nanoparticles by using *piper betle* leaf extract. In this paper, we report on the synthesis of silver nanoparticles using *piper betle* leaf, their characterization and their antibacterial activity.

EXPERIMENTAL DETAILS

Preparation of Leaf Extract

The fresh leaves of *piper betle* were collected from a retail shop in Tirupati, Andhra Pradesh, India. Silver nitrate (AgNO$_3$, 99.99%) was purchased from Sigma-Aldrich chemicals.10g of fresh leaves were washed thoroughly under the running tap water, while finely cut leaves were added with 50 ml of distilled water in a 250 ml Erlenmeyer flask, and then boiled for 10min, before decanting it. The extract was filtered and stored at 4°C for further experiments.

Synthesis of Silver Nanoparticles

The leaf broth with various concentration levels, ranging from 50 to 150 μl was added to 3 ml of 1mM aqueous AgNO₃ solution kept at room temperature. The bioreduced silver nitrate solution was monitored by periodic sampling of aliquots (0.3 ml). It wasdiluted to the ratio of 1:10 with distilled water, to avoid errors due to high optical density of the solution for measuring UV-Vis spectra.

Antifungal Activity of Silver Nanoparticles

The antifungal activity of the silver nanoparticles was checked against *Aspergillussps.* The pure cultures of the fungi were obtained by sub culturing. The culture slants were subjected to a 3 ml sterile distilled water containing 0.01 ml of TritionX-100. 100 μl of fungal spore   suspension was loaded into the Czapek-Dox agar medium plates. Later cavities of 0.5 cm diameter were made and filled with 100 μl of silver nanoparticle solution.

Antibacterial Activity of Silver Nanoparticles

The antibacterial property of silver nanoparticles was checked on both gram positive and gram negative bacteria by following the agar diffusion method. Gram positive bacteria like *Staphylococcus sps, Bacillus sps* and gram negative bacteria like *Escherichia coli (E.Coli) Psedomononassps*were used for the present study. The 24 hr active cultures of the above bacterial strains were seeded in the Agar plates by pour plate technique. Cavities of 0.5 cm diameter were made using a borer and the bottoms of the cavities were sealed. Each cavity was filled with 100 μl of silver nanoparticles solution and then incubated at 37°C in an incubator.

RESULTS AND DISCUSSION

UV-Visible Absorbance Spectroscopy

The concentration variation with bioreduced Ag⁺ ions, in aqueous component were measured with an UV-V is spectrometer, (Perkin-Elmer lambda 25)which operated at a resolution of 1nm in the range of 370800 nm. The progress of the reaction between the *betle* leaf broth and the metal ions were observed by UV-V is spectra of silver nanoparticles which are shown in Figure 1. A Bathochromatic shift in the surface plasmon resonance band of silver nanocolloid, with an increasing concentration of leaf extract and consequent color change was observed. From the spectrum, we observed that the peak blue shift was at 477440 nm while the amount of leaf extract was constantly increased. The reduction of silver ions and the synthesis of stable nanoparticles occurred with a concentration variation reaction, making it one of the smart phytofabricationmethods; in order to produce Ag nanoparticles reported nowadays (Dwivedi and Gopal, 2010; Gils et al., 2010; Konwarh et al., 2011; Philip and Unni, 2011).

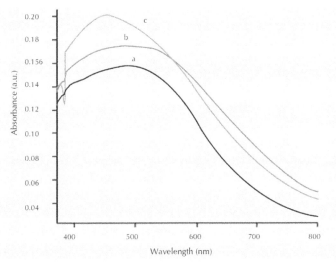

Figure 1. UV-Vis spectra of silver nitrate with *piper betle* leaf extract at different concentrations. a) 50 L, b) 100 μL and c) 150 μL.

X-Ray Diffraction Spectral Analysis

An X-ray diffraction (XRD) measurement of a thin film of the bioreduced silver ions' aqueous solution was drop coated onto a glass slide and carried out on an INEL X-ray diffractometer. The diffraction pattern was recorded by Co-kα₁ radiation with λ of 1.78A° in the region of 2θ from 20 to 90° at 0.02/min. and the time constant was 2 sec. The size of the nanoparticles was calculated through the Scherer's equation (Mulvaney, 1996). The Crystalline nature of Ag nanoparticles was studied with the aid of an X-ray diffraction (Figure 2).The diffracted peaks were observed at 37.6° and 44.4°

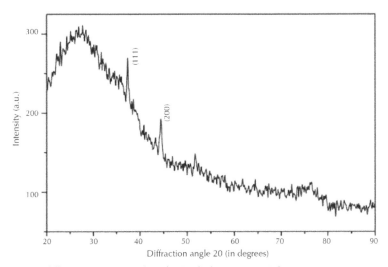

Figure 2. X-Ray diffraction spectrum of synthesized silver nanoparticles.

corresponding to the (111) and (200) facets of the face centered cubic crystal and the data was matched with the Joint Committee on Powder Diffraction Standards (JCPDS) file No.030921. The domain size of the phytofabricatedsilver nanoparticles is found to be 5.4 nm,by using the width of the (111) Bragg's reflection which was in consonance with the size of the particle, calculated from the TEM image.

Transmission Electron Microscopy Studies

The morphology and size of the silver nanoparticles were studied by the Transmission electron microscopy (TEM) image, by usingthe PHILLIPS TECHNAI FE 12 instrument.The TEM grids were prepared by placing a drop of the bio reduced diluted solution, on a carbon-coated copper grid and by later drying it under a lamp. The TEM image (Figure 3) was employed, so that the bio synthesized nanoparticles were in the size of 337 nm. They were spherical in shape and few nanoparticles were also agglomerated. Under careful observation, it is evident that the silver nanoparticles are surrounded by a faint thin layer of other materials. The histogram of fabricated silver nanoparticles is shown in Figure 4. It is evident that there is a variation in particle sizes and the estimated average size is 12 nm.The small sized nanoparticles were able to easily penetrate across the membrane; and similar results have been reported in literature (Jaidev and Narasimha, 2010; Pal et al., 2007; Morones et al., 2005).

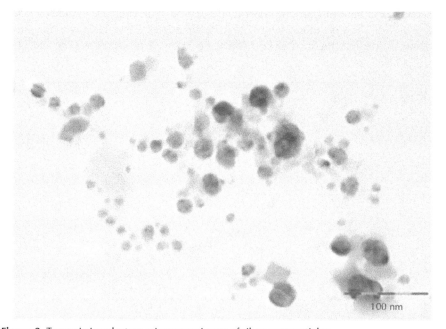

Figure 3. Transmission electron microscopy image of silver nanoparticles.

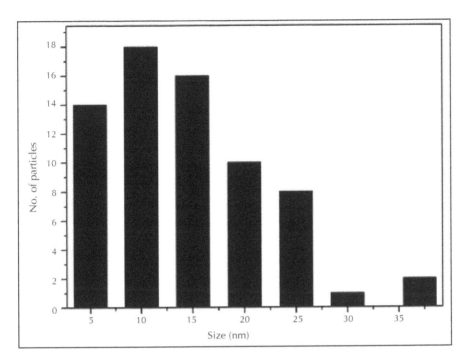

Figure 4. Histogram of synthesized silver nanoparticles.

Fourier Transformed Infra-Red Spectroscopy

For Fourier transformed infrared (FTIR) measurements, the bioreduced Ag$^+$ ion aqueous component was centrifuged at 10,000 rpm for 15 min. The dried sample was grinded with KBr pellets and analyzed on Thermo Nicolet Nexus 670 IR spectrometer which was operatedat a resolution 4 cm^1 in the region of 4,000400 cm^{-1}. The FTIR spectrum of synthesized silver nanoparticles by using *Piper betle* leaf extract is shown in Figure 5. It confirmedthe fact that to identify the bimolecular for reducing and efficient stabilization of the metal nanoparticles, the band at 3,419 cm^1 corresponds to O-H, as also the H-bonded alcohols and phenols. The peak at 2,920 cm^1 indicates carboxylic acid. The band at 1,640 cm^1 states primary amines. The band at 1,431 cm^1 corresponds to C-C stretching aromatics, while the peak at 1,378 cm^1 states C-H rock alkenes and 1,163, 1,113 and 1,058 cm^1 indicatethe C-O stretching alcohols, carboxylic acids, esters and ethers. Therefore, the synthesized nanoparticles were encapsulated by some proteins and metabolites such as terpenoids having functional groups of alcohols, ketones, aldehydes and carboxylic acids.

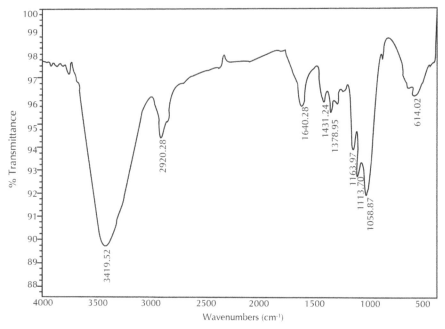

Figure 5. FTIR spectrum of green synthesized silver nanoparticles.

Table 1. Inhibitiory activity of silver nanoparticles (100μl) on bacterial strains.

S. No	Organism	Zone of inhibiton (cm)
1.	*Aspergillussps*	1.2
2.	*E.coli*	1.8
3.	*Pseudomonas sps*	1.12
4.	*Staphylococcus sps*	1.01
5.	*Bacillus sps*	0.89

*All values represented the in the table are average of conducted experiment.

The antifungal property of silver nanoparticles checked against the fungi *Aspergillussps.* was shown in Table 1. The Agar plate with fungal culture having the cavities filled with nanoparticles suspension showed a clear zone of diameter 1.2 cm. This indicates that silver nanoparticles have the antifungal activity and are very effective against the pathological fungi like *Aspergillus* which cause the disease Aspergillosis. Similar reports were made by Devendra, et al. 2009. According to his studies, papaya fruit extract mediated silver nanoparticles exhibited antibacterial activity against *E.coli* and *Pseudomonasaeruginosa*. The antifungal activity of silver nanoparticles could be disruption of transmembrane energy metabolism and membrane electron transport chain by formation of insoluble compounds in the cell wall; the formation of insoluble compound may be due to the inactivation of cell wall sulfhydryl group; silver ions can create mutation in fungal DNA by displacing the hydrogen bonds; silver ions can dissociate the enzyme complexes which are essential for respiratory chain and membrane permeability, disruption of membrane bound enzymes and lipids could cause the cell lysis(Velmurugan et al., 2009).

These bacterial strains in petriplate with the clearing zones around the cavities reveal that the silver nanoparticles inhibit the growth of the bacterial strains. The formation of inhibition zones around the wells containing silver nanoparticles against the test strains *Staphylococcus* sp. was measured as 1.01 cm, *Bacillus* sp. was 0.89 cm and *E.coli* was 1.8 cm (Table 1). This shows that the silver nanoparticles were more effective on *E.coli* (gram negative bacteria). Several studies have investigated and interpreted the interaction of the silver nanoparticles with bacteria. Similarly Sondi, et al. (2004) and Morones, et al. (2005), revealed that majority of the silver nanoparticles were localized on the membranes of treated *E. coli* cells. According to Lok et al. (2006), the treatment of *E.coli* cells with nanomolar concentrations of silver nanoparticles results in an immediate dissipation of the proton motive force, killing the cells. The gram positive and gram negative bacteria in antibiotic enhanced the action of silver nanoparticles and showed that the silver nanoparticles got bound to the DNA of the bacteria which caused their inactivation.

With reference to the above studies, the possible mechanism of the action of silver nanoparticles on both bacteria and fungi may be generalized as their accumulation in the cell membrane caused lysis of the cell by some unknown mechanism.

CONCLUSION

The bio synthesis of silver nanoparticles using leaf broth of *piper betle* provides an environment friendly, simple, cost effective and efficient route for the synthesis of benign nanoparticles. The size of the silver nanoparticles was estimated to be 337 nm. The reduced silver nanoparticles effectively inhibited the growth of microorganisms including bacterial and fungal strains which cause diseases in human beings. Further works needs to be conducted to investigate the cellular mechanism and toxicity of nanoparticles in microorganism.

KEYWORDS

- **Fourier transformed infrared**
- **Green chemistry**
- **Nanoparticles**
- **Transmission electron microscopy**
- **X-ray diffraction**

Chapter 8

Gold-peptide Nanoparticles Activation of Macrophages

Jagat R. Kanwar, Ganesh Mahidhara, and Rupinder K. Kanwar

MACROPHAGE BIOLOGY AND CYTOKINE ACTIVATION

Innate part of the human immune system tackles bacteria or foreign particle entry to the human body. As integral components, monocytes, and neutrophil granulocytes circulate in the bloodstream and readily eliminate pathogens or clear particles (Roslavtseva and Ivanova, 1975; Schwarzer et al., 1999). Monocytes are the parent cells for more stable and/or long lived macrophages or dendritic cells, which represent integral part of innate immune defense mechanism (Auffray et al., 2009). Macrophages are white blood cells that are mainly produced in bone marrow. Their primary function is immunity against bacteria and other pathogens. Macrophages also help the body to clean up cellular debris from organs through phagocytosis. They can act by a number of different mechanisms: directly, by destroying bacteria and pathogens' antimicrobial proteins, reactive oxygen species, and proteolytic enzymes (Cohen, 1994); indirectly by inducing certain pro-inflammatory cytokines [interleukin-1β (IL-1β), interleukin-6 (IL-6), tumor necrosis factor-α (TNF-α) and nitric oxide synthase-2 (NOS$_2$)] (Kanwar et al., 2009; Vadiveloo, 1999) which can activate other immune cells; and by repairing tissue damage (Vadiveloo, 1999). Macrophages originate in the bone marrow and are transported around the body *via* blood circulation. They can be differentiated after being modified with cytokines and resides in specific organs as a form of specific defense mechanism (Xaus et al., 2001). When they are required for inflammatory responses, macrophages need to be activated and become fully functional by interaction with the cytokine interferon-gamma (IF-γ), as well as its own growth factor macrophage colony-stimulating factor (M-CSF) (Mosser, 2003). Once they interact with these molecules they can either proliferate, become activated, differentiate into their stationary phases or die through apoptosis, if not needed. However, once they have been activated by M-CSF, proliferation is inhibited with further contact of IF-γ as well as the protein lipopolysaccharide (LPS) to be able to carry out their given functions (Vadiveloo, 1999). It was previously mentioned that macrophages indirectly induce this cytokine to activate other immune cells. Furthermore, there is conflicting data saying that instead of the growth factor M-CSF being a key role in activation, the other signal comes from TNF (Bastus et al., 2009a, 2009b). It can be concluded from the above observations that macrophage activation induces the different cytokines and their proliferation subsequently inhibited. In addition to the above mentioned phagocytic mechanisms, neutrophil granulocytes release structures into the extracellular space that mainly consist of DNA and protein and trap pathogens at infection sites (neutrophil extracellular traps (NETs) (Brinkmann et al., 2004). These structures contain a variety of antibacterial proteins from azurophilic granules. Recent reports have shown that the formation of extracellular traps is not restricted to neutrophils but they are formed as well by mast cells for entrapping pathogens (von Kockritz-Blickwede et al., 2008).

Synthesis of Nano Conjugated Peptides

There are a number of peptides used in the human body that acts as antigens, hormones, neurotransmitters in the brain and nervous system and as natural pain relievers by meddling the immune system (Bastus et al., 2009a). A recent study used the synthetic peptides LPFFDNH$_2$ and (VRLPPP)$_3$ (Bastus et al., 2009b), to tag gold nanoparticles to induce macrophage activation. The first one is an amyloid growth inhibitor peptide (AGIP). It has a number of amino acids that are in the same configuration as amyloid β protein associated with Alzheimer's disease (Bastus et al., 2009a, 2009b). This peptide when conjugated with gold nanoparticles (Kimling et al., 2006) can be selectively attached to the β-amyloid fibers, indicating its functions other than macrophage activation. It (VRLPPP)$_3$ is a non-toxic type peptide called sweet arrow peptide (SAP)—mainly used for cellular drug delivery that is attracted to the cell membranes. To compare the activation of macrophages in the presence of AGIP variants, LPDFFNH$_2$ (ISO1), and DLPFFNH$_2$ (ISO2), which have altered polarity were used. Changing the order of the amino acids produces a difference in overall charge, thus creating different polarities in the three species. All four species of peptide were synthesized by solid-phase peptide synthesis and characterized using TOF-SIMS spectrometry (Fernandez-Carneado et al., 2004). The gold nanoparticles used in this study were synthesized using the Turkevich method (Bastus et al., 2009b). Citrate stabilized nanoparticles that were conjugated to the amino acid cysteine were also used. The sulfur atoms in cysteine strongly bound covalently and were more strongly attracted to the peptides. To conjugate the gold nanoparticles (AuNPs) with the peptides, a solution of the peptides was added to the AuNPs and stirred for an extended period so as to coat the whole surface of the gold. Confirmation of the conjugation between the NP's and peptides was assured using a number of methods including UV-vis spectroscopy, dynamic light scattering (DLS), zeta potential, and electron energy loss spectroscopy (EELS). For UV spectrometry, the attachment of the peptides creates a shift in the surface plasmon resonance, producing a spectrum different to that of the single AuNP. High resolution TEM (HRTEM) and X-ray photo-electron spectroscopy were used in addition to EELS to characterize the morphology of the surface of the particles.

TLR-4 Dependent Activation of Macrophages

It has been observed that the recognition of the conjugates by the macrophages is mediated by toll-like receptor 4 (TLR-4) (Bastus et al., 2009a). The TLR-4 is also involved in the production of the pro-inflammatory cytokines IL-1β, IL-6, and TNF-α. These cytokines are used to analyze the response to addition of AuNPs. Experiments done with TRL-4 have used cell lines from mice with same genetic background to observe whether genetic makeup plays a role in macrophage mutation or inhibition. Mice were TLR-4 deficient and macrophage conjugations were injected to study the results of activation and proliferation. All the mice had a mutation of the TLR-4 that made them resistant to LPS—the surface molecule on the macrophages. This led the researchers to use LPS as the positive control in their experiments. Proliferation tests were carried out in the presence of polymixin B (Bastus et al., 2009a; 2009b), which binds to the lipid part of LPS and interferes with the production of TLR-4. Basically, the inhibition of proliferation by the AGIP and SAP conjugates was regressed in the absence of TLR-4. This data shows that TLR-4 is a major factor in inducing the signaling activated by the peptide conjugates. It is then mentioned that polymixin B restored the effects of M-CSF on proliferation of macrophages. Thus, TLR-4 was shown to be an important mediator in the immune-biology of macrophages in response to the peptide loaded gold nanoparticles. This would avoid any inflammation from the body not recognizing the particles, and then the molecules could accumulate in specific organs to induce phagocytosis of cellular debris and perform other functions (Bastus et al., 2009a). In another study, a significant increase in IL-6, reactive oxygen species (ROS) generation, nuclear translocation of nuclear factor-kappa B (NF-κB), induction of cyclooxygenase-2 (COX-2), and tumor necrosis factor-alpha (TNF-α) expression was observed in macrophages with maximum response found in cells exposed to AuNps for a prolonged time (Nishanth et al., 2011). More recently, 60 nm AuNPs, under the exposure conditions tested, are shown to be non cytotoxic, nor elicit pro-inflammatory responses. The localization of AuNPs in intracellular vacuoles suggests endosomal containment and an uptake mechanism involving endocytosis (Zhang et al., 2010). The Cy5.5-MMP-AuNPs are being developed for NIR fluorescence imaging of MMPs expressed in tumors, atherosclerosis, myocardial infarction, and other diseases. The peptide Gly-Pro-Leu-Gly-Val-Arg-Gly-Cys-NH$_2$ was found to be a MMP substrate and is cleaved between Leu and Gly residues. This sequence along with Cy5.5 has been used to attach to AuNPs to form fluorescence-quenched nanoparticles (Lee et al., 2008). It is well-known that nanoparticles are rapidly internalized by immune cells when the particle surface is not adjusted (for example, by surface grafting of poly(ethylene oxide) (PEO)) to minimize interaction (Gref et al., 1994). Thus, the interaction of gold nanoparticle library with primary human immune cells could be classified as macropinocytosis rather than phagocytosis.

Activation of Cytokine Response after Treatment with Conjugates

A set of experiments carried out by exposing the macrophages to the cytokines for 6 hr using the activation of LPS as a control shows that there was no response to Cys-AGIP or citrate-stabilized AuNPs as they produced similar results to the untreated tests. However, on addition of the conjugation, AuNP-CysAGIP, there was a definite pro-inflammatory response with an increase of cytokines, including IL-1β, IL-6, and TNF-α (Bastus et al., 2009a). Length of the peptide chains were compared to see if that has a marked affect on inducing cytokines. From the results of the AuNP-CysAGIP (6 amino acids) conjugation, they used AuNP, CysSAP, and AuNP-CysSAP (19 amino acids) for the same experiment. The results produced the same findings, suggesting that macrophage induction is independent of peptide length. Therefore, these studies were directed at another difference in peptide structure—polarity. For this purpose, they took the AGIP peptide and changed the configuration of amino acids to create change in polarity. These molecules, [LPDFFNH$_2$ (ISO1) and DLPFFNH$_2$ (ISO2)], also produced the same outcome as the AGIP and SAP tests (Bastus et al., 2009b)—that the non-conjugation of peptides had no affect on induction of macrophage response, whereas the conjugation to AuNPs showed significant induction. It is mentioned that induction was somehow dependent of peptide sequence, but do not explain how or to what extent. But in the experimental observations all the conjugates were found to induce TNF-α and IL-β, but only AuNP-CysAGIP stimulated the IL-6 cytokine. Also, that NOS2 levels were insignificant in the presence of AuNP-CysSAP. From this data, it could be concluded that the immune system could be adapted to produce certain immune response by simply changing the configuration of the peptides. The AuNPs alone were shown that they cannot induce macrophage activation but more so that different forms of peptides conjugated to gold could have varying affects on the immune response of macrophage and surrounding molecules.

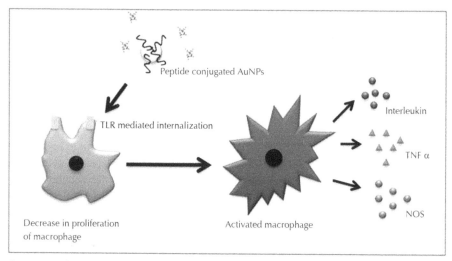

Figure 1. Outline of macrophage activation by using peptide loaded gold nanoparticles. Controlled activation of macrophages could be achieved by the conjugation of the oligopeptides, which otherwise could not be recognized by immune system.

Inhibition of Proliferation by Conjugates

As mentioned earlier, macrophages cannot proliferate without the addition of M-CSF. With the induction of cytokines, the separate peptide molecules do not have an effect until they are conjugated together. Tests using the AGIP or SAP conjugates showed that there was an inhibition of proliferation rate of 50% with just 0.3 μM of conjugate solution (Bastus et al., 2009a). It then mentions that higher doses up to 1 mM have no affect on inhibition. However, they fail to state reasons or as to why the increase in dosage has not affected the activation. It can be seen from the findings that anything above approximately 1 μM solution does not cause any inhibition to proliferation and/

or activation of macrophages. Thus, it could be concluded that conjugates of certain peptides have an effect on the macrophage biology by blocking cell cycle progression.

Internalization of Peptide Conjugates

Various experiments were carried out to study the phagocytic activity of macrophages in the presence of AuNPs and their peptide conjugates (Bastus et al., 2009b). A number of tests were undertaken with AuNPs alone, native peptides as well as the conjugates. The conjugate used was the AuNP-CysAGIP as it induced more pro-inflammatory cytokines (Bastus et al., 2009a). The macrophages were incubated with different treatments and scanned over a range of time periods ranging from 15 min to 24 hr. The samples were observed under TEM to assess the internalization of the nanoparticles (Bastus et al., 2009a). It was seen that the conjugations were initially internalized within 30 min and the internalization was maximum at 6 hr. However, at 12 hr there was not a good amount of nanoparticles observed within the macrophage (Bastus et al., 2009a). This was shown to be the case with using conjugations rather than separate molecules alone in accordance with other experiments. It seems to suggest that with a correlation to the pro-inflammatory response to the conjugates as mentioned earlier, internalization after a certain time frame shows that the macrophages detect the gold particles, which in turn induce particular cytokines that inhibit the macrophage proliferation. This prevents any further uptake of the conjugates, shown by minimal internalization after 6 hr. The results suggest that internalization is active via a certain receptor rather than the normal phagocytosis cycle (Bastus et al., 2009a, 2009b). Again, this highlights that not only are the AuNP conjugates used for activating macrophages, but altering the immunobiology of them to induce, activate or proliferate at any desired time.

CONCLUSION

Modern vaccines are usually produced by recombinant technology and do not replicate in the host. Unfortunately, isolated soluble components of viruses and other pathogens are often poorly immunogenic in the absence of nonspecific inflammatory stimuli. Gold nanoparticles seem to be promising carriers in this regard. Nanoparticles conjugated with peptides were shown to induce controlled activation macrophages. There were some minor findings that suggested other factors could be tested and used to advance the studies in other areas of macrophage activation. Various experiments conducted to study inhibition of proliferation by a number of peptide sequences, confirming the requirement of certain growth factors and cytokines in the induction of macrophages and the dependence of TLR-4 on activation. In addition to using the idea of increase in cytokine responses and activation of macrophages by gold nanoparticles, further study stemmed into new areas for the future, where peptide conjugates could lead with respect to drug delivery and integration or camouflage from the immune system. In addition to this, surface modifications of gold nano shells can minimize their RES uptake. Thus, conjugated AuNPs could have promising advantages in priming macrophages and there by enhanced immune response.

KEYWORDS

- **Extracellular traps**
- **Interferon-gamma**
- **Interleukin**
- **Lipopolysaccharide**
- **Toll-like receptor**
- **Tumor necrosis factor**

Chapter 9

Combating Infectious Diseases: Nanotechnology-based Drug Delivery

Zahoor Ahmad and Rajesh Panday

INTRODUCTION

Microorganisms are found in each part of our environment and they also colonize our skin, gastrointestinal tract and respiratory tract. Generally, these organisms live quietly with or without symbiotic existence on/and in our bodies, kept in check by a complex array of host defense mechanisms. Sometimes, however, a new microbe, or even one that had been living as part of our flora, attempts to invade or alter the host using various assaulting mechanisms. The resulting struggle between host and invader may present varied symptoms/signs constituting an "infectious disease" (Lambert, 1999). The outcome may range from complete resolution to death of the host, or chronic infection, either overt or latent. Since, the advent of penicillin (1929, 1940), there has been a steady development of antimicrobial chemotherapy, so that appropriate agents are now available and active against many infections. However, the evolutionary adaptability of microorganisms has been emphasized by the advance of antibiotic resistance, rendering many previously valuable drugs useless. Further, the targeting of chemotherapeutic agents is a key issue in the treatment of some stubborn intracellular infections. Nanoparticle-based drug delivery systems, as discussed below, form the crux of nanomedicine and are suitable for (but by no means limited to) targeting chronic diseases caused by mycobacteria, human immunodeficiency virus (HIV) and leishmania. These infections continue to share the majority of the "double epidemiological burden" (i.e., communicable plus non-communicable diseases) in developing countries (Laxminarayan and Jamison, 2010) and will be the focus of this chapter.

DRUG DELIVERY SYSTEMS

Advances in knowledge of disease pathogenesis especially at the molecular level, has allowed drug designing to flourish, not only as a science but also as an art. Drugs are hardly ever administered to a patient in an unformulated state. A drug dosage formulation consists of one or more active ingredients along with other molecules termed as excipients. It has been increasingly realized that the use of excipients is as important as the drug itself. Excipients facilitate the preparation and administration, enhance the consistent release of the drug and protect it from degradation. Thus, excipients are no longer considered to be inert substances because they can potentially influence the rate and/or extent of drug absorption and thus determine the bioavailability of the drug. The term bioavailability refers to the amount of drug available to the systemic circulation out of the total drug administered to a patient, and it is an important consideration in pharmaceutical dosage forms because the presence of the drug in the systemic circulation is essential to reach its target site and exert its therapeutic effect. A drug needs to be formulated as to extract the maximum therapeutic benefit out of it, and this is the underlying concept behind a drug delivery system. Out of the four "Ds" in a drug delivery system, drug, destination, disease, and delivery, the latter is the only variable parameter (Pandey and Khuller, 2004a). When a drug formulation is designed in such a way that the rate and/or place of drug release is altered, the formulation is called a modified release system. Alternative terms are in common usage including sustained/controlled/slow/extended/prolonged release etc. Modified release is generally achieved by means of encapsulation. Encapsulation technology finds extensive applications in the pharmaceutical industry for the controlled release of drugs. Polymers are extensively used, both as conventional excipients and more specifically as a tool in controlled drug delivery. Polymers are broadly classified as being synthetic or natural. Poly(DL-lactide-*co*-glycolide) (PLG), poly lactic acid (PLA), poly glycolic acid (PGA), poly anhydrides, poly methyl acrylates, carbomer, and so on are common examples of synthetic polymers used as drug delivery vehicles. On the other hand, natural polymers include alginic acid, chitosan, gelatin, dextrins, and so on. (Pandey and Khuller, 2004a). The drug release profile can be tuned depending on the choice of the drug carrier (Table 1). Among the most versatile polymers are PLG, alginic acid and chitosan. However, non-polymeric drug carriers, for example lipids in the form of solid lipid nanoparticles (SLNs) are also gaining importance. Whatever the carrier system, the ultimate aim is to improve the drug bioavailability by circumventing one or several of the possible factors known to affect the same (Pandey and Khuller, 2004a) (Table 2).

Table 1. Types of polymeric carriers used in drug delivery systems.

A. Natural carriers	B. Synthetic carriers
1. Proteins and polypeptides	1. Aliphatic polyesters and hydroxy acids
• Albumin	• Polylactic acid
• Fibrinogen/fibrin	• Polyglycolic acid
• Collagen	• Poly(lactide-co-glycolide)
• Gelatin	• Polyhydroxy butyric acid
• Casein	• Polycaprolactone
2. Polysaccharides	2. Polyanhydrides
• Alginic acid	3. Polyorthoesters
• Starch	4. Polyalkylcyanoacrylate
• Dextrans/dextrin	5. Polyamino acids
• Hyaluronic acid	6. Polyacrylamides
• Chitin	7. Polyalkylcarbonates
• Chitosan	

Table 2. Variables influencing drug bioavailability that are amenable to improvement by using an appropriate delivery system.

Parameters	Examples of drugs
Low shelf-life	Ethambutol
Unpalatability	Metronidazole
Extremes of pH	Rifampicin in presence of isoniazid in acidic pH
Interaction with food	Rifampicin
Interaction with other drugs	Rifampicin
Poor solubility in intestinal fluid	Danazol
Poor intestinal absorption	Streptomycin
Extensive first pass metabolism	Propranolol
Subtherapeutic levels in plasma	Clotrimazole
Short duration of stay	Azathioprine
Distribution to non-target organs	Anticancer drugs

TUBERCULOSIS: THE NEED FOR ANTITUBERCULAR DRUG DELIVERY SYSTEMS

Tuberculosis (TB) continues to be a leading killer disease worldwide. Although, an effective treatment regimen against TB is available, the fact that multiple antitubercular drugs (ATDs) known as first-line drugs need to be administered continuously for at least 6 months is responsible for patient noncompliance and treatment-related side effects. Misuse or mismanagement of these drugs also results in the emergence of multidrug resistant TB (MDR-TB). The MDR-TB takes even longer to treat with second-line drugs which are more expensive and have more adverse effects. When the second-line ATDs are misused (including the indiscriminate use of quinolones for ordinary non-mycobacterial infections), extensively drug resistant TB (XDR-TB) develops (Caminero et al., 2010; Sun et al., 2010). To make things worse, XDR-TB raises concerns of a future TB epidemic with limited therapeutic options and spoiling the achievements and progress made in TB control. Further, many countries lack the infrastructure to accurately diagnose MDR-TB and XDR-TB, hence TB mortality may alarmingly rise particularly in the face of co-existing opportunistic infections such as HIV. An ambitious TB control program referred to as directly observed treatment, short course (DOTS) was initiated by the World Health Organization (WHO) wherein, the administration of ATDs to a patient is directly supervised by a healthcare worker. However, practical difficulties in implementing the program especially in rural areas are yet to be solved. Obviously, if one could develop a system where it does not become necessary to administer ATDs on a regular basis, the strategy would certainly aid in improving patient compliance and avoid the drawbacks associated with the current chemotherapy. This is where the application of encapsulation technology (microencapsulation or nanoencapsulation) is likely to play its role by formulating ATDs into sustained release systems.

One of the early attempts toward preparing a sustained release ATD formulation was the incorporation of isoniazid (INH) in three different polymers, viz.

poly(methylmethacrylate), poly(vinyl chloride) and carbomer (Bulut-Oner et al., 1989). The primary objective of the study was to achieve sustained plasma INH levels in fast acetylators of the drug. Using another polymer, Eudragit RS 100, the encapsulation and detailed release kinetics of INH were studied in the early 1990s (Muhuri and Pal, 1991). The formulation, called spherical microcapsules, was not evaluated further. Soon it was realized that aliphatic poly (esters) such as PLA, PGA, and PLG (also abbreviated as PLGA, Figure 1) possess excellent biocompatibility, biodegradability, and mechanical strength (Jain et al., 1998). They are easy to formulate into various devices for carrying a variety of macromolecules and are approved by the US Food and Drug Administration (FDA) for drug delivery. Thus, with the reporting of PLG as a carrier for INH, the era of aliphatic poly (esters) as sustained release ATD carriers began (Gangadharam et al., 1991) and considerable progress was made in the next 10 years (Barrow et al., 1998; Dutt and Khuller, 2001; Gangadharam et al., 1994; Ul-Ain et al., 2003a).

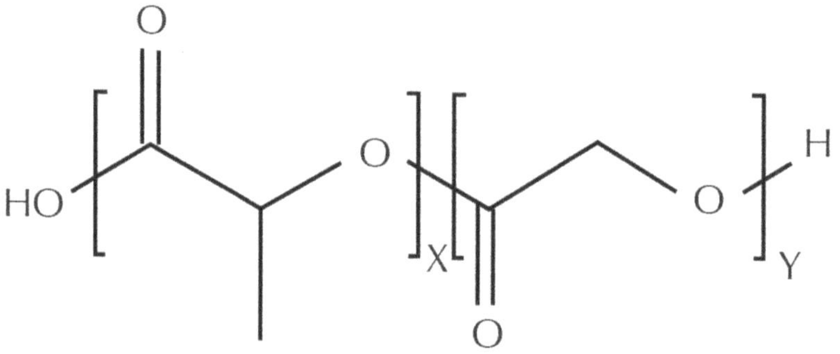

Figure 1. Structure of poly lactide-co-glycolide (PLG or PLGA).

With the foundation for controled release ATD-delivery systems laid, several pertinent issues needed to be addressed: would it be possible to achieve a higher drug encapsulation efficiency, drug loading into PLG, improve drug bioavailability and last but not the least, a further reduction in dosing frequency? Most of the answers were found in the concept of nanomedicine.

NANOMEDICINE AND TUBERCULOSIS

The importance of polymeric nanoparticles and their role in the development of drug delivery systems is well established (Table 3). The essential difference between microparticles and nanoparticles is not merely the size but also the ability of nanoparticles to achieve a higher drug encapsulation and enhance the bioavailability of orally administered drugs. Particles with large surface area per unit mass, such as nanoparticles may dissolve rapidly in the gastrointestinal tract which can increase drug uptake as the local concentration of drug may be higher than conventional dosage forms. Further, nanoparticles are known to cross the intestinal permeability barrier directly via transcellular/paracellular pathways which explain the better delivery of the encapsulated drugs into the circulation (Jiao et al., 2002). Several methods have been reported to obtain particles in the nano-range (Bala et al., 2004) (Table 4).

Table 3. Some important drugs reported to be incorporated in synthetic polymeric nanoparticles.

Drug	Category
Digitoxin	Cardiac glycoside (Guzman et al., 2000)
Rolipram	Anti-inflammatory (Lamprecht et al., 2001)
Heparin	Anticoagulant (Jiao et al., 2002)
Betamethazone	Corticosteroid (Horisawa et al., 2002)
Enalaprilat	Antihypertensive (Ahlin et al., 2002)
Octyl methoxy cinnamate	Sunscreen (Alvarez-Roman et al., 2004)
Cyclosporine	Immunosuppressant (Jaiswal et al., 2004)
Insulin	Hormone (Bilati et al., 2005)
Praziquantel	Anti-helminthic (Mainardes and Evangelista, 2005)
Clotrimazole, Econazole	Antifungal (Pandey et al., 2005a)
Moxifloxacin	Quinolone (Ahmad et al., 2008)
Gentamicin	Aminoglycoside (Imbuluzqueta et al., 2011)

Table 4. Various preparation techniques for PLG-nanoparticles.

Techniques	Merits/demerits
Emulsion/evaporation	Poor entrapment of hydrophilic drugs
Double emulsion/evaporation	Good entrapment of hydrophilic/hydrophobic drugs
Salting out	Lengthy purification process
Emulsification-diffusion	Quick process
Solvent displacement/nanoprecipitation	Poor entrapment of hydrophilic drugs
Emulsification-diffusion-evaporation	Better reproducibility of size/shape of nanoparticles

ORAL ATD-NANOMEDICINE

The feasibility of using ATDs in nanoparticle-based controlled delivery devices was begun to be explored almost 10 years back. Three front-line ATDs, that is RIF, INH, and PZA were co-encapsulated in PLG nanoparticles (PLG-NP) prepared by the double emulsion and solvent evaporation technique (Pandey et al., 2003a). The particle size ranged from 186–290 nm with drug encapsulation efficiency of 60–70% for all the drugs. Although, particle size distribution homogeneity was indicated by a polydispersity index of 0.38, the drug encapsulation procedure required optimization because several variables were found to influence the same (Table 5). The formulation was evaluated for its *in vivo* pharmacokinetic and pharmacodynamic potential at therapeutic drug doses, that is RIF 12 mg/kg + INH 10 mg/kg + PZA 25 mg/kg of body weight, or at sub-therapeutic doses (Sharma et al., 2004a). Following a single oral administration of drug-loaded PLG-NP to mice, the plasma drug levels were maintained above their minimum inhibitory concentration (MIC_{90}) for 6 to 9 days in the plasma, whereas no drug was detectable beyond 12 hr following the oral administration of free drugs (alone or mixed with drug-free PLG-NP) (Pandey et al., 2003a). In addition, the mice were sacrificed at different time points and the drugs were analyzed in homogenates of lungs, liver, and spleen. The drugs were detected above MIC in organs for up to day 9. Therefore, based on the tissue drug profile, the therapeutic schedule to be followed in infected animals comprised the formulation being administered every 10 days. It is known, however, that ATDs often result in dose dependent toxicity. Hence, it was important to determine whether or not oral dosing every 10th day would result in progressive drug accumulation in the tissues. To evaluate whether repeated administration of drug-loaded PLG-NP would result in any drug accumulation in the organs, studies were carried out in which tissue drug levels were monitored on every 10th day following the repeated administration of the formulation.

Table 5. The important variables influencing the encapsulation of ATDs in PLG-nanoparticles prepared by the double emulsion/evaporation technique.

Variable	Drug encapsulation efficiency (%)
1. Drug:polymer	
1:0.5	40–48
1:0.8	44–56
1:1	60–70
1:1.5	60–70
1:2	60–70
2. Concentration of polyvinyl alcohol (%w/v)	
0.5	45–55
1.0	60–70
1.5	60–70
2.0	54–66
3. Polyvinyl alcohol:dichloromethane (v/v)	
100:10	40–50
50:10	55–65
10:10	60–70
8:10	60–70
5:10	45–65

There was no evidence of any drug accumulation in the organs tested in the study, that is lungs, liver, and spleen. The chemotherapeutic evaluation of free drugs administered daily (46 doses) and drug-loaded PLG-nanoparticles administered every 10 days (5 doses) orally to *M. tuberculosis* infected mice showed nodetectable tubercle bacilli compared with a high bacterial load in lungs/spleen of untreated mice (Pandey et al., 2003a). It was also interesting to note that the results pertaining to the biodistribution, pharmacokinetics and chemotherapeutic efficacy of the formulation in mice were similar when carried out in a higher animal, that is guinea pigs (Sharma et al., 2004a).

In addition to reducing the dosing frequency, however, reduction in the overall duration of chemotherapy as well as the drug dosage are other key issues that need to be addressed for improving the patient's compliance during ATD treatment. Thus, WHO rightly recommends the addition of the bacteriostatic drug ethambutol (EMB) to the intensive phase of chemotherapy because the drug is known to hasten the rate of sputum conversion (Bastian et al., 2000). Hence, the chemotherapeutic potential of PLG-nanoparticle encapsulated EMB, when co-administered with the other three encapsulated front-line ATDs was evaluated. Following a single oral therapeuticdose of drug-loaded nanoparticles to mice, therapeutic drug concentrations were maintained in the plasma for 3 days, 6 days, and 8 days in the case of EMB, RIF, and INH/PZA, respectively (Pandey et al., 2006a). Free drugs, on the other hand, were not detectable in the plasma beyond 12 hr of intravenous/oral administration. There was a 1020-fold increase in the bioavailability of encapsulated drugs compared with free drugs, demonstrating the merits of nanomedicine. Furthermore, the concentration of RIF, INH, and PZA were maintained at or above MIC in the tissues (lungs, liver, and spleen) until day 9 as previously reported (Pandey et al., 2003a) while EMB was maintained until day 7.

Based on the pharmacokinetic and tissue drug biodistribution profile, ATD-loaded PLG nanoparticles were administered to *M. tuberculosis* infected mice every 10th day, while free drugs were administered daily. There was a significant reduction in bacterial load in all the treatment groups at 4 weeks post-chemotherapy. However, there was no detectable colony forming units (cfu) in those groups where ethambutol had been supplemented to the three-drug regimen. These observations translate into important conclusions (Pandey et al., 2006a). First, just three to four doses of the ATD-nanomedicine could replace 28 doses of conventional free drugs. Second, with the addition of EMB in the treatment regimen, four weeks of chemotherapy were sufficient to reach a state of undetectable bacilli, whereas in regimens involving the three-drug combinations, there was still a considerable bacterial burden. In fact, a further 2 weeks of treatment was required to reach a "no detectable bacilli" state in the case of the three-drug combination as reported previously (Pandey et al., 2003a). Thus, with the four-drug combination in PLG nanoparticles, it was possible to improve the drug bioavailability, to reduce the dosing frequency from daily to weekly/every 10 days and to reduce the number of doses from 28 to 34.

In the studies reviewed above, experimental infection had been established by the intravenous route. However, it was also important to evaluate the efficacy of the PLG-nanomedicine formulation in animals infected via the aerosol route because the latter is the natural mode of acquiring TB. In guinea pigs infected via the aerosol route, five oral doses of ATD-loaded PLG-NP and 46 doses of free drugs still proved to be equi-efficacious. This further strengthened the concept of ATD-nanomedicine (Johnson et al., 2005). Encouraging results have been obtained with ATD (particularly RIF) loaded in other synthetic polymer-based nanoparticulate systems such as poly butylcyanoacrylate (Oganesian et al., 2005) and poly ε-caprolactone (Moretton et al., 2010).

LIGAND-APPENDED ORAL ATD-NANOMEDICINE

The PLG nanomedicine was improved further by the addition of a mucosal ligand, that is lectin, to the PLG nanoparticles. It is known that the maximum duration of adhesion of a drug carrier to a mucosal surface is limited by the turnover time of the mucus gel layer, which is only a few hours for most mucosal surfaces. To circumvent this problem, polymeric drug carriers can be attached to certain cytoadhesive ligands that bind to epithelial surfaces through specific receptor mediated interactions. Lectins are appropriate candidates for this approach because they comprise a structurally diverse class of proteins found in organisms ranging from viruses and plants to humans (Lehr, 2000; Lis and Sharon, 1986). The specificity of lectins and their resistance to proteolytic degradation have advocated their use in pharmaceutics. Wheat germ agglutinin (WGA) is finding widespread applications in drug delivery because it is one of the least immunogenic lectins (Clark et al., 2000). Furthermore, WGA is known to have its receptors on intestinal as well as alveolar epithelium, thus potentiating its use for oral as well as aerosol drug delivery (Abu-Dahab et al., 2001). The sustained release profile of all the ATDs was improved as the drugs were detectable in tissues until day 15 in the case of the lectin-based ATD-nanomedicine against day 11 in the case of the uncoated formulation (Sharma et al., 2004b). In *M. tuberculosis* infected guinea pigs, three oral doses of ATD-loaded lectin PLG-NP spaced 15 days apart resulted in undetectable cfu against 46 conventional doses of oral free drugs.

PULMONARY DELIVERY OF ATD-NANOMEDICINE

Pulmonary TB is the commonest form of the disease and the respiratory route represents a novel means of delivering ATDs directly to the lungs. Inhalable nanoparticles stand a better chance of mucosal adherence, particle(s) delivery and hence net drug delivery to the lungs (Pandey and Khuller, 2005a). In addition, nanoparticles are known to be efficiently taken up by phagocytic cells (such as alveolar macrophages, the abode of *M. tuberculosis*), and subsequently release their payload (Gaspar et al., 2008). Inhalable PLG-nanoparticles co-encapsulating RIF, INH, and PZA, upon aerosolization, were found to possess a mass median aerodynamic diameter (MMAD, determined on a 7-stage Andersen Cascade Impactor) of 1.88 µm, suitable for deep lung delivery. It is known that high surface hydrophobicity can result in particle aggregation during nebulization, especially on a jet nebulizer. Because the PLG-NP were stabilized by PVA, thereby imparting hydrophilicity to the nanomedicine, particle aggregation was not a problem. A single nebulization of the formulation to guinea pigs was able to maintain therapeutic drug concentration in the plasma for 6 to 9 days and in the lungs for 9 to 11 days. There was a striking improvement in the half-life, mean residence time and bioavailability of encapsulated drugs compared with free drugs. It is emphasized that although one is aiming at pulmonary deposition of ATDs, the improvement in systemic bioavailability would still be advantageous following inhalation. The argument is that the enhanced bioavailability would lead to more of the drugs reaching the lungs by way of the circulation, that is the systemic spill-over could not be considered as drug wastage. In *M. tuberculosis* infected guinea pigs, 5 nebulized doses of the nanomedicine spaced 10 days apart resulted in undetectable cfu in the lungs replacing 46 conventional doses. This was the first report of an inhalable TB-nanomedicine (Pandey et al., 2003b). The advantage of the system over inhalable microspheres was clear; first, it was possible to co-administer multiple ATDs encapsulated in nanoparticles, and second, a better therapeutic response was elicited in the case of nanoparticles (Pandey and Khuller, 2005a). Further, repeated administration of the formulation failed to elicit hepatotoxicity as assessed on a biochemical basis (Pandey et al., 2003b).

Other research groups also reported the pulmonary delivery of PLG-NP encapsulated ATD especially RIF, with successful targeting to alveolar macrophages. Thus, RIF formulated into spray-dried PLG-NP and administered intra-tracheally to guinea pigs could maintain pulmonary drug levels for 8 hr in contrast to free RIF. Systemic levels were also attained with the nanoparticles for 68 hr (Sung et al., 2009a). Ohashi et al. (2009) employed yet another interesting approach wherein PLG-NP encapsulated RIF were formulated into mannitol microspheres. Following inhalation, efficient uptake of these microspheres by alveolar macrophages was demonstrated in rats in contrast to low uptake of simple RIF-PLG microspheres. Based on an *in vivo* imaging study, the authors concluded that the nanoparticles were cleared more slowly than the microparticles, resulting in their pulmonary retention.

As in case of oral PLG-NP, the formulation was further refined and improved by coupling it to lectin. With the knowledge that lectin receptors are widely distributed in the respiratory tract, it was worthwhile to evaluate the chemotherapeutic potential of lectin-functionalized PLG-NP, a somewhat similar approach to ligand-appended liposomes employed for lipid-based drug carriers (Vyas et al., 2004). Upon nebulization to guinea pigs, therapeutic drug concentrations were maintained in the plasma for 610 days and in the organs for 15 days. The bioavailability was enhanced compared with uncoated PLG-NP and free drugs. Most importantly, when nebulized to TB-infected guinea pigs every 2 weeks, three doses of the formulation produced undetectable cfu in the lungs as well as spleens (Sharma et al., 2004b). The series of experiments proved that 46 conventional doses could be reduced to five nebulized doses of PLG-nanomedicine and, further, to just three doses with lectin-PLG-NP.

Wet nebulization mandates that dried nanoparticles be reconstituted in isotonic saline just before pulmonary delivery because suspended particles are not stable as such. Further, the process is time-consuming, ranging from seconds to minutes depending on the amount of drug-loaded particles to be nebulized. The net drug delivered is also determined by the quality of the nebulizer and the inspiratory effort of the subject. Further, a part of the nebulized dose may be actually swallowed rather than inhaled, making it a confounding variable. Thus, pulmonary delivery of ATDs is a challenging task. Besides nebulization, however, there are other means to deliver ATDs to the lungs. This includes spray drying of drug-loaded particles to form inhalable powders followed by direct pulmonary deposition, a process called insufflation. Excellent work has been carried out in this area by some research groups. A promising anti-TB candidate molecule, PA-824 (a nitroimidazopyran), was formulated into dry powder porous particles stable at room temperature for 6 months and under refrigerated conditions for at least 1 year (Sung et al., 2009b). Insufflation to guinea pigs resulted in sustained drug levels in the lungs upto 32 hr which was significantly higher than oral PA-824. The lungs and spleens of *M. tuberculosis* infected guinea pigs receiving high doses of aerosolized PA-824 exhibited a lower cfu and tissue damage compared to untreated animals (Garcia-Contreras et al., 2010). The procedure was also suited for lower animals such as mice (where wet nebulization to an individual animal is difficult) and could be applied to other ATDs like capreomycin as well as vaccines (Fiegel et al., 2008; Morello et al., 2009; Pulliam et al., 2007). The technology is a stepping stone towards pulmonary delivery of ATDs in a quick (less time required compared with nebulization), efficient (in terms of net drug delivered to the lungs) and safe (minimizing local/systemic untoward reactions) manner.

INJECTABLE ATD-NANOMEDICINE

Intravenous administration of drugs results in all the drug molecules being instantly available to the systemic circulation, that is the bioavailability is absolute. The subcutaneous and intramuscular routes also provide bioavailability profiles close to the intravenous route. An important attribute of PLG-NP was a high chemotherapeutic efficacy following subcutaneous administration. A single injection of drug-loaded PLG-NP resulted in sustained drug levels in the plasma for 32 days and in the organs for 36 days. There was a complete bacterial clearance from the organs of TB-infected mice upon subcutaneous administration of a single shot of the formulation, demonstrating a better efficacy compared with daily oral free drug treatment (Pandey and Khuller, 2004b). Furthermore, the system was better than the injectable PLG microparticles previously reported because although the microparticulate system also demonstrated a significant reduction in bacterial load, it failed to result in complete tissue sterilization (Dutt and Khuller, 2001). Other advantagesof the nanoparticulate system over the microparticulate one are presented in Table 6. Recently, mannose-conjugated gelatin nanoparticles encapsulating INH were prepared by a two-step desolvation method. The particle(s) size ranged from 260 to 380 nm. Upon intravenous administration, the formulation achieved lung targeting in TB-infected mice leading to a significant reduction in cfu, besides minimal hepatotoxicity (Saraogi et al., 2011).

Table 6. Merits of PLG-nanoparticles over PLG-microparticles as ATD carriers.

Parameters	PLG microparticles	PLG nanoparticles
1. Particle size	10–12 μm	186–290 nm
2. Type of formulation	Separate formulations for each drug	Single formulation encapsulating multiple drugs
3. Drug encapsulation (%)	8–40%	55–73%
4. Drug:polymer	Varies with the drug	1:1 for each drug
5. Polymer consumption	High	Low
6. Sustained drug release in plasma following oral administration to experimental animals	3–4 days	6–9 days
7. Feasibility of nebulization	No	Yes

Table 6. *(Continued)*

Parameters	PLG microparticles	PLG nanoparticles
8. Increase in drug bioavailability	7–9 fold	9–53 fold
9. Schedule of oral therapy in experimental TB models	Weekly	Every 10–15 days
10. Therapeutic benefit	Partial	Complete

ALGINATE-BASED ATD-NANOMEDICINE

Alginic acid is a natural co-polymer of guluronic acid and mannuronic acid (Figure 2). Alginate, being approved by US FDA for oral usage, is already employed clinically for the supportive treatment for reflux esophagitis. It has diverse applications as a binding and disintegrating agent intablets, a suspending and thickening agent in water-misciblegels/lotions/creams, and a stabilizer for emulsions. Several attributes make alginate an ideal drug delivery vehicle (Table 7). These include a relatively high aqueous environment within the matrix, adhesive interactions with intestinal epithelium, a mild room-temperature drug(s) encapsulation process free of organic solvents, a high gel porosity allowing high diffusion rates of macromolecules, the ability to control this porosity with simple coating procedures using polycations such as chitosan or poly (L-lysine) (PLL), and dissolution/biodegradation of the system under normal physiological conditions (Hejazi and Amiji, 2003; Ravi Kumar, 2000; Tonnesen and Karlsen, 2002).

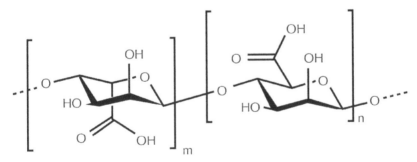

Figure 2. Structure of alginic acid.

Table 7. Alginate-advantages and favorable properties for use in drug delivery.

- A natural polymer
- Large-scale production economically
- Compatible with a variety of substances
- Simple drug encapsulation process
- Mucoadhesive
- Biodegradable
- Non-toxic
- Formulation of different delivery systems
- Sustained drug release
- Enhanced drug bioavailability
- Applications in biotechnology

Hence, it is not surprising that alginate has been used as a carrier for the controlled release of numerous molecules of clinical interest, for example indomethacin (Joseph and Venkataram, 1995), sodium diclofenac (Gonzalez-Rodriguez, 2002), nicardipine (Takka and Acarturk, 1999), dicoumarol (Chickering et al., 1997), gentamicin (Lannuccelli et al., 1996), ketoconazole (Cui et al., 2001), amoxycillin (Whitehead et al., 2000), insulin (Woitiski et al., 2010), anticancer drugs (Nanjwade et al., 2010) and ATDs (Lucinda-Silva and Evangelista, 2003; Pandey and Khuller, 2004c; Ul-Ain et al., 2003b). There are two broad types of alginate-based drug delivery systems the membrane system and the matrix system. In the membrane-reservoir system, the drug release from the inner reservoir core is controlled by the polymeric encapsulating membrane having a specific permeability. As the thickness of the coat/membrane increases, the release rate decreases. Moreover, the co-encapsulation of certain nonpolar substances may further reduce the release rates. This property was advantageously used in the encapsulation and controlled release of indomethacin, where the sudden release of the drug is highly undesirable because it is well known that indomethacin is an irritant to the gastrointestinal mucosa (Joseph and Venkataram, 1995). On the other hand, in the matrix system or more specifically the swelling-dissolution-erosion system, the drug molecules are dispersed in a rate controlling polymer matrix. The matrix swelling as well as dissolution/erosion occurring concomitantly at the matrix periphery are the factors that modulate drug release (Takka et al., 1998). Broadly speaking, factors related to the development of a particular formulation as well as factors encountered once the formulation is inside a living system can influence alginate-based drug delivery systems to agreat extent (Table 8).

Although, it is well-known that divalent cations induce the gelification of alginate, a critical adjustment in the relative proportions of Ca^{2+}/alginate allows the cation-induced rearrangement of the alginate molecules to form microdomains with high local concentrations of alginate instead of an infinite network of polymer. These microdomains are representative of a *pre-gel* state, that is alginate nanoparticles, which can be recovered by high-speed centrifugation.

Table 8. Factors influencing drug encapsulation/release from alginate-based systems.

- pH of the surrounding medium
- Relative proportion of G and M residues
- Molecular weight and viscosity of alginate
- Drug-polymer ratio
- Ionic nature of the drug
- Nature and amount of cross-linker
- Gelling time
- Variation in particle size
- Addition of regulatory molecules

Such formulations are suitable for intravenous administration, as has been shown for doxorubicin-loaded alginate nanoparticles (Rajaonarivony et al., 1993). Alginate exhibits satisfactory hemocompatibility and, being hydrophilic, avoids rapid clearance by the mononuclear phagocyte system on intravenous administration. This imparts a long circulation half-life to alginate nanoparticles. The system is certainly advantageous over the more traditional neutral polymers or liposomes that require the additional incorporation of hydrophilic co-polymers or polyethylene glycol fatty acid derivatives to enhance their hydrophilicity. Alginate nanoparticles have been prepared and stabilized with PLL/chitosan, encapsulating ATDs (RIF, INH, PZA, and EMB). The drug: polymer ratio was kept at 7.5:1 which is better compared with PLG-NP, where the ratio was 1:1. Thus, the alginate formulation allows more loading of the drug with lower consumption of the polymer.The formulation provides a sustained release for 711 days in plasma and 15 days in the organs following a single oral dose (Ahmad et al., 2006a). In *M. tuberculosis* infected mice, 3 oral doses of the formulation administered fortnightly led to complete bacterial clearance from the organs replacing 45 doses of free drugs (Ahmad et al., 2006b). Comparable results were obtained in guinea pigs by the oral (Ahmad et al., 2005a) as well as the respiratory route (Ahmad et al., 2005b). Therefore, alginate nanoparticles can certainlybe considered a better ATD-nanomedicine over PLG-NP (Ahmad and Khuller, 2008). Encouraging results have been obtained with ATD (particularly RIF) loaded in other natural carrier-based nanoparticulate systems. For example, Saraogi et al. (2010) prepared RIF-encapsulated gelatin nanoparticles by a two-step desolvation process resulting in 264±11.2 nm sized particles. In contrast to free drug, the RIF-gelatin exhibited significantly improved pharmacokinetics as well as pharmacodynamics in TB-infected mice. More recently, Verma et al. (2011) reported the encapsulation of mycobacterial proteins in chitosan nanoparticles.

SOLID LIPID NANOPARTICLES-BASED ATD-NANOMEDICINE

The SLNs are nanocrystalline suspensions in water, prepared from lipids which are solid at room temperature (Jenning et al., 2002). The SLNs are a new form of nanoparticulate carriers in addition to the more conventional ones such as liposomes, lipid emulsions, and polymeric nanoparticles. The SLNs possess good tolerability (due to their derivation from physiological lipids), scaling-up feasibility, the ability to incorporate hydrophobic/hydrophilic drugs, and an enhanced stability of incorporated drugs. Thus, SLNs are unique in the sense that they combine the virtues of traditional nanoparticles while eliminating some of their problems (Muller and Keck, 2004). It is not surprising that SLNs have been researched for formulation development and for the incorporation of drugs to improve their bioavailability as well as for targeted drug delivery (Kim et al., 2005; Prego et al., 2005; Yu et al., 2003; Zara et al., 2002a).

Several laboratory-scale methods for preparation of SLNs have been proposed (Jenning et al., 2002). For example, SLNs can be prepared by precipitation in oil-in-water emulsions. The lipophilic core material of SLNs is dissolved in water-immiscible organic solvent that is emulsified in an aqueous phase. Upon evaporation of the solvent, the lipid precipitates and forms solid nanoparticles. Another method entails preparing SLNs from warm oil in water microemulsions. The melted fatty acids or triglycerides are mixed with water, surfactant, and co-surfactant to form a transparent microemulsion which is quenched and dispersed in cold aqueous medium. The lipid solidifies and forms the nanoparticles. A more recent and popular method is the preparation of SLNs by high-pressure homogenization (Jenning et al., 2002).

The ATD-loaded SLNs have been prepared by the emulsion solvent diffusion technique to co-incorporate RIF, INH, and PZA. The chemotherapeutic potential of the formulation was evaluated via the respiratory route in guinea pigs. It was observed that a sustained drug release was maintained for 5 days in plasma and for 7 days in the organs. The pharmacokinetics was unaltered in healthy as well as TB-infected guinea pigs. Seven weekly doses of the formulation resulted in undetectable bacilli in the organs of TB-infected guinea pigs, replacing 46 conventional doses (Pandey and Khuller, 2005b). The possibility of administering this ATD-nanomedicine was also evaluated via the oral route and similar encouraging results were obtained (Pandey et al., 2005b).

ATD-NANOMEDICINE FOR SPECIAL SITUATIONS: CEREBRAL TB, DRUG-RESISTANT TB AND LATENT TB

Cerebral TB is perhaps the most feared form of extrapulmonary TB owing to the increased mortality associated with it (Katti, 2004). Several reports support the feasibility of nanoparticles (loaded with other drugs) localization to the brain in experimental models (Das and Lin, 2005; Joshi et al, 2010; Tosi et al., 2005), a process which is influenced by the targeting process (Kabanov and Batrakova, 2004) as well as by the surface charge on the nanoparticles; neutral particles (e.g., PVA-stabilized PLG) stand not only better chances of cerebral uptake but also a lower risk of toxicity to the blood brain barrier (Lockman et al., 2004). Hence, it was worth exploring whether ATD-PLG-NP could achieve brain tissue localization, keeping in view that following oral administration, nanoparticles are distributed to extrapulmonary sites including the liver and spleen (Pandey et al., 2003a; Sharma et al., 2004a). Indeed, a single oral dose of ATD-nanomedicine could attain drug levels in the brain for 9 days. In a murine TB model, 5 oral doses of the formulation administered every 10th day, resulted in undetectable bacilli in the meninges, as assessed on the basis of cfu and histopathology (Pandey and Khuller, 2006). These results certainly merit evaluation in a higher animal model.

As already mentioned above, poor patient compliance remains the main reason behind treatment failure and emergence of drug resistance including MDR-TB (Sosnik et al., 2010). Keeping in mind the rising incidence of MDR-TB and its deadly alliance with HIV (Ginsburg et al., 2003; Lalloo and Ambaram, 2010), it was thought that the concept of nanomedicine should be taken further to encapsulate second-line ATDs as well. Lopes et al. (2000) reported the nano-encapsulation of ethionamide and characterized the formulation but did not carry out *in vivo* studies. Ten years later, ethionamide-loaded PLG-NP were prepared and evaluated by a different research group (Kumar et al., 2011). A single oral dose of the formulation produced sustained release of ethionamide for 6 days in plasma whereas the free drug was cleared in 6 hr in mice. Ethionamide was detected in the organs for 57 days, suggesting a weekly therapeutic regimen in drug-resistant TB.

A more exciting development has been the nano-encapsulation of azole antifungals and fluoroquinolones (Ahmad et al., 2007; Kisich et al., 2007). Azole antifungals (clotrimazole, econazole) have potent anti-mycobacterial activity against drug-sensitive (Ahmad et al., 2005c; Ahmad et al., 2006c) and resistant (Ahmad et al., 2006d) strains of *M. tuberculosis* as well as latent bacilli (Ahmad et al., 2006e). Fluoroquinolones, especially moxifloxacin, also possess strong anti-mycobacterial activity and achieve prolonged, high concentrations in alveolar macrophages particularly following encapsulation. These important findings were reported by Kisich et al. (2007) who demonstrated that moxifloxacin encapsulated in poly (butyl cyanoacrylate) nanoparticles accumulated in alveolar macrophages 3 times more efficiently than free moxifloxacin. Further, the encapsulated drug was detected intracellularly for 6 times longer duration than free drug even at similar extracellular levels. An intracellular concentration of 0.1 μg/ml with encapsulated moxifloxacin was comparable to 1.0 μg/ml of free drug in terms of inhibiting mycobacterial growth (Kisich et al., 2007). In *M. tuberculosis* infected mice, 8 weekly doses of PLG-NP encapsulated triple-drug combination (moxifloxacin + econazole + rifampicin) resulted in complete bacterial clearance from the organs (Ahmad et al., 2008). Further, it has been documented that the addition of moxifloxacin has the potential to shorten the duration of treatment (Nuermberger et al., 2004). Studies with econazole encapsulated in alginate nanoparticles demonstrated that the system has an edge over the PLG-NP, both in terms of pharmacokinetics as well as pharmacodynamics, reducing the dosing frequency by 15-fold (Ahmad et al., 2007; Ahmad et al., 2008). The system is worth exploring for intermittent therapy against MDR-TB and latent TB.

Streptomycin has also been formulated into an oral dosage form by nano-encapsulation (Pandey and Khuller, 2007). Over the years, this antibiotic became less popular owing to the need for its parenteral administration and its potential for nephrotoxicity. However, it is one of the most cost-effective ATDs and is recommended in certain special cases, for example relapse/treatment failure, withdrawal of INH and RIF, TB meningitis, co-treatment with HIV protease inhibitors and certain cases of MDR-TB (World Health Organization, 2003). Streptomycin loaded in PLG-NP could not only be administered orally to mice but also exhibited an enhanced bioavailability, therapeutic efficacy and no nephrotoxicity in contrast to free drug (Pandey and Khuller, 2007). Reports of nanomedicine prepared with new anti-TB drugs, for example isoxyl (Wang and Hickey, 2010) or modified old drugs, for example fullerene-INH conjugate (Kumar et al., 2009) have also appeared.

POTENTIAL TOXICITY OF ATD-NANOMEDICINE

The standard ATDs have been used for several decades and PLG is also clinically popular for its use in surgical implants and sutures (Jain et al., 1998). However, a combination of PLG with a drug becomes a new chemical entity. Thus, ATD-loaded PLG-NP merit careful toxicological assessment, both short-term (single dose or acute toxicity to determine the median lethal dose, LD_{50}, that is the single dose that would produce mortality in 50% of the animals within 14 days) and long-term (multiple dose, that is sub acute toxicity for 28 days and chronic toxicity for 90 days).

The single dose acute toxicity in mice demonstrated the safety of the formulation since the LD_{50} could not be determined in contrast to free drugs. In fact, the free drugs were toxic at 80 times the therapeutic dose and above whereas the PLG formulation was non-toxic even at 150 times the therapeutic dose (it was technically not possible to administer further higher doses to mice by gavage owing to the bulk of the formulation). The data from acute toxicity studies formed the basis for the sub-acute and chronic toxicity studies wherein the PLG formulation was administered on every 10th day. No adverse effects were documented with either drug-loaded or drug-free nanoparticles in mice or rats. It is emphasized that the various analyses covered the essential organ function tests pertaining to the liver, heart, kidneys, pancreas, and bone marrow. The histopathology examination excluded the possibility of any minor changes in the organs that may have been too subtle to be manifested biochemically (Pandey et al., 2006b). It appears that polymeric nanoparticles, when applied to medicine, are less toxic compared with industrial production/exposure to nanoparticles (Dobson, 2007; Semete et al., 2010). The data should encourage researchers to further explore the safety profile of PLG that may expedite its approval for oral usage, besides undertaking toxicological evaluation in higher animal model as a prelude to clinical studies. Similar platform studies are also warranted with all forms of ATD-nanomedicine currently being explored.

ATD-NANOMEDICINE: UNRESOLVED AND UPCOMING ISSUES

There is compelling experimental evidence to declare ATD-nanomedicine as a promising alternative to the current practice of TB-chemotherapy although new drug carriers continue to be proposed, for example gold nanoparticles (Boisselier and Astruc, 2009). However, a critical appraisal reveals the as yet unachieved milestones including various shortfalls hindering human trials (Table 9). In the large-scale production of synthetic polymer-based ATD-nanomedicine, removal of residual organic solvents (e.g., dichloromethane used in preparing PLG-NP) could be a potential problem. Although, the problem could be solved by temperature-controlled vacuum drying, the process is likely to increase the cost of production. A natural polymer-based delivery system, such as alginate nanoparticles, is a suitable alternative.

Table 9. Shortfalls hindering ATD-nanomedicine from reaching human trials.

- Removal of residual organic solvents
- Cost of polymer/drug carrier
- Large-scale optimization of batch-to-batch drug loading
- Long-term stability studies
- Safety/toxicity profile of new chemical entities
- Efficient pulmonary delivery of a suitable dosage form (nebulization vs. insufflation)

Stringent quality control measures would need to be adopted to ensure an optimum batch-to-batch drug loading into the nanoparticles. Long term stability studies also need to be performed to assess the shelf-life of the formulation(s), keeping in view the bulk requirement of ATDs in rural areas of Asia and Africa with suboptimal drug storage conditions, besides the fact that PLG requires to be stored under cold conditions (48°C as per the manufacturer's instructions). It is worth mentioning here that alginate can be stored at room temperature. Further, despite the extensive animal-data available to support the sustained release kinetics and safety of ATD-nanomedicine, the exact dosing schedule to be followed in humans would be revealed only after the results of clinical studies become available.

Another point to be considered is the selection of the route of administration. Intermittent oral therapy would obviously be more patient-friendly, whereas treatment with inhalable or injectable ATD-nanomedicine would require supervision and medical expertise, at least during the initial few doses in adults and each time in children. Challenges to pulmonary delivery of ATDs including the issue of nebulization and insufflation were discussed above. Last but not the least; it is emphasized that the clinical success of ATD-nanomedicine, its marketing and post-marketing surveillance would not only require firm governmental commitment but also a keen interest from leading pharmaceutical companies even if it means a less profitable business.

PARTICLE ENGINEERING: PRESENT SCENARIO OF ATD-NANOMEDICINE

Most of the ATDs are commercially available as tablets or capsules requiring at least once a day dosing; injectable dosage forms such as streptomycin may be administered more intermittently. The active ingredient present in each of the conventional dosage forms gets widely distributed (hence diluted and metabolized) in the body so that the actual amount of drug reaching the desired target (e.g., alveolar macrophages in case of pulmonary TB) may be frequently suboptimal. This mandates the regular administration of ATDs for prolonged periods leading to noncompliance and chances of treatment failure, besides the emergence of drug resistance. In this regard, particle engineering (beginning with microparticles and re-enforced by nanoparticles) has resulted in alternative dosage forms with substantial success in animal models (Kurmi et al., 2010). The issue of precise drug targeting, however, is only partially solved since regional targeting within the lungs (e.g., airway versus alveoli and *vice versa*) are still unmet (Weers et al., 2010). Nevertheless, the possibility of weekly or fortnightly dosing remains the cornerstone of TB-nanomedicine.

NANOMEDICINE AND HIV INFECTION

The HIV is responsible for more than 2.5 million new infections worldwide each year (Khalil et al., 2011). Despite the availability of several drugs under "Highly Active Anti-Retroviral Therapy" (HAART), the problems of drug resistance and viral latency are far from being solved, warranting the need for better drug delivery systems (Kovochich et al, 2011; McNamara and Collins, 2011). There have been numerous studies evaluating the use of various polymeric nanoparticles for the delivery of antiretrovirals. Antiretroviral drugs whose mechanism of action requires that the drug reaching target cells must cross the mucosal epithelial barrier to exert their effect when administered by non-invasive routes such as oral, vaginal, or rectal delivery. Nanoparticles provide one strategy to traverse this mucosal barrier. In a study conducted by Ham et al. (2009), PLG nanoparticles were used for vaginal delivery of a chemokine receptor inhibitor. In these studies, the inhibitor was encapsulated into PLG nanoparticles via a double-emulsion, solvent-evaporation method. The nanoparticle system was produced to protect the active agent from the vaginal environment, and facilitate drug penetration into the vaginal and ectocervical tissue, allowing the drug to reach HIV target cells. The uptake of encapsulated drug by excised human ectocervical tissue as evaluated in an *ex vivo* model was 4.8 times greater than non-encapsulated drug during a 4 hr exposure time. Another application of this type of nanocarrier was demonstrated by Dembri et al. (2001). This study involved the preparation of poly(isohexyl cyanate) nanoparticles of zidovudine for the purpose of targeting the lymphoid tissue in the gastrointestinal tract. Use of this carrier system, when compared with aqueous drug solution, resulted in drug levels in the Peyer's patches being 4 times higher with the encapsulated drug form. Ina separate study, Lobenberg et al. (1998) formulated polyhexylcyanoacrylate nanoparticles for the delivery of zidovudine. *In vivo* studies in rodents demonstrated higher zidovudine levels in the body with the encapsulated drug compared with free drug solution after oral administration. However, when oral delivery of the nanoparticles was compared with intravenous administration using radio luminography, much of the orally administered nanoparticles were found to remain in the gastro intestinal tract.

Mucus, a dynamic layer present on the surface of the mucosal epithelium, is a major barrier for the delivery of antiretroviral drugs via non-invasive routes. Antiretroviral drugs must pass through mucus layers that may be up to a few hundred microns thick to reach the underlying epithelium and avoid clearance (Mrsny, 2009). Mucoadhesive nanoparticles can reduce the clearance of antiretroviral drugs from these sites and ensuretheir prolonged retention, resulting in improved absorption of poorly absorbable drugs. Several polymers, such as poloxamers, pectins, chitosans, polyacrylates, and their derivatives, have been used to impart mucoadhesive properties to the nanoparticles by surface coating (Mallipeddi and Rohan, 2010; Rekha and Sharma, 2009; Thirawong et al., 2008). In spite of extensive research on mucoadhesive nanoparticles for improving drug targeting to or through mucosal surfaces, several drawbacks limit their applications. The mucus turnover rate, influenced by a variety of factors including mucosal site, physiologic conditions, and presence of irritants affects the residence time of muco adhesive nanoparticles (Bernkop-Schnurch, 2005; Mallipeddi and Rohan, 2010). The second major limitation is that the mucoadhesive nanoparticles interact with and adhere to mucus and, hence, may be unable to reach the underlying epithelium or subepithelial tissues, making them inefficient as intracellular delivery systems (Lai et al., 2009a). Mucus-penetrating nanoparticles seem to be a better option for overcoming the mucosal barriers. Surface properties, such as net charge and hydrophilicity of the nanoparticles, play acrucial role in their ability to penetrate the mucus and reach the underlying epithelium (Lai et al., 2009a). Mucus is negatively charged due to the carboxyl and sulfate groups present on the mucinproteoglycans. Mucus has high densities of hydrophobic domains which entrap foreign materials by forming polyvalent, low-affinity, adhesive interactions (Cone, 2009; Lai et al., 2009b). These interactions pose a challenge, particularly in the design of polymeric nanoparticles, because most of the polymers used for this purpose are either hydrophobic or have a net charge. Mimicking viral surface properties may provide a way to enhance the diffusion of nanoparticles through mucus. Viruses capable of rapid transport in mucus possess hydrophilic surfaces that are densely coated equally with positive and negative charges, creating a net-neutral shell that minimizes hydrophobic and electrostatic adhesive interactions (Cone, 2009; Lai et al., 2009a). Successful engineering of neutral surfaces with such high densities of cationic and anionic charges, as in the case with viral proteins, has not been reported so far. Nanoparticles with hydrophobic groups which were masked from mucus interaction by covalently linked polyethylene glycol (PEG) moieties were designed by Lai et al. (2007). Surface modification improved the transport rates by several orders of magnitude. The nanoparticles with neutral surfaces were transported faster through human mucus compared with unmodified nanoparticles. The rate of transport was found to be dependent on nanoparticle size, density of surface coverage, and PEG molecular weight. Higher surface density and lower molecular weight of PEG resulted in better transport of the nanoparticles through mucus.

NANOPARTICLE TARGETING TO HIV-LADEN TISSUES

Lymphoid tissues such as lymph nodes, spleen, and gut-associated lymphoid tissue constitute major sanctuary sites for HIV. Approximately 99% of HIV replication occurs in activated and productively infected CD4 T cells of the blood and lymphoid tissues, primarily the lymph nodes. However, the viral load of lymphoid tissues is greater than the circulating blood, because only 2% of the lymphocytes are in the circulation at a given time, with the remaining being present in the lymphoid tissues, especially in lymph nodes (Gunaseelan, 2010). Lymph nodes are the sites of T cell activation and differentiation. They harbor a large number of T cells, antigen-presenting dendritic cells, and short-lived monocytes and macrophages. Hence, targeting antiretroviral drugs to the lymphoid tissues might help in better management of the viral infection compared with reduction of systemic viral load. Nanoparticles targeting macrophages and other cells of the mononuclear phagocytic system can be used to deliver antiretroviral drugs to the lymphoid tissues. The focus of the majority of the studies dealing with antiretroviral nanoparticles involves targeting the mononuclear phagocytic system, because these cells are responsible for harboring and dissemination of HIV virus to other anatomic sanctuary sites in the body, including lymph nodes. A host of published studies in this area demonstrate the superior ability of antiretroviral nanoparticles to deliver their payload to macrophages and monocytes *in vitro*. One example of the work in this area is the PLG nanoparticles containing multiple antiretroviral drugs (ritonavir, lopinavir, and efavirenz) which were fabricated by Destache et al. (2009) using a multiple emulsion solvent evaporation technique. The encapsulated antiretrovirals were detected intracellularly in peripheral blood mononuclear cells *in vitro* after 28 days. On the contrary, unencapsulated antiretrovirals could not be detected after two days. Lobenberg et al. (1998) studied the distribution of zidovudine-loaded poly(isohexyl cyanate) nanoparticles *in vivo* in rats. These studies revealed that encapsulation resulted in a higher concentration of drug in the cells of the reticuloendothelial system. Nanoparticle surface modification can alter biodistribution and circulation patterns. Shah and Amiji (2006) fabricatedpoly(ε-caprolactone) nanoparticles loaded with saquinavir for targeting the phagocytic mononuclear system. The surface of the nanoparticles was modified with poly(ethylene oxide) to prevent aggregation of the nanoparticles. Intracellular drug concentrations were found to be higher with encapsulated saquinavir compared with free drug solution. However, these studies did not include a performance comparison of the surface-modified versus surface-unmodified nanoparticles. Mainardes et al. (2009) studied the effect of surface modification in a methodical manner using zidovudine-loaded hydrophobic polylactide (PLA) and surface hydrophilic PEG nanoparticles. The concentration-dependent effects of PEG, used to modify the PLA nanoparticle surfaces, were studied. According to these studies, the uptake of zidovudine by macrophages and polymorphonuclear leucocytes was higher with unmodified PLA nanoparticles than with PEG-modified PLA nanoparticles. The PEG did not prevent the phagocytosis completely, even at higher concentrations, indicating a concentration-dependent steric effect. The CNS is the most important HIV reservoir site. However, this site offers limited access to drugs and drug-delivery systems. The HIV primarily infects the microglial cells of the brain and causes extensive neuronal damage, particularly in the frontal cortex, ultimately leading to dementia (Vyas et al., 2006). Antiretroviral drug transport across the blood-brain barrier (BBB) is essential to decrease or eradicate viral load. The BBB inhibits the transport of antiretroviral drugs to the brain by the presence of tight endothelial cell junctions and efflux transporters such as P-glycoprotein, multidrug resistance protein, and multispecific organic anion transporters (Rao et al, 2009; Shahiwala and Amiji, 2007). Nanoparticles are a means to overcome this barrier because they can cross the BBB by endocytosis/phagocytosis and can then release drug intracellularly. Kuo (2005) initially reported the loading of stavudine, a nucleoside analog reverse transcriptase inhibitor, into polybutylcyanoacrylate (PBCA) and methylmethacrylate-sulfopropylmethacrylate (MMA-SPM) nanoparticles for brain targeting. By using an *in vitro* brain microvascular endothelial cell model, Kuo and Chen (2006) further evaluated the effect of size of PBCA and MMA-SPM nanoparticles on the permeability of two reverse transcriptase inhibitors (zidovudine and lamivudine) across the BBB. The permeability of these drugs across the BBB was found to be inversely proportional to nanoparticle size. The permeability of zidovudine and lamivudine was 8–20-fold higher and 10–18-fold higher, respectively, with PBCA nanoparticles, whereas the MMA-SPM nanoparticles led to a 100% increase in the BBB permeability of both drugs. In a subsequent report, Kuo and Su (2007) studied the transport of stavudine, delavirdine, and saquinavir across the BBB when delivered as PBCA and MMA-SPM nanoparticles. The results revealed that the permeability of all three drugs increased about 12–16-fold with PBCA nanoparticles and 3–7-fold with MMA-SPM nanoparticles. In a further extension of their studies on nanoparticles, Kuo and Kuo (2008) studied the influence of electro magnetic field on the transport of antiretroviral nanoparticles across the BBB. The permeabilityof saquinavir-loaded PBCA and MMA-SPM nanoparticles across the BBB was enhanced significantly by the application of an electromagnetic field. Larger frequency, modulation or depth of amplitude modulation, or modulation or deviation of frequency modulation, resulted in greater permeability of the nanoparticles. Recently, emphasis is also being laid on RNA nanoparticles to deliver specific anti-HIV molecules (Zhou et al., 2011).

INORGANIC NANOPARTICLES

Inorganic materials such as gold, silver, iron, titanium, copper, silica, and zinc oxide have been fabricated as nanoparticles for several pharmaceutical applications, including cancer therapeutics (Porcel et al., 2010), cellular and biomolecular labels (Jain, 2003), and biosensors (Wang et al., 2010). Nanoparticles of noble metals like gold, silver, and platinum have been synthesized using a wide variety of methods such as bioreduction, hard template, and solution phase syntheses (Canizal et al., 2001; Yu et al., 1997; Zhou et al., 1999). Silver nanoparticles have received considerable attention as antimicrobial agents because they have been shown to be effective as antibacterial (Sondi and Salopek-Sondi, 2004) and antiviral (Lu et al, 2008; Sun et al., 2005) agents. Antimicrobial effectiveness was shown for both Gram positive and Gram negative bacteria (Sondi and Salopek-Sondi, 2004; Wei et al., 2009). Antiviral activity of silver nanoparticles has been demonstrated against several types of viruses, including hepatitis B, herpes simplex virus, respiratory syncytial virus, and monkey pox virus (Baram-Pinto et al., 2009; Lu et al., 2008; Rogers et al., 2008; Sun et al., 2008). Recently, several studies have demonstrated their antiviral activity against HIV-1 *in vitro* (Elechiguerra et al., 2005; Lara et al., 2010; Sun et al., 2005). Silver nanoparticles were shown to be effective against a wide range of HIV-1 strains *in vitro*, including laboratory strains, clinical isolates, M and T tropic strains, and resistant strains (Lara et al., 2010). The therapeutic index of silver nanoparticles was found to be 12 times higher than that of silver ions used as silver nitrate and silver sulfadiazine salts, indicating that higher antiviral efficiency was specific to silver nanoparticles (Lara et al., 2010). Silver nanoparticles act as viral entry inhibitors by binding to gp120 and thus preventing CD4-mediated viral membrane fusion to host cells and subsequent infectivity (Elechiguerra et al., 2005; Lara et al., 2010). They are also found to inhibit post-entry stages of HIV-1,70 indicating that silver nanoparticles act at multiple stages of the HIV life cycle. This would result in reduced risk for the development of viral resistance to silver nanoparticles. However, the *in vivo* antiviral activity of silver nanoparticles against HIV-1 has yet to be demonstrated. Another inorganic nanoparticulate system evaluated for antiretroviral drug delivery consists of gold nanoparticles. Bowman et al. (2008) used small molecule-conjugated gold nanoparticles as anti-HIV agents. The SDC-1721, a fragment of the potent HIV inhibitor TAK-779, was synthesized and conjugated to gold nanoparticles. Free SDC-1721 had no inhibitory activity in HIV infection. However, antiretroviral activity comparable with TAK-779 was observed when SDC-1721 was conjugated to gold nanoparticles. Gold nanoparticles transformed the biologically inactive SDC-1721 into amultivalent conjugate that effectively inhibited HIV-1 fusion to human T lymphocytes. Table 10 highlights some of the key advancements made in nanotechnology-based anti-HIV therapy.

Table 10. Important developments in nanotechnology-based anti-HIV therapy.

Targeted step in HIV life cycle	Active ingredient formulated into nanoparticles
Viral entry into host cell	Silver (Elechiguerra et al., 2005; Lara et al., 2010) Gold (Bowman et al., 2008)

Table 10. *(Continued)*

Targeted step in HIV life cycle	Active ingredient formulated into nanoparticles
Reverse transcription	Chemokine receptor blocker (Ham et al., 2009)
	Zidovudine (Dembri et al., 2001; Kuo and Chen, 2006; Lobenberg et al., 1998; Mainardes et al., 2009)
	Lamivudine (Kuo and Chen, 2006)
	Stavudine (Kuo, 2005; Kuo and Su, 2007)
	Delavirdine (Kuo and Su, 2007)
	Efavirenz (Destache et al., 2009)
Viral assembly	Saquinavir (Kuo and Kuo, 2008; Kuo and Su, 2007; Shah and Amiji, 2006)
	Ritonavir (Destache et al., 2009)
	Lopinavir (Destache et al., 2009)

POTENTIAL TOXICITY OF INORGANIC NANOPARTICLES

One drawback to the use of inorganic nanoparticles is potential toxicity. Toxicity of inorganic nanoparticles must be studied carefully before they can be clinically applied. Several studies have demonstrated the cytotoxic effects of these inorganic nanoparticles (Asharani et al., 2009; Braydich-Stole et al., 2005; Hussain et al., 2005; Kawata et al., 2009). In studies evaluating acute toxicity, silver nanoparticles were found to be highly cytotoxic to mammalian cells based on the assessment of mitochondrial function, membrane leakage of lactate dehydrogenase, and abnormal cell morphologies (Braydich-Stole et al., 2005; Hussain et al., 2005). Toxicity studies conducted on human lung fibroblast cells (IMR-90) and human glioblastoma cells (U251) revealed the generation of reactive oxygen species by cells exposed to silver nanoparticles (Asharani et al., 2009). The DNA damage and cell cycle arrest in the G(2) or M phase was observed. In studies by Kawata et al. (2009) using HepG2 human hepatoma cells, subacute exposure to silver nanoparticles resulted in abnormal cell morphology and increased cell proliferation possibly due to hormesis, that is, a stimulatory effect exhibited by low levels of potentially toxic agents. The incidence of micronuclei formation, indicative of chromosomal aberrations or breakage, was significantly higher in cells exposed to subacute levels of silver nanoparticles. Studies on rodents showed that silver nanoparticles accumulated in various organs including the lungs, kidneys, brain, liver, and testes (Kim et al., 2008). Furthermore, DNA microarray analysis indicated an induction of a large number of genes, particularly, stress associated genes coding metallothionine and heat shockprotein (Kawata et al., 2009). Similar studies on other inorganic nanoparticles, including gold and titanium dioxide, have indicated toxicity via DNA damage and cellular apoptosis (Goodman et al., 2004; Zhao et al., 2009).

DENDRIMERS

Dendrimers are a versatile class of regularly-branched macromolecules with unique structural and topologic features. Small size (typically less than 100 nm), narrow molecular weight distribution, and relative ease of incorporation of targeting ligands make them attractive candidates for drug delivery. Dendrimers have minimal polydispersity and high functionality. Similar to polymers, they are obtained by attaching several monomeric units, but unlike the conventional polymers, they have a highly branched three-dimensional architecture. Dendrimers are characterized by the presence of three different topologic sites, that is a polyfunctional core, interior layers, and multivalent surface (du Toit et al., 2010). The polyfunctional core, surrounded by extensive branching, has the ability to encapsulate several chemicalmoieties. Ammonia and ethylene diamine are two examples of core-synthesizing materials. The core may be surrounded by several layers of highly branched repeating units, such as polyethers, porphyrins, polyamidoamines, polyphenyls, and polyamino acids. The properties of the dendrimer are predominantly based on the multivalent surface, which has several functional groups that interact with the external environment. The precise physico-chemical properties of dendrimers can be controlled during synthesis by controlling the core groups, the extent of branching, and the nature and/or number of functional groups on the surface (Bosman et al., 1999; Svenson and Tomalia, 2005). Dendrimers can not only act as carriers of antiretroviral agents, but can also themselves act as antiretrovirals. Dendrimers with inherent antiretroviral activity can be synthesized by incorporating certain functional groups on their surface that can interfere with the binding of the virus to the cell. A diverse array of dendrimers with various patterns of biologic activity can be synthesized by making subtle changes, such as the type of initiator, branching unit type, dendrimer generation, linker, and surfaces (Gajbhiye et al., 2009). The inherent antiviral activity of dendrimers has been demonstrated against influenza virus (Oka et al., 2009), respiratory syncytial virus (Barnard et al., 1997), and HIV (Macri et al., 2009) *in vitro*. These dendrimers primarily act by blocking viral fusion to target cells and thus act as entry inhibitors in the early stages of viral infection, although secondary mechanisms of action at later stages of the viral life cycle have been reported (Oka et al., 2009; du Toit et al., 2010). Water-soluble dendrimers can be used as efficient carriers of antiretroviral agents which can be entrapped in the dendrimer architecture. The antiretrovirals or their prodrugs can also be grafted covalently onto the surface of the dendrimers, either alone or in conjunction with other molecules, such as targeting moieties and fluorescent tags. Multivalent dendrimeric systems have been of much interest in the field of antiviral therapy. Dutta et al. (2008) developed efavirenz-loaded, tuftsin-conjugated poly(propyleneimine) dendrimers for targeted delivery to macrophages. Tuftsin is a natural macrophage activator tetrapeptide which binds specifically to mononuclear phagocytic cells and enhances their phagocytic activity. These multivalent dendrimers showed reduced cytotoxicity compared with nonconjugated poly(propyleneimine) dendrimers *in vitro*. The free amino groups present on poly(propyleneimine) dendrimers are responsible for their cytotoxicity. Conjugation of tuftsin topoly(propyleneimine) dendrimers reduced the cytotoxicity of these dendrimers, possibly by shielding the positive charges and thus preventing their interaction with cell membranes. The tuftsin-conjugated poly(propyleneimine)dendrimers showed enhanced cellular uptake by mononuclear phagocytic cells and greater anti-HIV activity *in vitro*. The same research group loaded lamivudine into mannose-cappedpoly(propyleneimine) dendrimers and observed a significant increase in antiretroviral activity, cellular uptake, and reduced cytotoxicity (Dutta and Jain, 2007). The mannose conjugation enabled the targeted delivery of the lamivudine-loaded dendrimers to macrophages containing lectin receptors on their surface. Dendrimers have been used to transfect silencing RNA (siRNA) to reduce HIV infection *in vitro*. Amino-terminated carbosilane dendrimers were used to protect and transfer siRNA to lymphocytes *in vitro* (Weber et al., 2008). These dendrimers bind to siRNA via electrostatic interactions and protect it from RNase degradation. The V3 loop region of viral gp120 interacts with glycolipids, such as galactosylce-ramide, on the host cell for cell attachment and subsequent cell entry (Harouse et al., 1989, 1991). Anionic polymers and dendrimers through ionic interactions with the V3 loop of gp120 interfere with viral-host cell interactions (McCarthy et al., 2005 Moulard et al., 2000). One such anionic dendrimer is SPL7013, a poly-L-lysine den-drimer with naphthalene sulfonic acid terminations. It has a divalent benzhydrylamine amide of L-lysine as the core. Efficacy studies with 5% w/w SPL7013 as an aque-ous gel showed that a single intravaginal dose of the formulation protected pig-tailed macaques from intravaginal simian human immunodeficiency virus infection (Jiang et al., 2005). VivaGel® is anaqueous-based polyacrylic acid gel containing SPL7013 buffered to physiologic pH. VivaGel is the first dendrimer-based drug application that has been submitted to the USFDA as an investigational new drug (Rupp et al., 2007). Phase I clinical trials showed no systemic absorption following intravaginal dosing, indicative of the desired retention in the vaginal lumen. The safety profile of VivaGel was comparable with placebogel, indicating no toxicity (Patton et al., 2006). The an-tiretroviral activity of sulfated oligosaccharides is very low (Choi et al., 1996). How-ever, sulfated oligosaccharides when attached to a dendrimer show high antiretroviral activity due to cluster effects (Roy et al., 1993). Recently, Han et al. (2010) developed oligosaccharide-based polylysine dendrimers with sulfated cellobiose. These were shown topossess high anti-HIV activity, almost equivalent to dideoxycytidine, and low cytotoxicity.

Multivalent phosphorus-containing catanionic dendrimerswith galactosylce-ramide analogues were developed by Blanzat et al. (2002). The influence of the multi-functional core, the alkyl chains, and the surface properties of the dendrimerson their stability, cytotoxicity, and antiretroviral properties were reported by the same group in subsequent studies (Blanzat et al., 2005; Perez-Anes, 2010). Galactosylceramide has a high affinity for the V3 loop of thegp120 viral envelope protein of HIV-1, and subse-quently preventsviral fusion to the host cell membrane, thus acting as anentry inhibi-tor. Although, the galactosylceramide dendrimers showed good antiretroviral activity, a low therapeutic index associated with cytotoxicity is one of the issues that need to be addressed before these can be considered promising antiretroviral agents. Reports on dendrimer-based anti-HIV therapy continue to appear (Telwatte et al., 2011). Another strategy for oral delivery used cyclodextrins, cyclic hydrophilic oligosaccharides with a hydrophobic core, composed of glucose units joined through α-1,4-glucosidic bonds, widely used as drug absorption enhancers for drug delivery (Buchanan et al., 2007; Yang et al., 2008).

SOLID LIPID NANOPARTICLES

As already discussed above, SLNs containlipids in the solid state there by imparting greater drug stability and better control over drug-release kinetics. Zidovudine palmi-tate-loaded SLNs prepared by Heiatiet al. (1997) were the first reported antiretroviral

SLNs. Trilaurin was used as the lipid core in these systems. Dipalmitoylphosphatidyl-choline alone or in combination with dimyristoylphosphatidylglycerol was used as a coating. The resultant SLNs were either neutral or negatively charged. Drug loading was dependent on the outer phospholipid coat, with higher phospholipid content resulting in greater drug incorporation. In a subsequent study by the same group, the surfaces of these SLNs were modified by the attachment of PEG moieties, thus improving the plasma circulation half-life of the drug (Heiati et al., 1998). The SLNs have been widely used to overcome biological barriers, such as the BBB and blood-cerebrospinal fluid barrier. The use of SLNs for drug delivery to the brain was first proposed by Yang et al. (1999) and Zara et al. (1999) independently in the late 1990s in their studies of the pharmacokinetics of two anticancer agents, camptothecin and doxorubicin, respectively. Accumulation of the drug in the brain was observed after both oral and systemic administration of drug-loaded SLNs in rats. Since then, several studies were conducted on the ability of SLNs to improve the brain delivery of drugs. Kuo and Su (2007) prepared SLNs loaded with stavudine, delavirdine, and saquinavir independently and evaluated their ability to cross the BBB *in vitro* using human brain microvascular endothelial cells. The entrapment efficiency of the drugs followed their lipophilicity, with the more lipophilic saquinavir having the maximum entrapment efficiency, indicating the better suitability of SLNs to more lipophilic drugs. The permeability of the drugs was improved 4–11-fold when incorporated into SLNs. Chattopadhyay et al. (2008) used SLNs made of stearic acid for delivery to the brain of atazanavir, a highly lipophilic antiviral protease inhibitor. In this study, the SLNs were prepared by a microemulsion technique using Pluronic F68 as an emulsifier. *In vitro* studies using hCMEC/D3, a human brain microvessel endothelial cell line, showed a higher uptake of the drug when delivered in SLN form, as compared with free atazanavir. Atazanavir is a substrate for the adenosine triphosphate-binding cassette membrane-associated drug efflux transporters, such as P-glycoprotein. The activity of these efflux transporters results in lower intracellular accumulation of atazanavir. The authors hypothesize that SLNs circumvent P-glycoprotein mediated efflux and mask the drug from the membranebound P-glycoprotein efflux transporter, thus facilitating its intracellular accumulation.

Several surface modifications were studied to improvethe targeting ability of SLNs further. The PEG moieties attachedto the surface of SLNs impart stealth characteristics to the SLNs and improve their delivery to brain (Fundaro et al., 2000; Zara et al., 2002b). Surface charge modification is another approach that has been used to improve the targeted drug delivery of SLNs. Positively charged SLNs are found to deliver higher amounts of drugs to the brain than uncharged or negatively charged SLNs. Kuoand Chen (2009) prepared cationic SLNs loaded with the lipophilicprotease inhibitor, saquinavir. A blend of the nonionic lipids Compritol ATO 888 and cacao butter were used as corelipids. Stearylamine and dioctadecyldimethyl ammoniumbromide comprised the peripheral cationic lipids. Polysorbate80 was used as an SLN emulsifier/stabilizer. However, this study did not include any *in vitro* or *in vivo* demonstration of their improved ability to deliver the drug to the target sites. The modification of surface charge to enhance drug delivery to the CNS must be applied with caution because positively charged SLNs and high amounts of negatively charged SLNs were shown to increase the cortical cerebrovascular volume of rats significantly *in situ* in brain perfusion experiments, indicating a compromise in the integrity of the BBB (Lockman et al., 2004).

NANOMEDICINE AND LEISHMANIASIS

Leishmaniasis appears in different clinical manifestations-ulcerative skin lesions (cutaneous), destructive mucosal inflammation (muco cutaneous), and disseminated visceral infection (kala-azar) (Herwaldt, 1999). Drugs used in conventional treatments are poorly selective, or must be administered in repeated and high doses by parenteral routes (Thakur and Narayan, 2004). These facts undoubtedly contribute to the high toxicity and in most cases to the poor compliance and efficacy of current conventional medication used against all the clinical forms. Hence, as in case of tuberculosis and HIV infection, the need for a drug delivery system arises in case of leishmanias is supported by the success of liposomal Amphotericin B(AmB) (Meyerhoff, 1999).

SYNTHETIC BIODEGRADABLE PARTICLES

Primaquine loaded on polyalkylcyanoacrylate nanoparticles(PACA-NP) (Gaspar et al., 1992a) and polyisohexylcyanoacrylate nanoparticles(PIHCA-NP) (Gaspar et al., 1991) exhibited increased activity compared with free primaquine. However, empty PACA-NP was found to activate respiratory burst in macrophages in the absence of primaquine (Gaspar et al., 1992b) whereas PIHCA was toxic oninfected mice. Further, developments using these polymers were discontinued.

Primaquine loaded in (DL)PLA-NP was 3.3-fold more active in reducing liver amastigotes from experimental visceral leishmaniasis (*L. donovani*) than free primaquine (Rodrigues et al., 1994). Although, when diluted in circulation, primaquine loaded in (DL)PLA-NP is almost completely released from nanoparticle matrices, upon intravenous administration in healthy micethe LD_{50} was increased almost 2-fold compared with that of free primaquine (Rodrigues et al., 1995). Another hydrophilic drug, pentamidine (second-line treatment) also loaded on PLA-NP (Durand et al., 1997a) and in polymethacrylate-NP (Durand et al., 1997b) resulted in 3.3 and 6 times more activity than free drug (ED_{50} 0.17 and 0.32 mg/kg versus 1.05 mg/kg) in experimental visceral leishmaniasis (*L. infantum*). The natural antileishmanial agent 2',6'-dihydroxy-4'-methoxychalcone (DMC) loaded in PLA-NP reduced theamastigote number inside macrophages *in vitro*; and skinlesions were significantly reduced (60% the size of lesionsin control animals) upon two subcutaneous and two intraperitoneal administrations on experimental cutaneous leishmaniasis. Apparently, PLA-NP reach the parasite site in the parasitophorous vacuole before their degradation, suggesting that DMC may be discharged close to the parasites, improving its bioavailability. The slow biodegradation rate of PLA-NP can be related to the fact that nanoparticles remain inside the phagolysosome system while in transit, as occurs for all PLA-NP. Remarkably, the DMC PLA-NP effect was comparable to that of equivalent doses of glucantime. The particles were well tolerated by miceupon intravenous administration (Torres-Santos et al., 1999). Other polymeric nanoparticles such as poly(ε-caprolactone)-NP loaded with AmB were found to be 2 to 3 times more effective than free AmB in reducing parasite burden from experimental visceral leishmaniasis and also showed reduced side effects associated with AmB (Espuelas et al., 2002). Other experimental drugs such as the poorly hydrosolubledihydroindolo-(2,3a) indolizines incorporated in phospholipid microspheres prepared from a mixture of PLGA and pentamidine bearing a mannose arm were highly efficient in reducing spleen parasites (91%) (Medda et al., 2003). In another study, bassin acid incorporated in PLA-NP resulted in less toxicity and improved leishmanicidal activity than o/w microemulsions, both subcutaneously injected in experimental visceral leishmaniasis (Lala et al., 2006). An interesting recent development is the successful encapsulation of andrographolide, a potent antileishmanial drug in PLG-NP (Roy et al., 2010).

DRUG DELIVERY SYSTEMS FOR TOPICAL ADMINISTRATION

To date, no concrete strategy has been developed for topical treatment. Only a few attempts have been made to improve drug absorption. Using permeation enhancers like ethanol, significant improvements in lesion size on experimental cutaneous leishmaniasis (*L. major*) were observed upon topically applied dispersion of Amphocil and Abelcet insolution containing 5–25% ethanol, over animals treated with dispersed AmB (Frankenburg et al., 1998). Only *in vitro* permeation across rat skin studies were carried out with AmB loaded in different MLV matrices. Positively charged liposomes showed a high shelf life (1 year at 30°C), with a high flux of AmB across the stratumcorneum (58 ng/cm^2/h), being maximal in viable epidermis for negatively charged liposomes (23 ng/cm^2/h). The AmB loaded in liposomes is reported to be more stable than free AmB insolution and in powder forms (Manosroi et al., 2004). The highly hydrophilic antibiotic paromomycin associated to the permeation enhancer methyl benzethonium chloride (MBC, responsible for adverse reactions) is the most efficient topical formulation for treatment of cutaneous leishmaniasis. The skin permeation of paromomycin loaded in unilamellarliposomes (soybean phosphatidylcholine:cholesterol 1:1molar ratio) was increased compared with that of MBC aqueous solution of paromomycin (Ferreira et al., 2004).

DRUG DELIVERY SYSTEMS FOR ORAL ADMINISTRATION

Mucoadhesive nanosuspensions (hydrogels) containing chitosan were shown to adhere to the gastrointestinal mucosa, prolonging the contact time of released drugs. This property was formerly used for sustained drug release against *Cryptosporium parvum*, a parasite localised in the epithelial membrane of the gastrointestinal tract (Muller et al., 2001). In a furtherwork, nanosuspensions made of AmB in an aqueous solution of Tween 80, Pluronics F68, and sodium cholate were produced by a high-pressure homogenisation technique, showing long-term stability at 20°C, zeta potential of -36 mV and medium size of 620 nm. When orally administered against experimental visceral leishmaniasis (*L. donovani*), a significant reduction in the liver parasite load by nearly 29% occurred. Neither the oral administration of micronised AmB, or liposomal AmB significantly reduced liver parasiteload compared with untreated controls (Kayser et al., 2003).

Another strategy for oral delivery used cyclodextrins. Meglumine antimoniate is a highly hydrosoluble and low membrane permeability class III drug, hence complexes formed with cyclodextrins were not expected to be conventional, such as those in which hydrophobic drugs are trapped inside the cyclodextrin core (Loftsson et al., 2004). Meglumine antimoniate-β-cyclodextrin complexes were prepared by mixing β-cyclodextrins and meglumine antimoniate in distilled water at 1:1 cyclodextrin/Sb V molarratio and heating the mixture for 48 hr at 55°C. A final freeze-drying step seems to be the key to promoting the formation of supramolecular nano-assemblies between meglumine antimoniate and β-cyclodextrins, which act as asustained release system for meglumine antimoniate, following dilution in water. Plasma Sb V levels were about 3-fold higher for the complex than for the free drug upon oral administration in Swiss mice. Significantly, smaller skin lesions were developed on experimental cutaneous leishmaniasis (L. amazonensis) upon daily administration of the complex (32 mg/kg) than those treated with meglumine antimoniate (120 mg/kg) and control animals treated with saline. The effectiveness of the complex given orally was equivalent to that of the free drug given intraperitoneally at a 2-fold-higher Sb V dose (Demicheli et al., 2004; Frezard et al., 2008). An interesting approach used cochleates, stable phospholipid-cation crystalline structures consisting of aspiral lipid bilayer sheet with no internal aqueous space, which have the potential for oral administration of hydrophobic drugs. Cochleates containing AmB orally administered demonstrated similar activity as deoxycholate AmB administered by the intraperitoneal route in a mouse model of systemic candidiasis (Santiangelo et al, 2000). However, the antileishmanial activity remains to be determined.

Recently, miltefosine (hexadecylphosphocholine, HePC), a molecule that forms micelles in aqueous media, has been used to solubilise AmB (Menez et.al, 2007). The resulting mixed micellar system of 7 nm diameter and AmB in monomer form was less toxic toward mammalian cells than aggregated AmB (Gruda and Dussault, 1988). HePC enhances the paracellular permeability across the intestinal epithelium and could therefore improve the transport of co-administered therapeutic agents. *In vitro/ in vivo* toxicity as well as antileishmanial activity remain to be determined. Interestingly, encapsulation of specific proteins in SLNs for protection against leishmaniansis have also been reported (Doroud et al., 2011a, 2011b).

FUTURE PERSPECTIVE

The major drawbacks associated with new drug development includean input of immense research efforts, cost and time; difficulty in targeting drug-resistant and latent microorganisms; and uncertainty with respect to toxicity and resistance (Barry and Duncan, 2004). This is the driving force behind the search for alternative therapeutic strategies. By employing nanotechnology, synthetic/natural carrier-based controlled release nanomedicine formulations have been developed, encapsulating key drugs against tuberculosis, AIDS and leishmaniasis. Besides sustained release of drugs in plasma/organs, other potential advantages of the system include the possibility of selecting various routes of chemotherapy, reduction in drug dosage/adverse effects/drug interactions, targeting drug-resistant and latent microorganisms, and so on. On the other hand, the choice of carrier, large-scale production, stability and toxicity of the formulation are some of the major issues that merit immediate attention and resolution. Nevertheless, keeping in view the hurdles in new drug development, nanomedicine has provided a sound platform and a ray of hope for an onslaught against infectious diseases.

KEYWORDS

- Dendrimers
- Drug release
- Ethambutol
- Human immunodeficiency virus
- Microorganisms
- Poly glycolic acid
- Poly lactic acid
- Solid lipid nanoparticles
- Tuberculosis
- Wheat germ agglutinin

Chapter 10

Dendrimers in Biology and Medicine

Dzmitry Shcharbin, Volha Dzmitruk, Inessa Halets,
Elzbieta Pedziwiatr-Werbicka, and Maria Bryszewska

INTRODUCTION

The application of nanotechnology in biology and medicine led the appearance of new devices, supramolecular systems, structures, complexes and composites. An excellent example of nanotechnological composites are dendrimers (from Greek "dendron"– tree, and "meros"– branch). Dendrimers were first synthesized in laboratories of Tomalia, Newkome, and Vogtle (Fischer and Vogtle, 1999; Hawker and Frechet, 1990; Newkome et al., 1986; Tomalia, 1995, 1996). They are globular in shape with topological structure formed by monomeric subunit branches diverging on all sides from the central nucleus (Semchikov, 1998). The following features can be distinguished in dendrimers: (i) multivalent surfaces containing numerous potentially active sites, (ii) envelopes surrounding the nucleus, and (iii) nuclei with attached dendrons.

Since 1979, two main strategies have been used to synthesize dendrimers: the divergent method in which dendron growth begins from the nucleus (Bosman et al., 1999; Fischer and Vogtle, 1999; Hawker and Frechet, 1990; Newkome et al., 1985, 1986, 1998, 1999; Tomalia, 1986, 1995, 1996), and a convergent method in which preassembled dendrimer branches join the nucleus (Hawker and Frechet, 1990). According to the divergent method proposed by the Tomalia and Vogtle groups (Fischer and Vogtle, 1999; Tomalia, 1995, 1996), dendrimer synthesis includes association of monomeric modules in a radial structure, from one branch to another, following definite rules. According to the convergent method proposed by Hawker and Frechet (1990), branches that at the final stage of the process join the nucleus and form the dendrimer are first grown in dendrimer synthesis.

With regard to modifications, over 100 kinds of dendrimers have been synthesized (Bosman et al., 1999; Fischer and Vogtle, 1999; Hawker and Frechet, 1990, 1994; Majoral et al., 2002; Mansfield and Klushin, 1993; Matthews et al., 1998; Murat and Grest, 1996; Newkome et al., 1985, 1986, 1998, 1999; Ortega et al., 2006; Tomalia, 1986, 1995, 1996). Five of the most widespread families have been distinguished among them.

Polyamide amine (PAMAM) dendrimers (Tomalia et al., 1986) are based on a ethylenediamine nucleus, and their branches are based on methyl acrylate and ethylenediamine. Half generations of PAMAM dendrimers have surface carboxyls, while complete generations have surface amino groups. There is currently a great choice of PAMAM dendrimers with different types of surface groups. *Polypropyleneimine (PPI) dendrimers* (Bosman et al., 1999; Fischer and Vogtle, 1999; Frechet et al., 1994) are based on a butylenes diamine nucleus and polypropyleneimine monomers. Another popular abbreviation of these dendrimers, DAB (diaminobutyl; based on the name of the nucleus) are now commercially available. *Phosphorus dendrimers* are synthesized by Majoral and Caminade (2002). Phosphorus atoms are present in the nucleus and branches of these dendrimers. *Carbosilane dendrimers* are based on a silicon nucleus with ammonium or amino groups at the periphery (Ortega et al., 2006). *Polylysine dendrimers* based on lysine and have polylysine branches and surface groups (Vlasov, 2006) are also now commercially available.

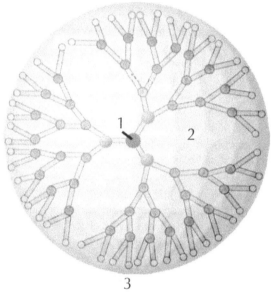

Figure 1. Dendrimer structure.
(1) Nucleus, (2) Internal cavities, (3) Surface groups.

The architecture and properties of dendrimers depend on their generation. Low generations of dendrimers have an open, flattened and asymmetric shape, but as the generation increases, the structure becomes globular and densely packed at the periphery. The insides of dendrimers are empty cavities. Another important feature of dendrimers is their monodispersity. The classical polymerization process is usually random and produces molecules of different sizes, whereas the size and molecular mass of dendrimers can be specifically controlled during synthesis. Finally, dendrimers possess many functional end groups that are responsible for high solubility and reactivity.

Because of their special and peculiar features, dendrimers have found their place in biology and medicine.

Dendrimers as new synthetic vectors for gene therapy. To understand the necessity of nucleic acid delivery systems, we shall briefly describe barriers to nucleic acid delivery within organisms. Introduction of free nucleic acid is accompanied in most cases by its enzymic degradation in the organism (Niven et al., 1998), which necessitates systems for plasmid nucleic acid packing and transport (Dufes et al., 2005). Viral and synthetic vectors are designed for this purpose. Additionally, vectors help in nucleic acid delivery to zones necessary for their localization and provide for efficient intracellular transport, usually to the nucleus (Eliyahu et al., 2005). Most often, the packing of nucleic acid is provided by electrostatic interaction of its anionic phosphate groups with positive charges of the synthetic vector, resulting in complex formation. Nucleic acid complexes with liposomes and different cationic linear polymers are now the most widely used non-viral vectors. Complexes with liposomes are called lipoplexes, and those with linear polymers are called polyplexes. Dendrimers with positively charged groups are also able to bind nucleic acid, and by analogy with lipoplexes and polyplexes, they are called dendriplexes (Eliyahu et al., 2005). This class of polymers has structural advantages for gene transport. Dendrimers are monodisperse and stable, characterized by relatively low viscosity at high molecular mass and numerous end groups that can be ionized, which allows them to bind efficiently a large amount of genetic material.

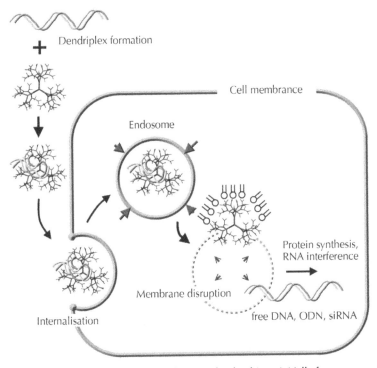

Figure 2. Genetic material transfer using dendrimers. The dendrimer initially forms a complex with nucleic acid *in vitro*. The complex is added to cells *in vitro* or introduced into animals *in vivo* or *ex vivo*. Dendriplexes can be delivered to their localization by the blood flow. The dendriplex becomes internalized by cells, and dendriplex-containing endosomes are formed. Deprotonation of dendrimer surface groups, dendrimer destruction and nucleic acid release occurs when the pH changes from 7.4 (extracellular value) to 5.5 (intracellular value). Simultaneously, the endosomes undergo lysis and free nucleic acid is released into the cytoplasm.

The patents on gene delivery by dendrimers can be found in (Florence et al., 1999; German and Szoka, 1998; Majoral et al., 2005; Matsunaga et al., 2008; Tomalia and Majoros, 2006; Uchegbu et al., 2005). The reviews on studying of efficiency of dendrimers for delivery of model genes of luciferase from firefly *Photinus pyralis* and β-galactosidase can be found in (Shcharbin et al., 2009, 2010). Also, dendrimers were successfully applied as gene carriers for *anticancer delivery* of genes of vascular endothelial growth factor (Kim et al., 2009), tumor necrosis factor receptor immunoglobulin (Hudde et al., 1999), tumor necrosis factor α (Dufes et al., 2005), Fas ligand of tumor necrosis factor superfamily (Nakanishi et al., 2003), herpes simplex virus type 1 thymidine kinase (Harada et al., 2000; Maruyama-Tabata et al., 2000; Tanaka et al., 2000) to the cancer cells; genes of IL-2 cytokine and a single chain IL-12 fusion protein (Balicki et al., 2000), human growth hormone (Eliyahu et al., 2002), bone morphogenetic protein-2 (Santos et al., 2009), angiostatin (Vincent et al., 2003), tissue inhibitor of metalloproteinase (TIMP-2) (Vincent et al., 2003), Na/I symporter (NIS) protein (Chisholm et al., 2009), Exendin-4, a glucagon-like peptide (GLP-1) analog (Ah Kim et al., 2009), brain-derived neurotrophic factor (Shakhbazau et al., 2010a, b) into different cells, including mesenchymal stem cells (Santos et al., 2009; Shakhbazau et al., 2010a,b). With respect to their efficiency as carriers, dendrimers showed in *anti-human immunodeficiency virus gene therapy* using anti-HIV olygodeoxynucleotides and siRNA for delivery of ANTITAR, GEM91, SREV oligodeoxinucleotides (Chonco et al., 2007; Pedziwiatr-Werbicka et al., 2011; Shcharbin et al., 2007), siGAG1, siP24, siNEF, siGAPDH (Jiménez et al., 2010; Shcharbin et al., 2011; Weber et al., 2008). The RNA interference mechanism was also used in *dendrimer-mediated delivery of anti-cancer siRNA and DNAzyme* to cancer cells: triplex-forming ODN and DNAzyme to *c-myc* oncogene (Pan et al., 2009; Santhakumaran et al., 2004; Tack et al., 2006a, b), survivin ODN to *survivine* oncogene (Pan et al., 2007), siGADPH, siP-EPCK, siOCT1 to GADPH, PEPCK, OCT1 genes (GADPH - glyceraldehyde 3-phosphate dehydrogenase, OCT1–organic cation transporter 1, PEPCK - phosphoenolpyruvate carboxykinase–enzyme of gluconeogenesis) (Inoue et al., 2008), siBCL-2 to mRNA of anti-apoptotic BCL-2 protein (Patil et al., 2009). The extremely important features of dendrimers include their possible conjugation with peptides that significantly increases penetration of dendrimers and dendriplexes into cells and nuclei (Han et al., 2010; Li et al., 2010; Szoka and Haensler, 1997; Vlasov, 2003). Conjugation of dendrimers with peptides also allows direct delivery of genetic material into cancer cells (Han et al., 2010; Li et al., 2010; Taratula et al., 2009). Using brain-penetrating peptides, genetic material can be delivered to the brain across the blood-brain barrier (Huang et al., 2007, 2009; Ke et al., 2009). By conjugating dendrimers and peptides, we can modulate the delivery of genes in brain.

Table 1. Dendrimers as new synthetic vectors for gene therapy.

Anticancer gene therapy using dendrimers	
vascular endothelial growth factor	Kim et al., 2009
tumor necrosis factor receptor immunoglobulin	Hudde et al., 1999
Fas ligand of tumor necrosis factor superfamily	Nakanishi et al., 2003

Table 1. *(Continued)*

tumor necrosis factor α	Dufes et al., 2005
herpes simplex virus type 1 thymidine kinase	Maruyama-Tabata et al., 2000; Harada et al., 2000; Tanaka et al., 2000

Dendrimer-mediated delivery of anticancer siRNA and DNAzyme

triplex-forming ODN and DNAzyme to *c-myc* oncogene	Santhakumaran et al., 2004; Tack et al., 2006a,b; Pan et al., 2009
survivin ODN to *survivine* oncogene	Pan et al., 2007
siGADPH, siPEPCK, siOCT1 to GADPH, PEPCK, OCT1 genes	Inoue et al., 2008
siBCL-2 to mRNA of anti-apoptotic BCL-2 protein	Patil et al., 2009

Anti - human immunodeficiency virus gene therapy

ANTITAR, GEM91, SREV oligodeoxinucleotides	Chonco et al., 2007; Pedziwiatr-Werbicka et al., 2011; Shcharbin et al., 2007
siGAG1, siP24, siNEF, siGAPDH	Weber et al., 2008; Shcharbin et al., 2011; Jiménez et al., 2010

Delivery of genes to stem cells using dendrimers

bone morphogenetic protein-2	Santos et al., 2009
brain-derived neurotrophic factor	Shakhbazau et al., 2010a,b

Dendrimers have shown their efficacy and efficiency in the field of *drug delivery*. Using non-covalent or covalent conjugation with dendrimers, one can significantly improve the direct delivery of drugs, notably in direct delivery of anti-cancer drugs (adriamycin (Kono et al., 2008), doxorubicin (Tan et al., 2009; Zhu et al., 2010), methotrexate (Kaminskas et al., 2009; Kono et al., 1999), fluorouracil (Tripathi et al., 2002; Zhuo et al., 1999), and cisplatin (Haxton and Burt, 2009; Malik and Duncan, 2004; Malik et al., 1999, 2006). These properties have been reviewed in detail in references (Bharali et al., 2009; Medina and El-Sayed, 2009; Sarin, 2009). Of importance and significance is the conjugation of dendrimers with folate receptors, resulting in the increase of recognition of such conjugates by folic receptors of cancer cells (Agarwal et al., 2008; Konda et al., 2000; Myc et al., 2008; Wiener et al., 1997). Using dendrimers as solubility enhancers, this significantly improves the delivery of hydrophobic drugs such as propranolol (D'Emanuele et al., 2004), naproxen (Najlah et al., 2007), indomethacin (D'Emanuele et al., 2004), niclosamide (Devarakonda et al., 2005), furosemide (Devarakonda et al., 2007), ketoprofen (Na et al., 2006), pilocarpine, tropicamide (Vandamme and Brobeck, 2005).

We believe that dendrimer-based drug delivery will replace such non-viral systems as liposomes.

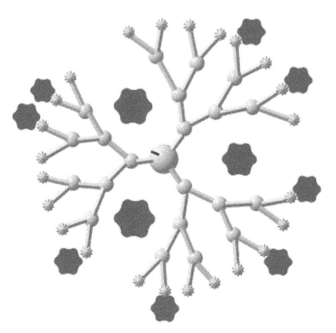

Figure 3. Drugs can be encapsulated into dendrimer or attached to the dendrimer surface.

Table 2. Dendrimers as drug delivery carriers.

Anticancer drug delivery using dendrimers	
Adriamycin	Kono et al., 2008
Doxorubicin	Zhu et al., 2010; Tan et al., 2009
Methotrexate	Kono et al., 1999; Kaminskas et al., 2009
Fluorouracil	Zhuo et al., 1999; Tripathi et al., 2002
Cisplatin	Malik et al., 1999; Malik and Duncan, 2004; Malik et al., 2006; Haxton and Burt, 2009
Dendrimers as solubility enhancers for hydrophobic drugs	
Propranolol	D'Emanuele et al., 2004
Naproxen	Najlah et al., 2007
Indomethacin	D'Emanuele et al., 2004
Niclosamide	Devarakonda et al., 2005
Furosemide	Devarakonda et al., 2007
Ketoprofen	Na et al., 2006
Pilocarpine, tropicamide	Vandamme and Brobeck, 2005

The extensive adaptability of dendrimer-based *contrast agents* is ideal for the molecular imaging of organs and other target-specific locations (Bourne et al., 1996; Kellar et al., 1997; Wiener et al., 1994). The ability of literally atom-by-atom modification on cores, interiors, and surface groups, permits the rational manipulation of dendrimer-based agents that can optimize their physical characteristics, biodistribution, receptor-mediated targeting and controlled release of their payload (Kim and Zimmerman, 1998; Kobayashi and Brechbiel, 2003, 2005). These modifications enable agents to localize preferentially to areas or organs of interest, facilitating target-specific imaging as well as assuming excretion pathways that do not interfere with desired applications. First, this concerns gadolinium salts of 2-(4-isothiocyanatobenzyl)-6 methyldiethylene-triaminepentaacetic acid (DTPA) or 1,4,7,10-tetraazacyclododecane tetraacetic acid (DOTA), which are used clinically, but quickly diffuse into the extravenous sites due to their low molecular mass. Therefore, both DTPA and DOTA are often conjugated with different macromolecules, such as polylysines, dextran, and polyethylene glycol polymers (Weissleder et al., 2001). Dendrimers showed themselves as excellent carriers for Gd based contrast agents (Kim and Zimmerman, 1998; Kobayashi and Brechbiel, 2003, 2005; New et al., 2010, 2011; Weissleder et al., 2001). They also improve visualization of vascular structures in magnetic resonance angiography (MRA) of the body by staying longer in the circulatory system instead of escaping through blood vessels walls (Kobayashi et al., 2001, 2003; Sato et al., 2001). This characteristic made dendrimer-based MRI contrast agents much more useful for assessing tumor angiogenesis. In addition, by taking advantage of the numerous attachment sites available on the surface of a single dendrimer molecule, new synthetic chemistry techniques have led to the development of multi-modality magnetic resonance, radionuclide, and fluorescence imaging agents for molecular imaging, such as Gd and Rhodamine green (Xu et al., 2007), Gd and Alexa Fluor 594 (Boswell et al., 2008).

Dendrimers have their own potentially *therapeutic activity against prion diseases* (Heegaard and Boas, 2006; Supattapone et al., 1999, 2001). Cationic dendrimers seem to accumulate together with PrP^{Sc} molecules in lysosomes, where the acidic environment facilitates dendrimer-mediated PrP^{Sc} disaggregation. Superfect, PPI dendrimers, phosphorus dendrimers have all made it possible to remove PrP^{Sc} from cells (Supattapone et al., 1999, 2001, 2009; Heegaard and Boas, 2006; Solassol et al., 2004). The strength of this action was dependent on dendrimer concentration and duration of exposure (Supattapone et al., 2009). Dendrimers may also be potential agents for the treatment of other *neurodegenerative disorders including Alzheimer's disease* since there is a similarity between these two pathologies. Alzheimer's disease is associated with the formation of amyloid aggregates. Klajnert et al. (2006a) compared the aggregation properties of the Alzheimer's peptide Aβ 1-28 with PrP 185-208, and how they were influenced by a third generation of PAMAM dendrimer. Later different generations of PAMAM dendrimers, PPI and phosphorus dendrimers were successfully used to disaggregate amyloid fibrils under different conditions (Klajnert et al., 2006b, c, 2007). Chafekar et al. (2007) studied the effect of 4 KLVFF peptides attached to the dendrimer (K(4)) on abeta aggregation. K(4) very effectively inhibits the aggregation of low-molecular-weight and protofibrillar Abeta (1-42) into fibrils, in a concentration-dependent manner, and far more potently than K(1). Thus, the conjugates might be useful as therapeutic agents for the treatment of Alzheimer's disease (Chafekar et al., 2007).

Dendrimers can be also used as therapeutic agents in other neurodegenerative disorders characterized by deposits of inappropriate protein aggregates, as in *Parkinson's disease* (Milowska et al., 2011; Rekas et al., 2009). The PAMAM dendrimers inhibited fibrillation of alpha-synuclein, an effect increased both with generation number and PAMAM concentration. The PAMAM also effectively promoted the breaking down of pre-existing fibrils of alpha-synuclein. In both processes of inhibition and disassociation of fibrils, PAMAM redirected alpha-synuclein to an amorphous aggregation pathway (Milowska et al., 2011; Rekas et al., 2009). It remains to be determined whether dendrimers will be of use as therapeutic agents in other neurodegenerative disorders characterized by deposit of inappropriate protein aggregates, such as multiple sclerosis. Dendrimers may help in preventing or delaying the onset of these diseases, where first symptoms can often be identified decades in advance of detectable neurologic or systemic dysfunction.

Dendrimers have very good proposects as *antibacterial agents* (Chen et al., 2000; Nishikawa et al., 2002; Tam et al., 2002). The antibacterial activity of dendrimers is due to their ability to bind and disrupt anionic bacterial membranes, resulting in lysis of bacteria such as *Staphylococcus aureus, Pseudomonas aeruginosa,* and *Escherichia coli* (Heegaard and Boas, 2006; Klajnert et al., 2006; Paddle et al., 2003). This is true for polylysine dendrimers and dendrimers with surface groups based on mannose and other sugars that are capable of binding with cell surface. Quaternary ammonium functionalized poly(propyleneimine) dendrimers were   affect both Gram-negative and Gram-positive bacteria (Chen et al., 2000). Mannose-terminating polylysine dendrimers inhibited the binding of *Escherichia coli* cells to blood cells (Nagahori et al., 2002). Some anionic or cationic dendrimer can have also *antimicrobial* or *autiprotozoan activity* (Cooper and Chen, 2002, 2003; Matthews and Holan, 2002). With anionic (e.g., neuraminic or sialic acid) modification of the 4-position by substitution with an amino, amido, cyano, azido or guanido group, dendrimers were able to inhibit bacterial, yeast, fungal, or parasitic infections in patients (Matthews and Holan, 2002). Balogh et al. (2001) proposed an antimicrobial agent involving a *silver compound distributed on or in a dendritic polymer.* Based on the dendrimer and the antimicrobial agent, a *fluid purification agent* (King and Hill, 2006, 2007, 2009) was proposed. Diallo proposed the *treatment of water by dendrimer-enhanced filtration* (Diallo, 2009). The process involves using dendritic macromolecules (dendrimers) to bind contaminants followed by a filtration step to produce water from which contaminants have been removed or modified.

Dendrimers *as antiviral agents.* Polyanionic (i.e., polysulfonate) dendrimers inhibit the replication of human immunodeficiency virus by interfering with both virus adsorption and some later steps (reverse transcriptase/integrase) in the replicative cycle (Kensinger et al., 2004; Witvrouw et al., 2000). Pérez-Anes et al. (2010) is developing dendrimers with multivalent catanionic galactosylceramide (GalCer) for inhibiting HIV-1 entry into host-cells, based on the not so obvious approach of treating epithelial cells lacking of CD4 receptors. Based on dendrimers, Starfarma put forward the commercial product - VivaGel®, which protects against sexually transmitted diseases and also human immunodeficiency virus (HIV) (McCarthy et al., 2005). Dendrimer-based conjugates have been successfully used against human respiratory syncytial virus (RSV) (Gazumyan et al., 2000; Razinkov et al., 2001), herpes symplex virus (Bernstein et al., 2003; Gong et al., 2002, 2005), Ebola-pseudotyped viral model (Rojo and Delgado, 2004), human influenza viruses (Oka et al., 2008, 2009), human papilloma viruses (Donalisio et al., 2010), and Japanese encephalitis (Nazmi et al., 2010).

Table 3. Dendrimers as antiviral agents.

Human immunodeficiency virus	VivaGel®, Pérez-Anes et al., 2010
Sexual transmitted infections	VivaGel®
Human respiratory syncytial virus (RSV)	Gazumyan et al., 2000; Razinkov et al., 2001
Herpes symplex virus	Gong et al., 2002; Bernstein et al., 2003; Gong et al., 2005
Ebola-pseudotyped viral model	Rojo and Delgado, 2004
Human influenza viruses	Oka et al., 2008, 2009
Human papilloma viruses	Donalisio et al., 2010
Japanese encephalitis	Nazmi et al., 2010

Dendrimers and detoxication. Lipopolysaccharides (LPS), otherwise termed 'endotoxins', are outer-membrane constituents of Gram-negative bacteria that play a key role in the pathogenesis of 'septic shock', a major cause of mortality in critically ill patients. Polyamidoamine dendrimers, with the surface amines sub-stoichiometrically derivatized with alkyl groups, bind LPS with high affinity, neutralize LPS-induced inflammatory responses *in vitro*, and gave protection in a murine model of endotoxic shock (Cromer et al., 2005). Galactose-containing dendrimers with long spacer arms inhibited cholera toxin binding as strongly as the natural ganglioside GM1 oligosaccharide (Branderhorst et al., 2007). Oligosaccharide-derivatized dendrimers inhibited the adherence of cholera toxin and the heat-labile enterotoxin of *Escherichia coli* to cell surfaces (Thompson and Schengrund, 1998). Dendrimers bind hydrophobic toxins and transport them in water-soluble form that decreases their toxic effect (King et al., 2004; Shcharbin and Bryszewska, 2006; Shcharbin et al., 2003). This opens the possibility of using dendrimers in *hemodialysis*.

It is very important to take notice of the development of dendrimer-based drugs in *photodynamic therapy* (Battah et al., 2001; Gillies and Fréchet, 2005; Nishiyama et al., 2003). Encapsulation of 5-aminolevulinic acid and porphyrin in a dendritic shell leads to increase in their distribution in tissues, and to disrupting the effect of radicals generated at irradiation by light of the porphyrin molecule. The second application is a porphyrin- based dendrimer in *oxygen sensing in biological systems* (Dunphy et al., 2002; Lebedev et al., 2009; Vinogradov and Wilson, 1998). Oxygen can quench porphyrine phosphorescence; based on this effect, it is possible to measure the concentration of oxygen in tissues using porphyrin-based dendrimers. The third application of dendrimer-photosensitizer complexes is *photo-triggered release of active substances from dendrimer-photosensitizer complexes* (Albrecht et al., 2005) in which compositions of dendrimer-photosensitizer complexes include therapeutic molecules; methods for their synthesis and use have been disclosed. The therapeutic molecules and photosensitizers are covalently and randomly attached to dendrimers at the end-groups. Upon exposure to radiation of a suitable wavelength, the photosensitizers are activated to break up the dendrimer structure and thus release the therapeutic molecules.

Dendrimers can serve as *mimetics of enzymes*. Encapsulation of catalytic center into core of dendrimer and its defense by dendritic branches can lead to chemical catalysts with an efficiency of activity comparable with that of enzymes. According to the patent (Kubota, 2002), dendrimer constructs and metal complexes with superoxide dismutase activity were proposed for medicine. This dendrimer construct has a generally globular shape, and the branched chains nearer the surface are sufficiently densely packed to restrict the movement of larger biomolecules into the dendritic construct toward the metal active sites. Smaller molecules, such as the superoxide anion ($O_2^{\cdot-}$), move freely from the milieu into the dendritic complex and to the metal active sites, where the dismutation of superoxide to hydrogen peroxide is affected. Smaller molecules, such as hydrogen peroxide, move freely out from the dendritic complex to the milieu (Kubota, 2002). Florence et al. (2001) proposed *peptide dendrimers as multiple antigenic peptides.* A dendritic compound comprises two dendrons, each comprising dendritically linked amino acid units, preferably lysines, joined to a focal group. One of the dendrons has terminal branches including anchor groups of hydrophobic units, and the other has terminal branches that are (or may be) linked to active ligands or sugar moieties.

In contrast to dendrimers having some mimetic properties of proteins, other dendrimers can have an *inhibitory effect on enzymes*. Starfarma proposed the dendrimer-based drug, SPL7013, for the *treatment of rheumatic arthritis*. The preparation reputedly inhibits excessive activity of hyaluronidase, the enzyme that breaks down hyaluronic acid. This substance is widely distributed in the body, functioning as a lubricant, a cushion for joints and a retainer of moisture in the skin. Dendrimers also can serve as *agonists and antagonists of G-protein coupled receptor superfamily* (Jacobson et al., 2009). This invention provides a conjugate comprised of a dendrimer and at least one ligand, which is a functionalized congener of an agonist or antagonist, or a receptor of the G-protein coupled receptor (GPCR) superfamily. The invention also provides pharmaceutical compositions and methods for treating various diseases.

Dendrimers can serve as effective *immunostimulating components (adjuvants)* that increase significantly the efficiency of vaccines (Heegaard et al., 2010; Toyokuni et al., 1994; Wright, 1998). They can complex with small molecules of immuno-stimulators or antigens. Starburst dendrimers, primarily the poly(amidoamine) starburst dendrimers, can be used as an adjuvant for influenza antigen and similar materials. Their mid-generations are preferred and yield high antibody titer levels with reduced antigen dosage (Wright, 1998). Being monodisperse polymers, dendrimers offer the possibility of producing molecularly defined adjuvants, combining very specific immunomodulating activities with targeting to relevant tissues (e.g., mucosal surfaces) and antigen transportation. The resulting macromolecular constructs are expected to behave as highly immunoactive and specific adjuvant/carrier compounds. Thus, dendrimers are useful generic platforms for developing defined and safe vaccines with new properties and application potentials. They will also be useful for basic investigations of the mechanisms behind the induction and control of immunity (Heegaard et al., 2010).

Dendrimers can also be used in methods of *assay and detection on a microarray* (Getts, 2002; Lin et al., 1999; Moll et al., 2000; Singh et al., 1999) for binding cDNA, formation of prehybridized cDNA-dendrimer complex, and interaction of this complex with nucleotide sequence of microarray. According to the patent (Spangler and Spangler, 2006), *biosensor utilized dendrimer-immobilized ligands* are proposed. The present invention is directed at methods and compositions useful as biosensors that specifically interact with various pathogens and other target analytes.

Dendrimers are capable of being a new type of antioxidant. According to the patent (Migdal, 1990), the polyisobutenyl succinimide-polyamidoamine dendrimer has been proposed as an antioxidant, showing an antioxidant score of 20.7 (according to Bench Oxidation Test) that characterise antioxidants. Dendritic polyphenols were also antioxidants (Lee et al., 2009, 2011), showing strong activity according to the 1,1-diphenyl-2-picrylhydrazyl (DPPH) radical assay. The syringaldehyde dendrimer was twice and 10-times stronger than quercetin and Trolox, respectively. The vanillin-based dendrimer and its more hydrophobic iodinated derivative were also more potent antioxidants than quercetin and Trolox. All three dendrimers also protected human LDL from free-radical attack in a dose-dependent manner (Lee et al., 2009). In this (Esumi et al., 2004) gold-dendrimer nanocomposites were prepared in the presence of the poly(amidoamine) (PAMAM) dendrimer. The catalytic activities of these nanocomposites on elimination of hydroxyl radicals formed in an $H_2O_2/FeSO_4$ system were examined by the spin-trapping method. They showed high catalytic activities, which were hardly affected by the concentration and the generation of the dendrimer - except PAMAM dendrimer 3.5. The highest activity for the gold–PAMAM dendrimer 3.5 nanocomposites was 85 times that of ascorbic acid.

Dendrimers and the treatment of stroke. A stroke is a medical emergency and can cause permanent neurological damage, complications, and death. It is the leading cause of adult disability in the United States and Europe, and the second leading cause of death worldwide (Feigin, 2005). About 87% of strokes are caused by ischemia, and the remainder by hemorrhage. Johnson et al. (2010) reported the therapeutic potential of S-nitroso-*N*-acetylpenicillamine-derivatized generation-4 polyamidoamine dendrimers (G4-SNAP) for reducing ischemia/reperfusion (I/R) injury in an isolated, perfused rat heart. The unique combination of G4-SNAP dendrimer and glutathione trigger represents a novel strategy, with possible clinical relevance toward salvaging ischemic tissue. Another approach–neuroprotection in the post-ischemic brain by biodegradable PAMAM ester (e-PAM-R)-mediated HMGB1 siRNA delivery-was proposed by Kim et al. (2010). They showed that e-PAM-R successfully delivered HMGB1 siRNA into the rat brain, wherein HMGB1 expression was depleted in >40%

of neurons and astrocytes of the normal brain. Moreover, e-PAM-R-mediated HMGB1 siRNA delivery notably reduced infarct volume in the post-ischemic rat brain, generated by occluding the middle cerebral artery for 60 min. These results indicate that e-PAM-R, a novel biodegradable nonviral gene carrier, offers an efficient means of transfecting siRNA into primary neuronal cells and in the brain and of performing siRNA-mediated gene knockdown (Kim et al., 2010). The N-Acetyl cysteine (NAC) is an anti-inflammatory agent with significant potential for clinical use in the treatment of neuroinflammation, stroke and cerebral palsy. There is a need for delivery of NAC, which can enhance its efficacy, reduce dosage and prevent it from binding plasma proteins (Kurtoglu et al., 2009). For this purpose, a poly(amidoamine) dendrimer-NAC conjugate was synthesized and tested for its release kinetics in the presence of glutathione, cysteine, and bovine serum albumin at physiological and lysosomal pH. The conjugates showed an order of magnitude increase in antioxidant activity compared to free drug, and can be used for in vivo studies (Kurtoglu et al., 2009).

Dendrimers are new kind of displacers in protein displacement chromatography. According to the patent (Cramer et al., 1995), dendrimers were proposed as new kind of displacers for protein displacement chromatography. In the author's opinion, dendrimers do not require extensive regeneration of the column and can be readily removed from the product protein.

Dendrimers can serve as *tissue coatings*. Hubbell et al. (2008) presented the multifunctional polymeric tissue coatings based on dendrimer structure. When the copolymer is in the form of a brush copolymer, the polycationic block is polyethylene imine, wherein the block copolymer is applied to the surface to form a coating by ionic binding of the cationic charges to the surface, and wherein the non-tissue binding block prevents or minimizes the attachment of proteins or cells to the surface (Hubbell et al., 2008; Jimenez and Moll, 2005). Duan et al. (2007) proposed dendrimers with YIGSR, as a model cell adhesion peptide, for incorporation into collagen scaffolds. The YIGSR incorporation into the bulk and its modification of the surface promoted the adhesion and proliferation of human corneal epithelial cells, as well as neurite extensions from dorsal root ganglia (Duan et al., 2007).

Dendrimers can serve as *dental and medical polymer composites and compositions* (Vallittu et al., 2008). The invention relates to polymerizable multifunctional polymer composites and compositions, which are suitable for dental and medical applications, such as dental prostheses, filling materials, implants and the like. It also relates to a method for the manufacture of such polymerizable multifunctional polymer composites and compositions, and to their use in dental and medical applications.

Thus, dendrimers are nanomaterials of the future. Despite a variety of potential applications, there is at present only one product based on dendrimers on the market. This product, VivaGel® (Starpharma, Australia), protects again sexually transmitted diseases and human immunodeficiency virus. To speed up translational studies and improve the pace of developing new drugs based on dendrimers, systematic studies on dendrimers are needed.

Table 4. Additional applications of dendrimers.

Dendrimers as detoxication agents	Cromer et al., 2005; Branderhorst et al., 2007; Thompson and Schengrund, 1998; King et al., 2004; Shcharbin et al., 2003; Shcharbin and Bryszewska, 2006
Dendrimer-based drugs for photodynamic therapy	Battah et al., 2001; Nishiyama et al., 2003; Gillies and Fréchet, 2005
Porphyrine based dendrimers in oxygen Lsensing in biological systems	Vinogradov and Wilson, 1998; Lebedev et al., 2009; Dunphy et al., 2002
Dendrimer as mimetic of superoxide dismutase	Kubota, 2002
Peptide dendrimers as multiple antigenic peptides	Florence et al., 2001
Dendrimer-based drug SPL7013 for treatment of rheumatic arthritis	Starfarma news
Dendrimers as agonists and antagonists of G-protein coupled receptor superfamily	Jacobson et al., 2009
Dendrimers as immunostimulating components (adjuvants)	Wright, 1998; Toyokuni et al., 1994; Heegaard et al., 2010
Dendrimers as antioxidants	Migdal, 1990; Lee et al., 2009, 2011; Esumi et al., 2004
Dendrimers for treatment of stroke	Kurtoglu et al., 2009; Johnson et al., 2010; Kim et al., 2010
Dendrimers as tissue coatings	Hubbell et al., 2008; Jimenez and Moll, 2005; Duan et al., 2007

KEYWORDS

- **Dendrimers**
- **Dendriplexes**
- **Diaminobutyl; based**
- **Liposomes**
- **Polyamide amine**
- **Polypropyleneimine**
- **Resonance angiography**

Chapter 11

Capsules Based on Lipid Vesicles: Potentiality for Drug Delivery

Brigitte Pépin-Donat, Francois Quemeneur, Marguerite Rinaudo, and Clément Campillo

---

INTRODUCTION

The method by which a drug is delivered can have a significant effect on its efficiency. Therefore, the design and development of advanced drug delivery systems has emerged last four decades in order to improve their biocompatibility (Kocsis et al., 2000), controlled release (Gibbs et al., 1999; Uhrich et al., 1999), active targeting in tissues (Vasir et al., 2005; Yokoyama, 2005), and stimuli response (MacEwan et al., 2010). The strategy used to develop smart drug cargos is based on interdisciplinary approaches that combine polymer science, pharmaceutics and molecular biology.

Among a large variety of colloidal drug delivery carriers (e.g., micelles, polymer nanoparticles, vesicles), we focus here on lipid vesicles (also referred as liposomes), which consist in self-closed lipid bilayers (lipid membranes) (Lipowsky and Sackmann, 1995). Depending on the method of preparation, it is possible to produce vesicles with different sizes ranging from nanometers to tens of micrometers in diameter. Small unilamellar vesicles (SUVs; 20–100 nm) and large unilamellar vesicles (LUVs; 100–500 nm) are generally used as protective capsules in pharmaceutical and cosmetic domains (Barenholz, 2001; Edwards and Baeumner, 2006; Malmsten, 2003) and usually compared to cellular organelles (vesicles of secretion, of transport) (Alberts et al., 2002), while giant unilamellar vesicles (GUVs; 0.5–100 μm) are generally regarded as over-simple models of biological cells (Lim et al., 2006; Liu and Fletcher, 2009; Noireaux and Libchaber, 2004).

Nevertheless, the simple structure and poor resistance of vesicles to external stresses limit their applications for drug delivery or their relevance to mimic real cells. In order to improve structural and mechanical properties of vesicles, composite polymer vesicles have been developed by modifying either their internal medium (Jesorka et al., 2005; Markström et al., 2007; Osinkina et al., 2010; Stauch et al., 2002a) or their lipid membrane (Nikolov et al., 2007; Ringsdorf et al., 1993; Simon et al., 1995). Such polymer vesicles may find applications as drug carriers because (i) the polymer internal medium may improve their resistance to external stresses and confer to the vesicles responsive mechanical properties (changes of mechanical and structural properties triggered by an external parameter such as temperature) (Kiser et al., 1998) and (ii) the polymer coating of the membrane may improve their biocompatibility, enhance their *in vivo* lifetime (Drummond et al., 1999) and confer specific targeting character, in particular for cancer therapy (Kaasgaard and Andresen, 2010; Peer and

Margalit, 2004; Surace et al., 2009). Interaction of polymers with lipid membranes has been extensively studied, both experimentally (Frette et al., 1999; Kawakami et al., 2001; Tribet and Vial, 2008; Tsafrir et al., 2001, 2003) and theoretically (Bickel et al., 2000; Brooks et al., 1991; Clément and Joanny, 1997; Lipowsky, 1997; Shafir and Andelman, 2007).

In the present chapter we report the preparation and structural, mechanical and responsive properties of vesicles with either modified internal medium or membrane. The internal medium of the vesicles of the first category is modified by encapsulating thermo-responsive polyNIPAM systems (solutions or gels). The membrane of the vesicles of the second category is in gel phase while that of the third category is coated by a polyelectrolyte (chitosan or hyaluronan). These original vesicles exhibit some characteristics required for smart drug carriers: biocompatibility, controlled release and specific shapes.

VESICLES ENCAPSULATING POLYNIPAM SYSTEMS

The interest of using vesicles as drug carriers is strongly enhanced when these vesicles are combined with responsive polymers to prepare responsive composite vesicles. Indeed, a responsive polymeric gel inside a vesicle or a polymeric scaffold linked to its membrane allows a controlled delivery of drugs encapsulated inside the vesicle upon an external stimulation. We have encapsulated polyNIPAM solutions or gels in vesicles with the aim to get responsive systems (section 2.1). PolyNIPAM is a very widely used thermo-responsive polymer (Schild, 1992), and thus a good candidate for the preparation of responsive vesicles since temperature appears as a convenient stimulus for *in vivo* applications. Actually, PolyNIPAM exhibits a Low Critical Solution Temperature (LCST): $T_c = 32°C$; above this temperature, polyNIPAM chains collapse leading either to small aggregates formation in dilute solutions (local demixion of the solution) or to a global volume transition of all the chains in the case of highly concentrated solutions (strongly entangled polyNIPAM chains) or covalent gels (covalently cross-linked polyNIPAM chains) (see Figure 1).

Several works are devoted to the preparation of vesicles coupled with polyNIPAM either as a bulk gel that fills the vesicles lumen (Stauch et al., 2002a) or as a cortical layer linked to the vesicle's membrane (Ringsdorf et al., 1993; Stauch et al., 2002b). In the latter case, the transition of the polyNIPAM chains changes the diffusion of the polymer chains in the bilayer as well as the equilibrium shape of the membrane (Simon et al., 1995). The encapsulation of non-reticulated polyNIPAM chains inside giant vesicles is also a way to control their internal structure (Jesorka et al., 2005; Markström et al., 2007; Osinkina et al., 2010).

The originality of our work is to control and measure the mechanical properties of composite responsive vesicles (section 2.2) and to control their thermo-responsive behavior through the composition of their polyNIPAM internal medium (section 2.3).

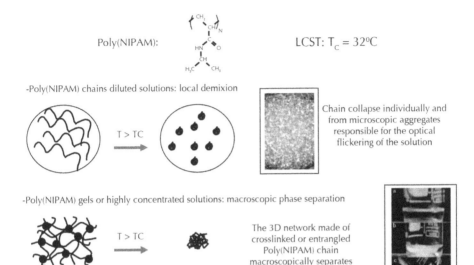

Poly(NIPAM):   LCST: $T_C = 32°C$

-Poly(NIPAM) chains diluted solutions: local demixion

T > TC

Chain collapse individually and from microscopic aggregates responsible for the optical flickering of the solution

-Poly(NIPAM) gels or highly concentrated solutions: macroscopic phase separation

T > TC

The 3D network made of crosslinked or entangled Poly(NIPAM) chain macroscopically separates

● :Crosslinks or entanglements

Figure 1. (a) polyNIPAM structure, (b) Thermal transition of polyNIPAM solutions resulting in local chain demixion, and (c) Thermal transition of highly concentrated solutions or gels resulting in a global volume transition (due to the presence of entanglements with a life time greater than the duration of the thermal transition or of cross-links).

Preparation of Vesicles Enclosing PolyNIPAM Systems

We have prepared vesicles from 1–2 dioleoyl sn-glycero 3-phosphocholine lipids (DOPC) or from a mixture of 99% DOPC and 1% of fluorescent-labeled (rhodamine or fluoresceine) DOPC for fluorescence observation, using the standard electro-formation method (Angelova et al., 1992): briefly, a solution of lipids (1 mg/ml in chloroform) is spread onto two conductive glass plates, the solvent is removed and the electro-formation chamber is formed by the two plates facing each other and separated by a Teflon spacer. The solution to be enclosed in the vesicles is injected in the chamber. Vesicles are formed by the application of an alternative potential between the two plates. Vesicles containing polyNIPAM solutions (so called "sol-vesicles") are easily obtained by injecting in the chamber a so called "pre-sol" solution (containing NIPAM monomers and photo-initiators at the required concentration) and illuminating (Ultra Violet-irradiation) the electroformed vesicles to photo-polymerize their internal "pre-sol" medium and get the vesicles containing polyNIPAM solutions freely moving in the same polyNIPAM solution. As far as elastic vesicles (so called gel-vesicles) are concerned, the preparation is not so easy: a "pre-gel" solution (water + NIPAM monomers + cross-linker + photo-initiator + possible drugs) is injected in the electro-formation chamber. Polymerization is also induced by UV irradiation but the challenge is to prevent gelation of the external solution, which would trap unusable gel-filled vesicles in an external macroscopic polyNIPAM gel. This challenge can be achieved by a selective control of the polymerization kinetic, which allows preparing gel-vesicles easy to handle and moving freely in the external solution. For experimental details, see (Faivre et al., 2006).

Resistance to External Stress

The NIPAM gel-vesicles are strongly resistant to external stresses: for example, the mechanical resistance of the membrane to an applied pressure was tested for unmodified and polyNIPAM sol and gel-vesicles using the micropipette aspiration technique. The membrane tension σ is determined from the imposed micropipette suction pressure ΔP by the Laplace law, $\sigma = \dfrac{\Delta P \, Rp}{2(1 - Rp / Rv)}$, where R_p and R_v are respectively the internal micropipette and vesicle radii (Olbrich et al., 2000) (see Figure 2).

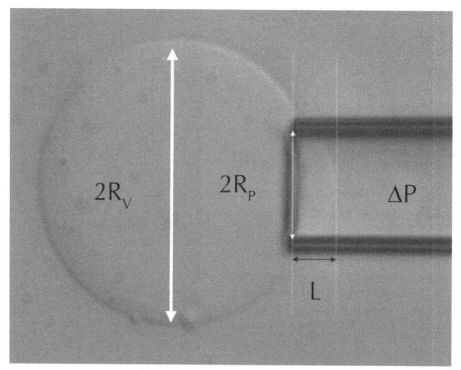

Figure 2. Video-micrograph of the micropipette aspiration of a polyNIPAM gel-vesicle.

For unmodified vesicles and NIPAM sol-vesicles, we find that the membrane is disrupted at tensions of the order of 0.7 ± 0.4 mN/m. In the case of gel-vesicles, pressures as high as $\Delta P = 1000$ Pa, can be applied without disrupting the membrane, which corresponds to a tension σ = 15 mN/m, well above the disruption tension measured for unmodified and sol-vesicles (Campillo et al., 2007). This may be interpreted in terms of strong membrane-polyNIPAM gel interaction energy (W). This assumption is confirmed by estimating the gel-membrane adhesion energy, W = 4 × 10⁻⁴ J, using the technique of membrane nanotubes extrusion (Kremer et al., 2008): this value is ten times larger than that observed for red blood cells. Because of this strong gel-membrane interaction, vesicles encapsulating a polyNIPAM gel can be regarded as homogeneous elastic spheres covered by a biological membrane. We have measured the Young modulus of these elastic capsules by the micropipette aspiration technique and shown that we are able to adjust it in a controlled way between 0.5 and 25 kPa (Campillo et al., 2007) by controlling the cross-link ratio of the internal gel. This range of Young moduli is pertinent to mimic mechanical properties of internal media of some real cells (Hoffmann et al., 1997).

Thermoresponsive Vesicles

Due to the strong gel-membrane interaction, we observe a sharp global volume transition for vesicles containing polyNIPAM gels when the temperature is raised up to 32°C, with a release of 98% of the internal solution (see Figure 3). During the collapse, the phospholipids membrane remains confined to the gel surface. The transition is fully reversible and the membrane remains undamaged after few collapse-swelling cycles (Campillo et al., 2008). The temperature of collapse can be varied from 32 to 20°C by varying the internal glucose concentration from 0 to 5 mol/l. The same global volume transition is observed for vesicles encapsulating highly concentrated polyNIPAM solutions: this phenomenon is interpreted in terms of entanglements with a life time greater than the duration of the thermal transition, playing the role of cross-links. These systems look promising as drug carriers with thermo-controlled release.

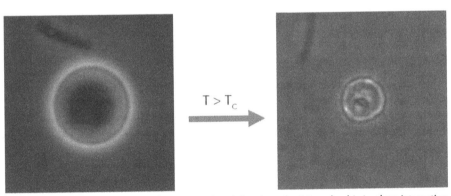

$T > T_c$

Figure 3. Global transition in a polyNIPAM gel vesicle where the internal gel is in close interaction with the membrane (the same phenomenon is observed in vesicles containing highly concentrated polyNIPAM solutions).

Another interesting point is that we are able to get multiphase capsules by decreasing the interaction between the membrane and highly concentrated polyNIPAM solutions. In order to decrease the polyNIPAM-membrane interaction, we firstly encapsulate a solution of low polyNIPAM concentration in the vesicle, then we osmotically deflate the vesicle, thus increasing the internal polyNIPAM concentration, and finally we increase the temperature in order to cross the polyNIPAM transition. This procedure allows us to get partial demixion of the polyNIPAM system (instead of the global demixion), leading to a micro-compartmentalization of the capsule, made of a hydrophobic poly(NIPAM) phase and a hydrophilic phase (see Figure 4).

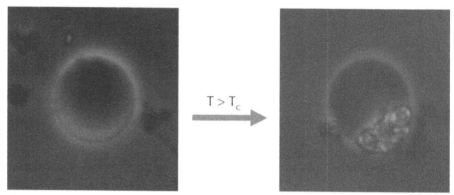

Figure 4. Micro-compartments in vesicles containing highly concentrated polyNIPAM solutions in low interaction with the membrane.

These thermo-responsive bio-compatible polyNIPAM vesicles present potential applications as *in vivo* thermo-responsive drug carriers, for example their membrane could be covered with adhesive molecules to target a specific organ and liberate encapsulated drugs in response to temperature changes. In addition, this type of composite vesicles may also be regarded as hydrophobic/hydrophilic macroscopically compartmentalized capsules.

VESICLES WITH MEMBRANE IN GEL-PHASE

When the temperature is decreased below the main transition temperature T_m, lipid membranes exhibit a structural phase transition from a liquid disordered phase to an ordered gel phase (Luzzati and Husson, 1962). It appears that, upon phase transition, the structural and mechanical properties of lipid membranes are dramatically affected (Charitat et al., 2008; Dimova et al., 2000). We now address the question of the role of such structural and mechanical changes on the vesicles behaviors under external stresses.

Morphological changes of liquid-phase vesicles under deflation induced by osmotic pressure have been largely studied: vesicle shapes are governed by the bending energy, the spontaneous curvature and by the area difference between the two monolayers of the membrane (Döbereiner, 2000; Döbereiner et al., 1997; Helfrich, 1973). It is not the case for gel-phase vesicles for which only very few studies have been reported (Antunes et al., 2009; Knorr et al., 2010). However, in the gel-state, due to the new mechanical properties of the membrane, different vesicle shapes are expected to be generated. This is indeed observed in the model of red blood cells made of coupled bilayer-cytoskeleton (Mukhopadhyay et al., 2002) and in actin-coated (Helfer et al., 2001) and gel-phase vesicles (Delorme and Fery, 2006). Here, we show that deflation due to isotropic osmotic pressure induces buckling on gel-phase vesicles, leading to unusual faceted like-shaped vesicles, which may find application as drug carriers of specific shapes.

Vesicles with membrane in gel-phase are made of DMPC (1,2-dimyristoyl-sn-glycero-3-phosphocholine) self-closed bilayers in the rippled gel phase P_β. (Kaasgaard et al., 2003). The GUVs are prepared by electroformation (Angelova et al., 1992) above the main acyl chain crystallization temperature (T_m = 23.6°C (Koynova and Caffrey, 1998)) in a 100 mM sucrose solution. Then the temperature is slowly decreased down to 15°C with a cooling rate of 0.05°C/min. In order to prevent lipid membrane breaking at the transition, vesicles in the fluid phase are osmotically deflated to compensate the 28% loss of surface between the fluid and the rippled phases (Needham and Evans, 1988) by controlled sucrose addition in the external solution. Gel-phase vesicles obtained with this protocol are spherical. The GUVs which are then subjected at 15°C to controlled deflation by addition of glucose in the external solution, and observed by phase contrast microscopy.

The purpose here is not to report an extensive characterization of the faceted shapes but to show that capsules with original shapes can be obtained in this way (see Quemeneur et al., 2011) for extensive structural and mechanical studies of these gel-phase vesicles), which may be considered as potential shape-controlled drug carriers. Figure 5 presents a non extensive panel of the final shapes that can be obtained in this way. These regular concave polyhedra-like shapes are reached around 40 min after the beginning of the deflation, and, thereafter, no shape modification is observed over several hours, when temperature and osmolarity are kept constant. Some of these shapes reproduce biological objects such as virus (Lidmar et al., 2003), red blood cells (Lim et al., 2008) or desiccated pollens (e.g., mahonia, ligustrum) (Katifori et al., 2010).

A interesting perpective should consist in preparing strongly resistant responsive vesicles with controlled specific shapes whatever the phase of the lipid membrane (and consequently whatever the temperature) by encapsulating polyNIPAM gels.

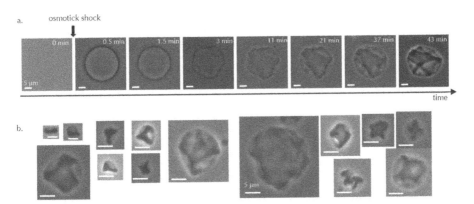

Figure 5. Faceted shapes obtained by osmotic deflation of DMPC vesicles in the gel-phase at 15°C. (a) Time sequence of a GUV deflation and (b) Equilibrium shapes observed for vesicles of different initial radius. The scale bars represent 5 μm.

POLYELECTROLYTE-COATED VESICLES

It is well known that polymer coating may improve the structural stability of liposome's, biocompatibility and drug delivery efficiency (Xu et al., 2007). As an alternative to neutral poly(ethylene glycol) which in particular enhances liposome circulation time under *in vivo* conditions (Drummond et al., 1999), various polyelectrolytes are used to improve drug carriers efficiency. In the following, we consider two polyelectrolytes: the chitosan, a positively charged polymer in acidic conditions (pH < 6.5), and the hyaluronic acid (hyaluronan), a negatively charged polymer at pH > 2.0, interacting with DOPC lipid membranes.

Chitosan (Chit) is a pseudo-natural polyelectrolyte obtained by deacetylation of chitin extracted from crustaceous shells and cell walls of some fungi (Brugnerotto et al., 2001; Rinaudo, 2006). It is a linear random copolymer of D-glucosamine and N-acetyl-D-glucosamine (Figure 6(a)). Thanks to its biocompatibility, biodegradability, mucoadhesivity, non toxicity, and because it exhibits wound healing properties, chitosan finds many applications in biomedical domains such as surgical sutures, dental implants, encapsulating material (Khor and Lim, 2003; Pospieszny et al., 1994; Rinaudo, 2006).

Adsorption of chitosan on lipid DOPC membrane is proposed to be mainly of electrostatic origin (Henriksen et al., 1994). The additional contribution of hydrogen bonding and hydrophobic interactions, due to the chemical structure of chitosan (e.g, -CH groups on the glucopyranose unit (Mazeau and Vergelati, 2002)), have been proposed in the literature (Pavinatto et al., 2010) to justify the higher bioactivity of chitosan if compared to that of other polycations.From a drug delivery point of view, adsorption of chitosan on membranes (i) induces changes in lipid organization (Elsabee et al., 2009) increasing thus the liquid to gel phase transition temperature of the phospholipid bilayer and leading to higher thermal stability (Mertins et al., 2008), (ii) enhances the drug entrapment efficiency (Guo et al., 2003) by decreasing the membrane permeability (Filipovica-Grcï et al., 2001; Henriksen et al., 1997), (iii) stabilizes the coated liposome suspension and increase their resistance to surfactants (Mady et al., 2009). Chitosan coated liposomes are proposed for oral (Thongborisute et al., 2006), ocular (Zhang and Wang, 2009), nasal (Ding et al., 2007) or cutaneous applications (Perugini et al., 2000).

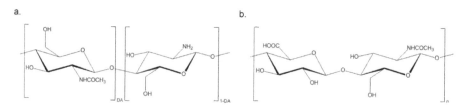

Figure 6. Chemical structure of the two polyelectrolytes studied: (a) Chitosan, positively charged polymer in acidic conditions (pH < 6.5) due to protonation of the –NH$_2$ groups; (b) Hyaluronan, anionic polymer at pH > 2.0 in relation with dissociation of carboxylic groups.

Hyaluronan (HA) is a linear alternated copolymer of repeating disaccharide units of β(1-4) D-glucuronic acid and β(1-3) N-acetyl-D-glucosamine) (Figure 6(b)) belonging to the glycosaminoglycan family (Rinaudo, 2009). It is a component of the synovial fluid, cartilage, vitreous humor, and extracellular matrices, where it plays important structural and biological roles (Kogan et al., 2007). The HA is a highly biocompatible polysaccharide, naturally present in the body, and often used for biomedical applications including viscosupplementation in joint diseases, because of its good viscoelastic properties. Films have also been developed for tissue engineering. Many data are available in (Kennedy et al., 2002) which concern the biological activity and the biomedical applications of HA. Complexes with polycations are proposed for controlled drug release. The HA is also used in dermatology and cosmetic industries (preserve tissue hydratation), or in drug delivery (Rinaudo, 2008).

As for chitosan, the interaction between HA and lipid DOPC membrane is assumed to be mainly of electrostatic origin (Taglienti et al., 2006).

In spite of the numerous biomedical and industrial applications of HA for cancer therapy (Kaasgaard and Andresen, 2010; Peer and Margalit, 2004; Surace et al., 2009), only few physico-chemical studies deal with hyaluronan-coated vesicles: published studies mainly discuss various techniques to prepare chitosan- or hyaluronan-coated vesicles and membrane-polyelectrolyte interaction, origin and stability.

We focus here on the quantitative study of both chitosan and hyaluronan adsorbtion; on the polymer conformation at the surface of the membrane and on the coating-effect on vesicle mechanics and resistance under various stresses.

Preparation of the Coated Vesicles

Studied polyelectrolyte-coated vesicles (LUVS and GUVs) are obtained by incubation of already formed DOPC vesicles, filled with a 200 mM sucrose solution, in chitosan and HA solutions at the desired pH during 30 min at room temperature. The LUVs are obtained by extrusion of a suspension of GUVs produced by electro-formation (Angelova et al., 1992), through a 0.2 μm filter. Chitosans with different weight-average molecular weights (MW; from 5×10^4 to 5×10^5 g/mol) and degrees of acetylation (DA; from 5 to 20%), and HA with different Mw (from 1.14×10^4 to 1.8×10^6 g/mol) are used. Solutions of HA are prepared at 0.4 g/l by dissolving the polymer in 200 mM sucrose solution at pH = 6.0 while dissolution of cationic chitosan requires addition of stoichiometric amounts of HCl on the basis of $-NH_2$ content in the chitosan (final pH around 3.5). The solutions of polyelectrolyte are stirred for one night at room temperature until complete solubilization. The solutions of polyelectrolyte are diluted for vesicles' incubation and range between 0.1 and 0.01 g/l in a solution of 200 mM sucrose at pH = 3.5 or 6.0 and are directly used. The exact lipid concentrations are determined in each vesicles sample by *in situ* fluorescence measurement in relation with the labeled lipid content (1,2-dioleoyl-sn-glycero-3-phosphoethanolamine-*N*-(lissamine rhodamine B sulfonyl) (ammonium salt) (18:1 Liss Rhod PE) and 1-oleoyl-2-[12-[(7-nitro-2-1,3-benzoxadiazol-4-yl)amino]dodecanoyl]-sn-glycero-3-phosphocholine (18:1-12 : NBDPC)). For the reported results, lipid concentrations range between 3 and 5×10^{-3} mg/ml for LUVs suspensions and 10 and 30×10^{-3} mg/ml for GUVs suspensions. For fluorescence experiments, chitosan and HA are respectively labeled with fluorescein and rhodamine. The adsorbed amount of polyelectrolyte on the lipid membrane is determined from ζ-potential measurements. We assume as usual that, upon addition of very small amounts of polyelectrolyte into a vesicle suspension (with a membrane of opposite charge if compared to that of polyelectrolyte), the polyelectrolyte is fully adsorbed on the outer leaflet of liposomes and we relate the variation of ζ-potential to the amount of ionized groups (i.e., NH_3^+ and COO^- for chitosan and hyaluronan, respectively) fixed on the membrane. This allows calculation of the amount of polyelectrolyte adsorbed taking into account the protonation degree (controlled by pH) and acetylation degree (DA) in the case of chitosan (Quemeneur et al., 2008a). For more experimental details on the preparation and the experimental methods, see (Quemeneur, 2010) and references therein.

Characterization of the Polyelectrolyte Coating

Using complementary techniques on LUVs (such as electrophoretic mobility (ζ-potential measurements) and Dynamic Light Scattering) and on GUVs (optical microscopies), we have studied the mechanism of chitosan and HA adsorption on lipid membranes. We have revealed the electrostatic origin of the interaction between polyelectrolytes and zwitterionic lipid membrane, showing the role of their respective charge densities (both tuneable by pH) on the amount of adsorbed polymer (Quemeneur et al., 2008a). This result is confirmed by recent studies (Mertins et al., 2010; Mertins and Dimova, 2011). Because of the zwitterionic nature of DOPC lipids, polyelectrolyte adsorbs whatever the respective global sign of the membrane and the polyelectrolyte. Nevertheless, we observe that the amount of adsorbed polymer is higher in the case of membrane and polymer opposite charge signs (Quemeneur et al., 2010) (Figure 7(a)).

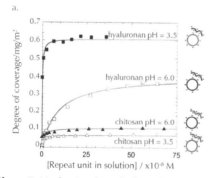
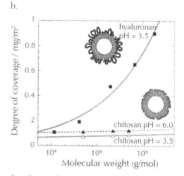

Figure 7. Mechanism for polyelectrolyte adsorption on lipid membrane. (a) Degree of coverage (in mg/m²) for chitosan (MW = 5×10^5, DA = 0.20; triangles) and HA (MW = 6.63×10^5; squares) as function of the repeat unit concentration of polyelectrolyte free in solution. Sketches illustrate the respective charge signs of the membrane and polyelectrolytes. The dotted lines are added to guide the eye and have no physical meaning. (Quemeneur et al., 2010) - Reproduced by permission of The Royal Society of Chemistry and (b) Influence of the molecular weight (MW) on the maximum amount of chitosan and HA adsorbed on the DOPC membrane.

We have demonstrated that the chemical structure of polymer controls the adsorbed polyelectrolyte chain conformation at the vesicle surface (chitosan adsorbs flat while hyaluronan forms loops and trains), and consequently the amount of adsorbed polymer (Figure 7(b)). We have shown that the global charge of the coated vesicle can be modified in a controlled way by changing the adsorbed amount of polymer, the pH or the nature of the polyelectrolyte. We have also demonstrated that it is possible to adjust the sign and the thickness of the coating by absorbing successive layers of HA and chitosan on the membrane surface (Quemeneur et al., 2008b).

We have determined the role of the polyelectrolyte sorption on LUVs and GUVs suspensions state. A reversible aggregation of LUVs is observed upon progressive addition of both polyelectrolytes when membrane and polyelectrolyte charges are of opposite sign. A maximum in size of particles is reached when the global charge of the lipid vesicles is compensated by the adsorbed oppositely charged polyelectrolyte (i.e., at the isoelectric point). On addition of excess of polymer, adsorption still occurs but vesicle aggregates are progressively dissociated with charge inversion to finally obtain isolated overcharged vesicles exhibiting the same dimension than that of vesicles in the bare state (Figure 8(a)). Such aggregation phenomenon is also reported for LUVs prepared with other lipids and coated by other polyelectrolytes: DPPG-LUVs/poly(L-lysine (Volodkin et al., 2007), DOTAP-LUVs/polyacrylate (Cametti, 2008) or DOPC + DOPG-LUVs/chitosan (Mertins and Dimova, 2011).

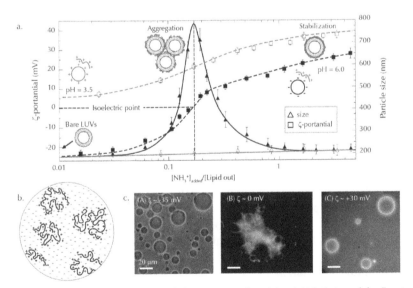

Figure 8. Formation of finite aggregates of chitosan-coated vesicles. (a) Variation of the ζ-potential (squares) and the particle diameter (triangles) of LUVs upon addition of chitosan at pH = 6.0 and pH = 3.5. Lines are added to guide the eye and have no physical meaning, (b) Possible arrangement (patch-like) of adsorbed polycations on a particle with low negative surface charge density (Gregory, 1972), and (c) Similar aggregation-dissociation process is highlighted by microscopy observations on DOPC GUVs incubated, at pH = 6.0, with chitosan at different molar ratios. The scale bars represent 10 µm. (Quemeneur et al., 2010) –

Source: Reproduced by permission of The Royal Society of Chemistry.

We interpret this aggregation-disaggregation process assuming a patch-like structure of the coated membrane where domains of stuck charged polymer (i.e., with a local charge excess) alternate with domains of bare surface as illustrated in Figure 8(b) (Dobrynin et al., 2000; Gregory, 1972) and using the extended DLVO model proposed by (Velegol and Thwar, 1984). Within this model, particles association mainly results from short range electrostatic attraction between oppositely charged patches of two approaching vesicles, while aggregates dissociation, upon further polyelectrolyte addition, is attributed to long range electrostatic repulsion between overcharged vesicles.

We have observed the same aggregation-disaggregation phenomenon for GUVs suspension in the presence of oppositely charged polyelectrolyte: Figure 8(c) shows the direct observation by optical microscopy of bare GUVs (A), GUVs aggregation at isoelectric point (B) and isolated highly coated GUVs (C) (corresponding to the maximum adsorbed amount reported in Figure 7(a)), which result from aggregate dissociation. The interesting conclusion is that, in excess of polyelectrolyte, coated vesicles are isolated in solution which allows testing their intrinsic physicochemical properties with classical techniques (micropipette aspiration, atomic force microscopy...).

We stress that these finite-size liposome clusters open interesting perspectives as "multi-compartments" vectors for simultaneous and independent multi-drug delivery at the same location as proposed by (Bordi et al., 2009).

We have already discussed the mechanism of adsorption, and estimated a coverage degree for both polyelectrolytes at equilibrium (i.e., at a given polymer concentration in solution). We now address the question of coating stability under modification of the external solution where the coated vesicles are suspended: does the polyelectrolyte desorb when its concentration is decreased upon dilution or when the pH or salt concentration is varied?

Using a combination of ζ-potential measurements on LUVs and fluorescence microscopy observations on GUVs, we have demonstrated that chitosan coating is stable over 4 days when the polyelectrolyte concentration in the external solution remains constant. If now, the polyelectrolyte concentration is decreased (upon dilution), desorption slowly occurs. Coating is reversible upon dilution: the degree of coverage obtained at the equilibrium (typically reached after 2 days) corresponds to the one expected by the direct incubation of bare vesicles at this polyelectrolyte concentration. Nevertheless, due to slow desorption kinetic, coating is stable during few hours (Quemeneur et al., in preparation), which allows us to assume that no polymer desorption occurs during the time scale of the experiments (~ 1–2 hr) we report just after. This slow desorption also allows to use polyelectrolyte coated vesicles as drug carriers.

Behaviors under External Stresses

We now focus on the polyelectrolyte-coated GUVs responses to various external stimuli such as osmotic pressure, pH, salt shocks or compression (atomic force microscopy (Fery and Weinkamer, 2007; Liu, 2006). Results are discussed in comparison with those obtained for bare vesicles in order to assess polyelectrolyte coating effect on membrane properties.

Firstly, we have studied the response of bare and polyelectrolyte coated vesicles submitted to changes in osmotic pressure induced by glucose shocks (Figure 9(a)). For bare vesicles, a large panel of deflated shapes are obtained (Döbereiner, 2000) while for polyelectrolyte coated vesicles only spherical deflation with tube ejection are observed. We have demonstrated the presence of polyelectrolyte on the ejected tubes (Kremer et al., 2011). This behavior can be interpreted taking into account the spontaneous curvature (C_0) induced by the asymmetric polyelectrolyte coating on the external surface of the membrane. We have confirmed this interpretation by performing membrane tethers extrusion experiments (Kremer et al., 2011) and estimated the spontaneous curvature $C_0 = 9.4 \pm 0.6 \ 10^{-3} \, nm^{-1}$.

Secondly, we have applied salt shocks (Figure 9(b)); for bare vesicles, systematic explosion was observed within 2 min, whereas for coated vesicles we observed only spherical deflation with invaginations (Quemeneur et al., 2007).

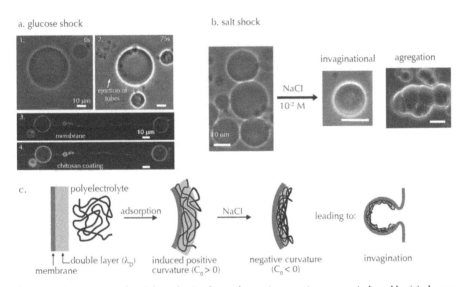

Figure 9. Chitosan-coated vesicles submitted to a change in osmotic pressure induced by (a) glucose shocks, (b) NaCl shocks at pH = 6.0. The lipid membrane (3) and the polyelectrolyte coating (4) are successively visualized by fluorescence confocal observations. The scale bars represent 10 μm. (Kremer et al., 2011; Quemeneur et al., 2007, 2008a), and (c) Schematic figures of membrane bending induced by polyelectrolyte adsorption and of invaginations formation upon addition of salt and related spontaneous curvatures (C_0) as proposed by (Kim and Sung, 2001).
Source: Reproduced by permission of The Royal Society of Chemistry.

The formation of invaginations under salt shocks can be also explained by the spontaneous curvature (Figure 9(c)). Indeed, when polyelectrolyte adsorbs on the membrane, it tends to bend it, inducing the previously evoked positive spontaneous curvature. Upon salt addition, the intra and inter-chains electrostatic repulsions are repressed inducing the polymer collapses, hence causing a negative spontaneous curvature and consequently invaginations. At this point, we would like to stress that we can control the sign of the spontaneous curvature and consequently the response of coated vesicles submitted to stresses by modifying the electrostatic screening: when osmotic deflation is applied, some excess area of membrane becomes available and regarding the sign of the spontaneous curvature can lead to the ejection of tubes (when curvature is positive) and the apparition of invaginations (when curvature is negative).

Thirdly, we have observed the behaviors of the polyelectrolyte-coated GUVs under pH shocks. Bare GUVs experiments are realized at pH = 3.5 and 6.0; similar behaviors being observed in both cases, therefore, we only report here results obtained at pH = 6.0. Figure 10 sums up observations at the equilibrium state (~ 30 min after injection of HCl or NaOH), obtained for bare GUVs (line a), chitosan-coated GUVs (line b) and hyaluronan-coated GUVs (line c) as a function of pH. First of all, under basic conditions, for pH > 10.0, polyelectrolyte-coated GUVs remain stable and exhibit osmotic spherical deflation with tube ejection. Secondly, under acidic conditions, for pH between 2.0 and 1.5, spherical deflation is also observed but it is not possible to clearly show evidence of tube ejection. On the contrary, bare GUVs burst quickly under acidic conditions for 2.0 < pH < 3.0 or deflate to complex shapes (e.g., budding previously reported by (Lee et al., 1999)) under basic conditions for pH > 10.0. The conclusion is that contrary to bare GUVs, chitosan or hyaluronan-coated vesicles are stable in extreme pH conditions, confirming thus that polyelectrolytes remains adsorbed on the membrane. Such stabilization in extreme pH conditions opens applicability in particular for drug delivery in the gastrointestinal tract and may explain the observed efficiency of liposomes modified with chitosan (Takeuchi et al., 2005).

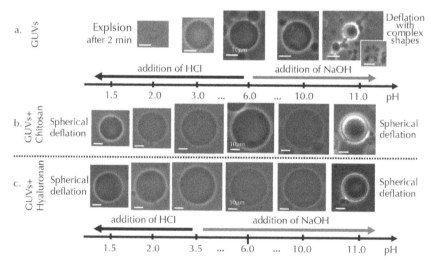

Figure 10. Behavior of non-coated GUVs (a) and chitosan, (b) or HA, and (c) coated GUVs as a function of pH. The scale bars represent 10 µm.

Finally, we have applied anisotropic compressions by performing AFM experiments on chitosan-coated GUVs. We show that chitosan-coating induces an increase of the membrane stretching modulus, in good agreement with recent measurements published for lipid monolayer in contact with chitosan (Pavinatto et al., 2010). We show that AFM experiments allow probing global mechanical properties of composite GUVs (Dubreuil et al., in preparation).

CONCLUSION

We have developed polymer composite vesicles, which are promising as drug carriers because they present enhanced resistance to various stresses of biological interest (pH, salt shocks, osmotic pressure, point acting force) or (and) interesting structural (specific shapes) and (or) mechanical properties (for example spontaneous curvatures inducing invaginations or tethers ejection) or (and) responsive properties if compared to standard liposomes.

Vesicles enclosing polyNIPAM-gels are thermo-responsive: they present a sharp volume transition during which they release more than 98% of their internal content. By functionalizing these gel-vesicles with specific membrane receptors and adjusting their transition temperature close to 37°C by NIPAM copolymerization, we should obtain smart drug vectors capable to specifically deliver therapeutic molecules in response to a temperature increase.

Vesicles coated by biocompatible and biodegradable chitosan and HA can be regarded as interesting drug cargos because of their strong resistance to osmotic pressure, pH and salt shocks. They also hold promise for new potential applications such as multi-compartment carriers because of their ability to form well-defined finite aggregates when suspended in external polyelectrolyte solution at specific concentration.

The study finally offers interesting insights into the structured, reproducible and stable polyhedral-like shapes that can be obtained through the deformation of simple gel phase vesicles.

KEYWORDS

- **Acetylation degree**
- **Drug carriers**
- **Hyaluronan**
- **Polymer vesicles**
- **Polymerization**
- **PolyNIPAM**

ACKNOWLEDGMENTS

Francois Quemeneur thanks IRTG "Soft Condensed Matter: Physics of Model Systems", DAAD, UFA-DFH Saarbruucken and Universities of Konstanz, Strasbourg and Grenoble for funding.

Chapter 12

A Simulation Study on the Transport of Ions Through Ion Channels

Keka Talukdar and Apurba Krishna Mitra

INTRODUCTION

Ions can be transported inside our body through cell membrane or through ion channels (Hille, 2001) which may be selective for a specific ion. The function of the cells depends on the functioning of ion channels as they balance the concentration of the electrolytes inside and outside the cells. The channel proteins are surrounded by lipid membrane which separates its internal medium from the external medium and the passage of ions through the ion channel is regulated by the potential difference across the membrane, called membrane potential. Ionic currents perpendicular to the membrane is opposed by a longitudinal current which closes the channel pore after a certain interval. It appears due to the difference of concentration of the ions inside and outside the membrane. There are some specialized proteins which carry ions through the channels. The main groups of ion channels are voltage gated channels, extracellular ligand-activated channels and intracellular ligand-gated ion channels. The main exploration of the ion propagation as a result of action potential was possible by the studies of Hodgkin and Huxley (1952a, 1952b, 1952c, 1952d) with the squid giant axon. Besides these experiments and some other experimental techniques (Doyle et al., 1998; Neher and Sakmann, 1976; Zhou et al., 2001) that revealed the transport mechanism and channel structure, latest development on mathematical models and simulation is observed which relate the molecular structure of channel components to the physiological properties of ion channels. In 1998, Molecular Dynamics (MD) simulation was performed by Zhong et al. (1998) for a synthetic ion channel consisting of four α-helical peptides. Millar et al. (2005) developed a self-consistent particle simulation of ion channels using Poisson and Langevin equations which described the simulation of ion behavior in extremely small pores. An algorithm was developed combining kinetic lattice grand canonical Monte Carlo (MC) simulations and mean field theory by Hwang et al. (2007). The molecular switching mechanism of ion channels can be exploited in the construction of novel biosensors (Christine, 2008; Cornell et al., 1997; Joseph et al., 2003; Krishnamurthy et al., 2010; Urisu et al., 2008).

To study the nature of transport of ions in a sodium or potassium ion channel, we have used the software (Hwang et al., 2006, Radak et al., 2011) developed on Poisson-Nernst-Planck (PNP) model. The transport properties of ion channels are similar to that of semiconductors for which PNP equations have proved to be successful simulation models. Also, MC simulation is performed to simulate ion flow through a channel and hence to find when and where ion scattering occurs. The MC simulation is done using the software developed by Straeten et al. (Straeten et al., 2005). However, the detection of a particular ion can be done using a biosensor (Ahn et al., 2010; Chiu and Huang, 2009; Kim et al., 2005; Maxwell et al., 2002; Ooe et al., 2008; Wanekaya et al., 2006) with required geometry. Mathematical modeling and simulation for devising high performance nanobiosensor is reported in different literatures (Baronas et al., 2010; Nair and Alam, 2007, 2008; Tan et al., 2006). Here, we have briefly described the performance of a silicon nanowire biosensor and a nanosphere biosensor for efficient detection of charged biomolecules even in a very low concentration of analyte.

MATHEMATICAL MODEL

The PNP model approximates proteins as cylindrical tubes embedded in a lipid membrane (Hwang et al., 2006). Finite difference method is used to solve PNP equations simultaneously and self-consistently. The ions, lipids, protein, and water molecules are all described as dielectric continuums. Complex boundary conditions are applied to model an ion channel. Monte Carlo methods are used to simulate the flow of ion (Papke et al., 2009; Straeten et al., 2005). This helps to find out when ion scattering takes place from ion-water interactions. Alpha helical protein structure is simulated in each case. The theoretical model of a biosensor is based on self-consistent solutions of Diffusion-Capture model (for the settling time response), Poisson-Boltzmann, and drift-diffusion equations (for electrolyte screening and conductance modulation) and the statistical properties of biomolecule adsorption (Selectivity).

RESULTS AND DISCUSSION

PNP Model

First of all simulation is performed for a peptide channel of radius 3.5 Å using PNP cyclic ion channel simulator. The alpha helical peptide structure is shown in Figure 1 (Drummond et al., 2010). In PNP theory, proteins, membranes, ions, and water molecules are considered as continuum dielectric materials and the structure of proteins and lipids are not taken into consideration. As there exists a concentration gradient across the lipid membrane, the ions can pass through the channel sometimes which is generally impossible through the lipid bilayer. The thermal motion of the ions changes their probability of crossing the pore. Once the channel is opened it allows the ions to flow through it until the potential difference across the membrane balances the flow of ions in the upward and downward direction. This equilibrium potential is called Nernst potential.

Ion channels help to establish a voltage gradient in neurons by regulating the influx of sodium and potassium ions. Sending rapid electrical signal in neurons is possible for the presence of these channels. Generally sodium channels are too narrow and so the incoming of a potassium ion is restricted by this channel.

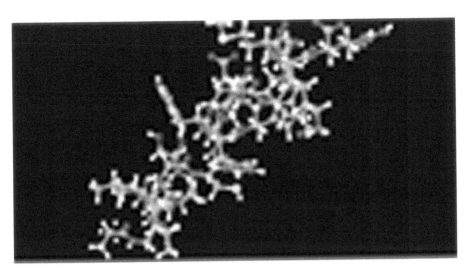

Figure 1. α-Helical peptide structure.

The channel is sensitive to Na^+ and Cl^- ions where diffusion coefficients of Na^+ and Cl^- ions in bulk water and in the channel are 2×10^{-5} m²/s and 1×10^{-5} m²/s respectively. Obviously, the diffusion coefficients inside the channel are lesser than that of the coefficients outside the channel. For this, narrow channel cation and anion currents are obtained as 0.000453845 pA and 5.56853 pA respectively. Three more simulations are run with 4 Å, 4.5 Å, and 5 Å channel radii. Cation and anion current are found as-

Channel radius = 4 Å

Cation current = 0.00124441 pA

Anion current = 1.0661 e^{-05} pA

Channel radius = 4.5 Å

Cation current = 0.00160074 pA

Anion current = 2.36111 e^{-05} pA

Channel radius = 5 Å

Cation current = 0.00151038 pA

Anion current = 3.12194 e^{-05} pA

The potential profiles and anion concentrations for different channel radii are shown in Figure 2 and Figure 3, Figure 4 and Figure 5 give the potential profile at channel radius 3.5 Å and cation concentration at channel radius 5 Å.

The radii of Na^+ and Cl^- ions are 102 pm and 181 pm respectively. So, with the increase of channel radii, the anion current increases with slight increase of cation current. The ions cross the channel in such a way that when positive ion crosses the channel, the negative ions face a potential barrier. The charge separation across the lipid membrane will build up a potential. The potential increases until a balanced condition is reached. This potential is called the membrane potential and it depends on the concentration of all the permeable ions present there.

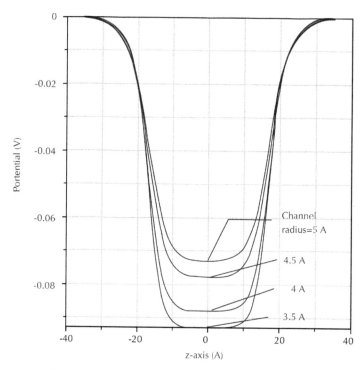

Figure 2. Variation of potential along z-axis different channel radii.

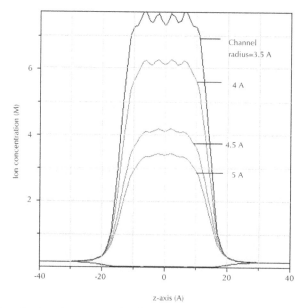

Figure 3. Variation of anion concentration for along z-axis for different channel radii.

However, due the unpredictability of the opening and closing of the channel, it cannot be definitely said when the channel is really close. It depends on the thermal motion of the protein molecules that decide the fact. The membrane potential changes the probability of opening or closing of the channel. These channels are known as voltage-controlled channels. Such channels (Na and K) are mostly present in neurons. For K^+ and Cl^- ions, the voltage current relationship and potential are given in Figure 6 and Figure 7. The ion channels show voltage-current relationship same as that of diodes and transistors. Figure 8 shows the ion concentration along z-axis at two different potentials (0 Volt and 0.1 Volt).

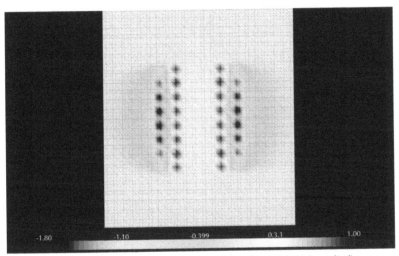

Figure 4. Potential profile in the ZY plane with channel length 3.5 E (0 Volt applied).

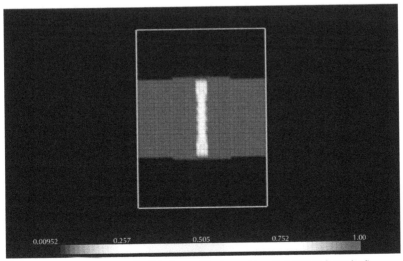

Figure 5. Cation concentration in the ZY plane with channel length 5 E (0 Volt applied).

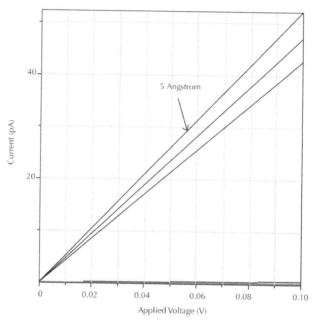

Figure 6. Voltage-current relationship for different channel radii.

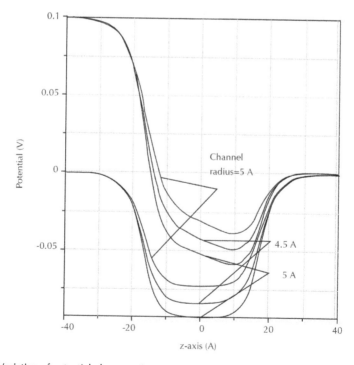

Figure 7. Variation of potential along z-axis.

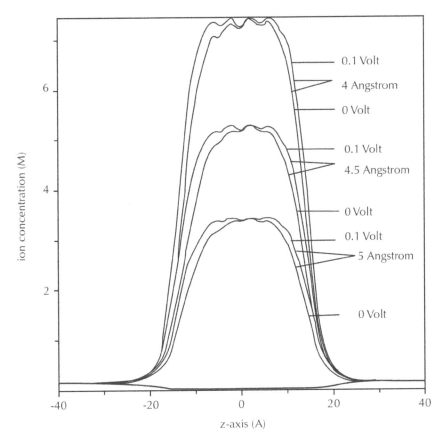

Figure 8. Ion concentration along z-axis.

Monte Carlo Simulation

In this model, water and lipid are treated as background dielectric materials but ions and proteins are treated discretely. First of all map generator sets up appropriate 3D simulation box. Then the protein is wrapped to set lipid boundaries and radius. The lipid is treated as a slab of material having a uniform dielectric constant. The lipid covers the protein very tightly. Boundary force potential can be calculated which is the potential energy profile of a point charge while passing through the channel. Then, MC simulation is performed and forces on each particle are calculated. After running the map generator, the channel structure is obtained as Figure 9 and Figure 10 gives the channel structure after wrapping the peptide with lipid. Again, the boundary force potential changes by changing the dielectric constants of the protein, lipid, and water. The change of this potential takes the form of Figure 11 and Figure 12, where dielectric constants are 20, 5, and 80 (Protein, lipid, bulk water in order) and 10, 2, and 80 respectively.

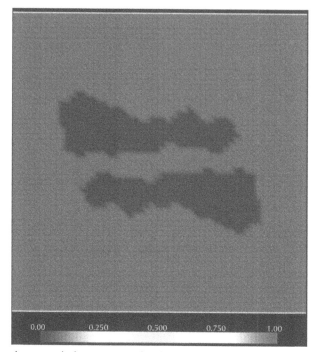

Figure 9. Channel structure before wrapping the channel with lipid.

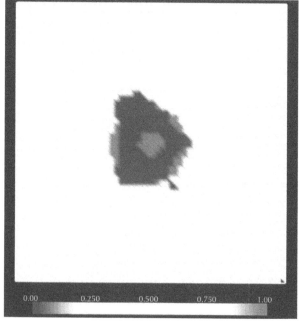

Figure 10. The structure of the channel after wrapping the channel with lipid.

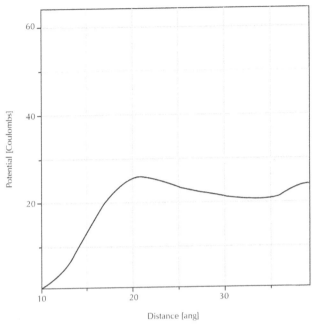

Figure 11. Boundary force potential for protein, lipid and water dielectric constant as 20, 5, and 80 respectively.

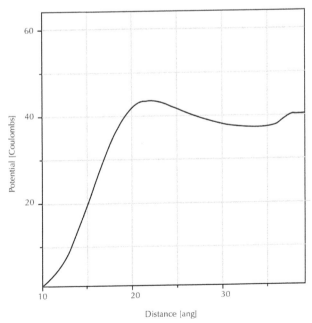

Figure 12. Boundary force potential for protein, lipid and water dielectric constant as 10, 2, and 80 respectively.

The MC simulation gives the equilibrium properties of the ions in the channel and can work with numerous numbers of atoms. Some simulation results showing different ions crossing the channel, their charge, mass, radius, thermal velocity, diffusion coefficient, and rate of scattering are shown in Table 1.

Table 1. Results of MC simulation showing different properties of the ions crossing the channel and their scattering rate.

Charge of the species	Mass(Kg)	Radius (Å)	v-therm (m/s)	Diffusion coefficient (m²/s)	Scattering rate (/s)
0	3.81761e-26	0.95	525.628	1.334e-09	8.13318e+13
-1	5.8872e-26	1.81	423.272	2.032e-09	3.46238e+13
1	6.49314e-26	1.33	403.038	1.957e-09	3.25958e+13
2	3.81761e-26	0.99	525.628	7.9e-10	1.37337e+14
2	3.81761e-26	0.65	525.628	7e-10	1.54995e+14

Maximum energy of the ions is found as 1.26105e + 11 V/m where,

Domain dimensions:

X: -22.823 22.17,7 Y: -22.5 22.5, Z: -25.921 19.079 and aqueous volumen = 6.58028e-26 m³, channel volumen = 1.62295e-27 m³ protein volumen = 4.56975e-27 m³, lipid volumen =2.07525e-26 m³

Volume of the left bath, 2.6584e-26 m³ and right bath 3.75958e-26 m³

Poisson equations are solved in every 100 time steps for the system and forces on each particle are calculated. In MC simulation, unphysical movement of ions can also be simulated. But here unphysical movements are restricted that is no two ions overlap or no ion overlap with protein. So, close range calculations are performed. So, the influx of ions through in channels can be regulated using suitable gate voltage, channel radius, and several other different factors.

The Importance of a Biosensor and its Relation to Ion channel

As stated earlier, biosensors can be devised depending on the function of an ion channel, at the same time the analyte detected by a biosensor, in the reverse way can be controlled to enter into the cell through ion channel. Biomolecules carrying charges can be detected by a nanobiosensor. It can be made up with nanowire or nanosphere which is previously functionalized with some receptor molecules of known identity. When the biomolecule (like DNA) enters into the sensor volume it get attached with the receptor. The excess charge after catching can be measured by the electrical circuit of the sensor. Thus, the presence of some specific disease causing antigens can be detected if their charge be known. In the same way, ions can also be detected. Here, we have shortly described how a DNA molecule (Figure 13) can be detected using a silicon nanowire and nanosphere sensor.

The device geometry is shown in Figure 14. Firstly, we have varied the radius of the nanowire and found that when the settling time is 3 hr, the minimum analyte density that can be detected is 1.5×10^{-14} M for a wire of radius 50 nm. When the radius decreases, the sensor becomes more sensitive and the minimum analyte concentration approaches 10^{-15} (Figure 15). However, the sensor activity does not depend on the length of the wire and a fixed length of 80 nm is used. Here, lower and upper values of analyte concentrations are $1e^{-15}$ M and $1e^{-06}$ M respectively. In these studies, we have considered that the test fluid of volume 10 c.c. is injected into the sensor via pipette drop.

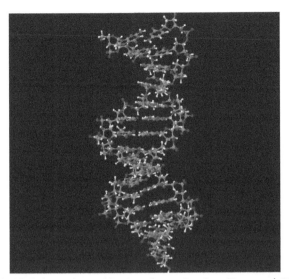

Figure 13. DNA double helix as obtained by the software Geneious (Drmmond, 2010).

A nanosphere sensor shows the variation of settling time similar to a nanowire sensor. But, it can detect minimum analyte concentration for a lower incubation period (Figure 16). The lower line is for a nanosphere of diameter 5 nm. For a quantum dot of diameter 5 nm, the sufficient decrease of settling time is observed. A minimum analyte concentration of 1.08×10^{-14} M can be detected in only 10.08 s. For a given incubation time, sensitivity predicts the surface coverage due to receptor molecules and the Signal-Noise Ratio due to the physisorption of parasitic molecules on the sensor surface [Figure 17].

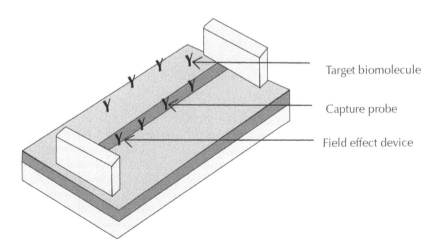

Figure 14. Cylindrical nanowire sensor geometry.

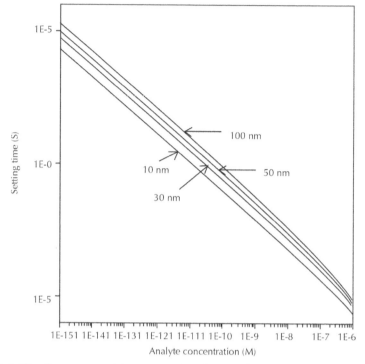

Figure 15. Settling time versus analyte concentration of a nanowire sensor.

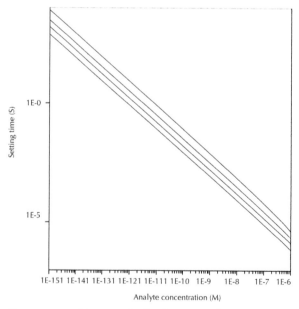

Figure 16. Settling time versus analyte concentration for a nanosphere sensor.

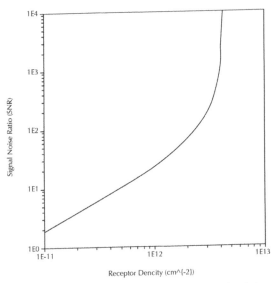

Figure 17. Selectivity of the sensor (signal noise ratio versus receptor density).

So, biosensor efficiently detects charged biomolecules near the sensor surface by electrostatic interaction. The settling time is found to vary with radius of the nanosphere or the nanowire. Sufficient reduction of settling time is reported for a nanosphere of dimension 5 nm. So, *in vivo* detection of charged biomolecules is efficiently done by adjusting the device parameters properly by the above technique. Connecting the transducer part of a biosensor to the ion channel, the controlled influx of the detected molecule can be achieved.

CONCLUSION

The importance of ion channels in sending fast electronic signals in the nervous system is the motivation behind the considerable research progress in the field of biology and biophysics. Also detection of different biomolecules is of vital importance in the field of nanomedicine. These two processes can be coupled together to regulate the transport of detected analyte to different cells of our body, especially to the nervous system. Rather than an ion channel biosensor, we have discussed about the "regulation after detection" in this work.

KEYWORDS

- **Diffusion-capture model**
- **Electronic signals**
- **Ion channels**
- **Molecular Dynamics**
- **Monte Carlo simulation**
- **Poisson-Nernst-Planck model**

Chapter 13

Effects of Intranasal Administration of Interferon-alpha on Rat Behavior

Loginova N. A., Sarkisova K. Yu., Kurskaya O. V., and Loseva E. V.

INTRODUCTION

Nasal drug administration is commonly used for the treatment of local ailments like cold, cough, rhinitis, and so on. (Ali et al., 2010) The nasal administration seems to be a primary route to circumvent the obstacles of blood–brain barrier, allowing the direct drug delivery to the central nervous system (CNS) (Pires et al., 2009), such as, for example, some vaccines and large molecules (Ozsoy et al., 2009; Yuki and Kiyono, 2009). Intranasal administration of insulin used for the treatment of cognitive impairments prevents peripheral side effects (Benedict et al., 2010; Hallschmid et al., 2007). Thorne and colleagues have demonstrated that intranasal administration of cytokine resulted in rapid, widespread targeting of nervous tissue (Thorne et al., 2008). The authors suggested that both interferon-beta and interferon-alpha (IA), which share the same receptor, may bind with relatively high affinity in the same brain structures.

The IA is a cytokine with neuroimmunomodulatory properties. The IA consists of 166 amino acid residues with molecular weight 18 kDa (Khaitov et al., 2000). Structure of IA and its type 1 receptors are well known (Bekisz et al., 2004; Chill et al., 2003; Kontsek, 1994). Systemic administration of high doses of IA is commonly used for treatment of oncological and viral diseases. However, in patients in stressful conditions provoking increased anxiety this treatment quite often give rise to neurological or psychiatric disorders including depression (Raison et al., 2005). At the same time, chronic systemic treatment with low doses of IA does not result in development of depression in humans or animals. On the contrary, it activates some functions of the neuroimmunoendocrine complex (Loseva et al., 2008, 2009a). In particularly, low doses of IA have been shown to reduce the defensive behavior and anxiety level in unstressed rats (Loseva et al., 2007a, 2007b, 2009b). Intranasal administration of IA is usually used for prophylaxis and treatment of influenza and cold. However, it is practically unknown, the effects of different doses of IA on the functions of the nervous system, particularly on behavior. It is known that similar cytokine, for example interferon-beta after intranasal administration penetrates into the brain much deeper in comparison with other ways of application (Thorne et al., 1995). We suppose that intranasal administration of different doses of IA might exert unequal influence on behavior of stressed and unstressed rats. As a model of stress, social stress was used. Unfavorable living conditions, including overcrowding, quite often give rise to social stress followed by the development of elevated anxiety and depression (Daniels et al., 2000). Overcrowding is known to suppress immune system, increase anxiety and lead to development of depression in animals (Naitoh et al., 1992). Therefore, a search for medicines based on physiologically active substances without side effects has a great importance for prophylaxis and treatment of social stresses.

The goal of the present study was to investigate the behavioral effects of high and low doses of IA after chronic intranasal treatment of rats, living in overcrowded and standard conditions.

MATERIALS AND METHODS

For behavioral experiments, 60 mature male rats (180–200 g) were used. Rats were housed in cages with free access to food and water, and maintained in a room temperature of $24 \pm 2°C$ with a 12 hr light-dark cycle. During the first 5 days, rats were kept in standard conditions that is 5 animals per cage. Low (50 IU/kg, n = 10) or high (8000 IU/kg) doses of human IA (Lockferon, "Biomed", Russia) in 100 µl of saline were administered intranasally. Control rats received 100 µl of saline. On the 6 day, rats from 3 cages, receiving different doses of IA or saline, were placed together in one cage and kept there until the end of the experiments (10 days). Two cages with overcrowded rats were formed (n = 15 in each) as according to some researchers, number of rats in one cage should be more than 12 for the development of overcrowding stress-induced differences in behavior (Botelho et al., 2007).

There were three experimental groups (10 rats per each) kept together in overcrowded conditions (low IA dose, high IA dose and saline, five rats from each group in one cage), and three corresponding control groups (10 rats per each) kept in standard conditions (low IA dose, high IA dose and saline).

Animals were tested in the "open field" a day before drug application and on the second day of overcrowding. The following behavioral parameters were registered for 5 min: the number of squares crossed (locomotor activity) and rearing (vertical activity), freezing time, grooming time. Rats were tested in the "light-dark" choice test on the third day of overcrowding. Latency of entering the dark box (s), the time spent in the light and dark compartment (s) was measured for 5 min in this test. "Elevated plus maze" was used on the day 6 of overcrowding. The number of squares crossed (locomotor activity) and rearings (vertical activity), the time and number of grooming reactions (s), the time of freezing (s), the number of entries into the open and close arms, the time spent on each arm and central square of the maze, the number, and duration of head dips were recorded for 5 min. Rats were tested in the forced swimming test on the tenth day of overcrowding (Sarkisova and Kulikov, 2006; Sarkisova et al., 2003). The duration of passive swimming (immobility), the duration of the first episode of active swimming (s), and duration of swimming (s) were registered for 5 min.

Statistical analysis of data was carried out using nonparametric Mann-Whitney U-test for two independent samples, nonparametric Wilcoxon test for two dependent samples or Student's t-test. Software packages STATISTICA 6.0 and STATGRAPHICS 6.1 were used. All values reported in the text are mean ± standard error of mean. The statistical threshold was set at $p < 0.05$ and $p < 0.1$ as a tendency.

DISCUSSION

The IA is a cytokine with the neuroimmunomodulatory properties. It is increasingly used for treatment of some virus infections and several malignancies. Expression of IA in the brain is induced in neurons and glial cells in response to viral infection or occurrence of a tumor.

The IA receptors (IAR) are mainly located on glial cells, but in case of pathology they can be expressed on neurons (Dafny and Jang, 2005; Yamada and Yamanaka, 1995). The increase of IA level in the CNS during viral infections or neuro-oncological processes stimulates expression of the type 1 specific transmembrane IAR in the brain cells. Interaction of IA with two IAR subunits results in activation of the universal signaling pathway the Janus activated kinase-signal transducer and activator of transcription (JAK-STAT).

The JAK-STAT triggers a cascade of reactions leading to expression of IAR proteins, anti-inflammatory cytokines and other signals. In mild cases, this can help to cope with a viral infection or tumor. In severe cases, however, the amount of naturally produced IA is insufficient. Therefore, such patients are treated with IA-containing drugs. However, treatment with high doses of human IA quite often causes unfavorable side effects such as elevated anxiety and depression both in animals and in humans, therefore clinical usage of this drug is problematic (Raison et al, 2005; for review see Loseva et al., 2008).

Mechanisms of IA-induced psychiatric side effects, including depression are not well understood. There are several putative ways of depression development during IA therapy. The first way might be mediated by hyperactivity of the corticotropin-releasing hormone (CRH). The CRH activates both the hypothalamic-pituitary-adrenal axis and sympathetic nervous system, which is widely recognized as the principal contributor to the mammalian stress response (Capuron et al., 2003; Owens and Nemeroff, 1993). The second mechanism of depression development during IA therapy could be associated with serotonergic neurotransmission in the CNS. The IA is believed to induce activation of the enzyme indoleamine 2,3-dioxegenase (IDO), which shunts the metabolism of tryptophan away from serotonin toward kinurenine. Since tryptophan is not synthesized in the body, IDO-induced tryptophan depletion results in reduced availability of serotonin (Capuron et al., 2003). Peripheral administration of IA can activate IDO in concert with central cytokine responses, resulting increases in the brain KYN and QUIN, which correlates with depressive symptoms (Raison et al., 2010).

Animal studies have demonstrated that IA alters activity of the opioid, dopaminergic, and noradrenergic systems in the CNS. Like other inflammatory stimuli, IA also appears to increase free radical and glutamate production, which, in turn, promote neuronal damage (Schaefer et al., 2003). The neurogenesis in the hippocampal dental gyrus decreases after IA treatment, and this can lead to cognitive disorders (Kaneko et al., 2006). Recent study shows, that depressive symptoms following IA therapy may be mediated by immune-induced reductions in brain-derived neurotrophic factor in serum (Kenis et al., 2010). Interestingly, transgenic mice with CNS expression of IA did not develop depression or anxiety as measured by Porsolt's forced swim test and elevated plus-maze respectively in comparison with wild-type animals. Authors suggested that factors other than IA may be involved in the development of psychiatric complications following IA therapy in patients (Zhang et al., 2010).

On the other hand, in contrast to high doses administration, depression does not develop in most patients treated with low doses of IA (Raison et al, 2005). Moreover, in patients with myeloproliferative disorders, long-term therapy with low to intermediate doses of IA does not seem to impair neurological functions; on the contrary, such treatment enhances muscle power, attention and memory (Mayr et al., 1999). However, effects of low doses of human IA on animal behavior are still unknown.

In the present study, it has been shown that in groups, kept in standard conditions, high dose of IA increased (elevated plus maze) or did not change (open field, light-dark choice) baseline level of anxiety. Low IA dose did not change (open field) or decreased (light-dark test, elevated plus maze) anxiety level. Put into other words, the present research confirms our previously obtained data concerning effects of low dose of human and rat IA on anxiety level in rats (Loseva at al., 2007a, 2009b). Our findings are also in line with the data indicating depression-provoking effects of high doses of IA in rats (Sammut et al., 2001) and humans (Lotrich, 2009; Raison et al., 2005), although low dose of IA in our investigation also increased the level of depression in the forced swimming test. It is possible that the development of depressive-like state depends on duration of intranasal administration of IA and has cumulative effect (Moriyama and Arakawa, 2006). For example, IA treatment decreased the time spent immobility in the forced-swimming test after a single intraperitoneal injection at 2 x 10(6) IU/kg (Wang et al., 2009).

Here, we confirmed that overcrowding increases the level of anxiety and depression. Our results are in agreement with the data of literature that overcrowding results in increase of anxiety (in the elevated plus maze test) and depression (in the forced swimming test) (Botelho et al., 2007, Naitoh et al., 1992).

In our experiments, in overcrowded conditions, low dose of IA normalized behavior of rats in all tests, whereas high dose of IA had either no influence on behavior (open field, light-dark choice test) or it was mixed.

In the forced swimming test, both low and high doses of IA induced increases in depressive-like behavior in rats, kept in standard conditions, and decreases in overcrowded rats. This immobility-reducing effect was more pronounced when low dose of IA was administered. Thus, in all tests that characterize the level of anxiety (open field, light-dark choice, elevated plus maze), dose-dependent effects of intranasal administration of IA on the behavioral parameters have been revealed in groups of rats, kept both in standard and overcrowding conditions. In the forced swimming test, which characterizes the level of depression, IA administration caused behavioral changes both in stressed and unstressed rats, effects were not dose-dependent in unstressed groups but dose-dependent (greater effect at low IA dose) in case of stressed group.

We hypothesize that upon treatment of different illness with high doses of IA, the excess of IA is not bound by IAR and is capable to bind with other receptors in the brain. This may prevent effects of some intrinsic agonists to these receptors. For instance, IA can act in the brain via μ-opiod receptors changing the balance of neurotransmitter systems (Makino et al., 2000a). High doses of IA can trigger the same processes in the healthy brain, where there are not enough previously expressed IARs. Therefore, high doses of IA can result in direct or indirect binding of this cytokine not only to IARs but to other receptors as well, for example μ-opioid, serotonin, and corti-cotrophin releasing factor receptors (Cai et al., 2005; Makino et al., 2000b; Sato et al., 2006; Wang et al., 2008; Yamano et al., 2000), that can deplete the receptive fields for corresponding substances necessary for normal CNS function. This misbalance can re-sult in depressive disorders, mediated by impairments of opioidergic and serotonergic systems as well as hypothalamo-pituitary-adrenal system.

In contrast, low doses of IA are expected to stimulate additional expression of IAR and other IA-binding receptors. This can take place with or without preliminary stimu-lation by antigens and activation of the intrinsic interferonergic brain system. In this case, anti-viral and anti-tumor IA effects can be amplified by an additional activation of protective biochemical cascades via JAK-STAT signals or other systems. Besides, one can expect functional facilitation of brain systems due to modulatory effects of IA through corresponding receptors, resulting in suppression of possible depressive disorders. This assumption is supported by our research (Loseva et al., 2007a, 2007b) and other published data.

RESULTS

"Open field" Test

In the standard conditions, intranasal administration of IA did not significantly change any of the parameters measured (Figure 1). However, the number of squares crossed in the groups "IA, 50 IU/kg" and "IA, 8000 IU/kg" had a tendency to be lower (36.9 ± 7.8 and 42.1 ± 5.6 respectively) in comparison with "vehicle" group (59.4 ± 10.5) (Figure 1(A)).

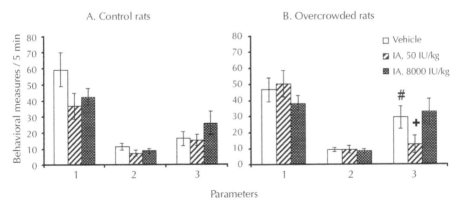

Figure 1. Behavioral measures in the "open field" test in the control (A) and overcrowded (B) rats.

Values are the mean ± SEM 1 – the number of squares crossed; 2 – the number of rearings (vertical activity); 3 – time of grooming (s). Vehicle – intranasal administra-tion of the saline; IA, 50 IU/kg – intranasal administration of the IA in dose of 50 IU/

kg; IA, 8,000 IU/kg – intranasal administration of IA in dose of 8,000 IU/kg # – p < 0.05 – in comparison with control rats, + – p < 0.1 – in comparison with "vehicle" group (Mann-Whitney U-test for independent samples).

In the overcrowded conditions, locomotor (Figure 1(B, 1)) and vertical (Figure 1(B, 2)) activities did not differ significantly in any of the experimental groups compared with the respective control groups, living in standard conditions. At the same time, overcrowding caused increases in grooming time (29.5 ± 7.0 s) in comparison with the respective control group, housed in standard conditions (16.4 ± 4.3 s) (p < 0.05) the IA treatment (50 IU/kg, but not 8,000 IU/kg) induced a tendency to decrease the grooming time (12.8 ± 5.5 s) compared with the overcrowded "vehicle" group (29.5 ± 7.0 s) (Figure 1(B, 3)).

Thus, intranasal administration of IA did not cause changes in behavioral measures of rats housed in standard conditions. Overcrowding resulted in increase of grooming time and only low dose of IA decreased grooming time up to 'normal' level.

"Light-dark" Choice Test

Intranasal administration of low (50 IU/kg) dose of IA induced increases in the time spent in the light box compared with "vehicle" group both in the standard (36.4 ± 7.1) and overcrowded (26.1 ± 7.2) conditions (p < 0.1 – tendency) (Figure 2). Number of crossings and vertical activity did not change in any of the groups. Overcrowded conditions did not change any behavioral parameters in the "vehicle" or IA groups.

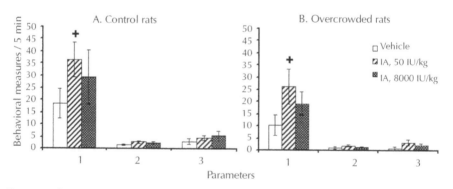

Figure 2. Behavioral measures in the "light-dark" choice test in the control (A) and overcrowded (B) rats.

Values are the mean ± SEM 1 – the time spent in the light box (s); 2 – the number of transitions between compartments; 3 – the number of rearings (vertical activity) + – p < 0.1 – in comparison with "vehicle" group (Mann-Whitney U-test for independent samples) other designations as in Figure 1.

Thus, low dose of IA caused decreases in anxiety measure both in standard and overcrowded conditions, whereas large dose of IA did not affect the anxiety level. In this test, overcrowding did not change any behavioral parameters.

"Elevated plus maze"

Following parameters were recorded to assess rat's behavior: vertical activity (number), grooming time, number of crossed squares, freezing (number and duration), and entrances into the open and close arms of the maze. All data is presented in the Table 1 (see below).

The IA in the dose 8,000 IU/kg had influence on the most part of behavior of rats housed in standard conditions. Number of crossed squares decreased in the group "IA, 8,000 IU/kg" (45.8 ± 6.7) in comparison with groups "vehicle" (64.2 ± 4.2) ($p < 0.05$) and "IA, 50 IU/kg" (59.6 ± 3.6) ($p < 0.1$) (Table 1) housed in standard conditions. Time of immobility in the groups "IA, 50 IU/kg" and "IA, 8,000 IU/kg" increased (10.7 ± 4.1 and 18.0 ± 16.0) in comparison with "vehicle" group (5.9 ± 4.1) ($p < 0.2$ – tendency).

The rats from group "IA, 8,000 IU/kg" were found in the center of the maze less often than other animals. Time spent in the center decreased in the group "IA, 8,000 IU/kg" (17.1 ± 3.9) in comparison with group "vehicle" (34.2 ± 3.3) ($p < 0.2$) and group "IA, 50 IU/kg" (31.2 ± 7.8) ($p < 0.05$) (Table 1).

Duration of staying in the close arm of the maze in the group "IA, 8,000 IU/kg" was longer (237.7 ± 20.4) than in the group "IA, 50 IU/kg" (190.4 ± 11.5) ($p < 0.2$ – tendency).

Time spent in the open arm in the group "IA, 50 IU/kg" increased (76.6 ± 7.7) in comparison with group "vehicle" (49.7 ± 12.1) ($p < 0.1$ – tendency). At the same time, this parameter in the group "IA, 8,000 IU/kg" was smaller (43.7 ± 17.5) than in the group "IA, 50 IU/kg" (76.6 ± 7.7) ($p < 0.2$ – tendency).

Time of grooming increased in group "IA, 50 IU/kg" (16.5 ± 7.6) in comparison with control "vehicle" group (7.3 ± 5.1) ($p < 0.2$ – tendency). However this parameter decreased in group "IA, 8,000 IU/kg" (2.7 ± 1.7) in comparison with group "IA, 50 IU/kg" (16.5 ± 7.6) ($p < 0.1$ – tendency).

Duration of head dips increased in group "IA, 50 IU/kg" (12.6 ± 1.2) in comparison with "vehicle" control group (5.1 ± 2.1) ($p < 0.05$).

Latent period of the first entrance into the close arm of the maze in the group "IA, 50 IU/kg" increased (47.2 ± 5.9) in comparison with group "vehicle" (27.9 ± 13.4) ($p < 0.2$ – tendency) and group "IA, 8,000 IU/kg" (25.3 ± 7.4) ($p < 0.05$). Intranasal introduction of the IA in the dose 8,000 IU/kg resulted in increase of anxiety behavior.

Overcrowding influenced some behavioral parameters. Overcrowded conditions resulted in the decrease of the number of rears (18.6 ± 2.9) in comparison with "vehicle" group (24.2 ± 2.7) ($p < 0.2$ – tendency). Furthermore, number of crossed squares decreased (42.2 ± 8.6) in comparison with "vehicle" group housed in standard conditions (64.2 ± 4.2) ($p < 0.2$ – tendency). Time spent in the center decreased (15.9 ± 6.4) in comparison with "vehicle" (34.2 ± 3.3) ($p < 0.1$ – tendency). Time of immobility increased in the overcrowded "vehicle" group (21.1 ± 11.0) in comparison with control "vehicle" group (5.9 ± 4.1) ($p < 0.2$ – tendency).

Administration of IA altered most behavioral parameters in rats housed in overcrowded conditions. Number of rears decreased in the group "IA, 8,000 IU/kg" (18.2

+ 3.2) in comparison with "vehicle" control group (24.2 + 2.7) (p < 0.2 – tendency) (Table 1).

The IA administration in the dose of 50 IU/kg led to increase in number of crossed squares (60.6 ± 7.7) in comparison with "IA, 8,000 IU/kg" group housed in standard conditions (45.8 ± 6.7) (p < 0.2 – tendency). This parameter was smaller in the overcrowded "IA, 8,000 IU/kg" group (47.2 ± 7.7) than in the control "vehicle" (64.2 ± 4.2) and control "IA, 50 IU/kg" (59.6 ± 3.6) groups (p < 0.2 – tendency).

Time of staying in the close arm of the maze decreased in the overcrowded "IA, 8,000 IU/kg" group (201.4 ± 16.1) in comparison with overcrowded "vehicle" group (242.1 ± 20.4) (p < 0.2 – tendency). Similarly, time spent in the open arm of the maze increased in the group "IA, 8,000 IU/kg" (76.7 ± 14.0) compared to overcrowded "vehicle" group (41.3 ± 15.1) (p < 0.2 – tendency).

Number of groomings decreased in the group "IA, 50 IU/kg" (2.2 ± 1.0) in comparison with overcrowded "vehicle" group (5.2 ± 1.4) (p < 0.1 – tendency). This parameter also decreased in the group "IA, 8,000 IU/kg" (1.4 ± 0.7) in comparison with control "vehicle" (3.8 ± 1.4) and "IA, 50 IU/kg" (2.8 ± 0.7) groups (p < 0.2 – tendency) and overcrowded "vehicle" group (5.2 ± 1.4) (p < 0.05) (Table 1).

Number of head dips increased in the overcrowded group "IA, 8,000 IU/kg" (9.6 ± 1.5) in comparison with overcrowded "vehicle" group (6.4 ± 2.2) (p < 0.2 – tendency). Duration of the head dips increased in the overcrowded group "IA, 8,000 IU/kg" (12.1 ± 2.3) in comparison with control "vehicle" (5.1 ± 2.1) and overcrowded "vehicle" (4.6 ± 1.7) groups (p < 0.2 and p < 0.05 accordingly).

The latency of the first entrance into the close arm of the maze decreased in the group "IA, 50 IU/kg" (18.3 ± 7.5) compared to control "IA, 50 IU/kg" group (47.2 ± 5.9) (p < 0.05). The latency of the first entrance into the open arm of the maze increased in the overcrowded "IA, 50 IU/kg" group (8.9 ± 7.0) in comparison with control "IA, 50 IU/kg" group (3.9 ± 0.4) (p < 0.2 – tendency) and decreased in comparison with control "IA, 8,000 IU/kg" group (58.5 ± 54.8) (p < 0.1 – tendency) and overcrowded "vehicle" group (38.7 ± 34.1) (p < 0.1 – tendency).

Table 1. Behavioral measures in the "elevated plus maze" test in the control and overcrowded rats.

Behavioral parameters	Control rats			Overcrowded rats		
	Vehicle	IA, 50IU/kg	IA, 8000IU/kg	Vehicle	IA, 50IU/kg	IA, 8000IU/kg
Rearings (number)	24,2±2,7	20,2±0,9	20,8±2,8	18,6±2,9 *	23,6±3,1	18,2±3,2 *
Squares crossed (number)	64,2±4,2	59,6±3,6	45,8±6,7 ***$$	42,2±8,6 *$$	60,6±7,7 ^	47,2±7,7 *$
Time on central square (sec)	34,2±3,3	31,2±7,8	17,1±3,9 *$$$	15,9±6,4 **$$	16,5±4,6 *$$$	19,3±5,3 *$
Freezing (sec)	3,2±1,1	3,1±1,3	9,3±6,9	1,0±0,6 *	0,0±0,0 ***$$$^^^###	0,23±0,23 ***$$^

Table 1. *(Continued)*

Behavioral parameters	Control rats			Overcrowded rats		
	Vehicle	IA, 50IU/kg	IA, 8000IU/kg	Vehicle	IA, 50IU/kg	IA, 8000IU/kg
Immobility (sec)	5,9±4,1	10,7±4,1 *	18,0±16,0 *	21,1±11,0 *	12,9±8,2	28,7±12,3 *$
Time in closed arms (sec)	210,4±17,7	190,4±11,5	237,7±20,4 $	242,1±20,4 $	209,9±26,2	201,4±16,1 #
Time in open arms (sec)	49,7±12,1	76,6±7,7 **	43,7±17,5 $	41,3±15,1 $	66,4±20,4	76,7±14,0 #
Grooming (number)	3,8±1,4	2,8±0,7 *$$	1,4±0,4 $^^^	5,2±1,4 $^^^	2,2±1,0 ##	1,4±0,7 *$###
Grooming (sec)	7,3±5,1	16,5±7,6 *	2,7±1,7 $$	35,2±26,3 ^	13,3±6,3	18,9±10,7
Head dips (number)	8,6±2,3	11,2±0,8	6,8±1,8 $$	6,4±2,2 $	13,8±4,2	9,6±1,5 #
Head dips (sec)	5,1±2,1	12,6±1,2 ***	11,2±5,1	4,6±1,7 $$$	11,1±4,1	12,1±2,3 *###
Latency of entering the closed arm (sec)	27,9±13,4	47,2±5,9 *	25,3±7,4 $$$	25,2±12,8 $	18,3±7,5 $$$	41,3±18,9
Latency of entering the open arm (sec)	10,0±3,9	3,9±0,4	58,5±54,8	38,7±34,1	8,9±7,0 $^^##	10,8±4,0

Values are the mean ± SEM Vehicle – intranasal administration of the saline; IA, 50 IU/kg – intranasal administration of the IA in the dose 50 IU/kg; IA, 8,000 IU/kg – intranasal administration of the IA in the dose 8,000 IU/kg * – $p < 0.2$, ** – $p < 0.1$, *** – $p < 0.05$ – in comparison with control "vehicle" group, $ – $p < 0.2$, $$ – $p < 0.1$, $$$ – $p < 0.05$ – in comparison with control "IA, 50 IU/kg" group, ^ – $p < 0.2$, ^^ – $p < 0.1$, ^^^ – $p < 0.05$ – in comparison with control "IA, 8,000 IU/kg" group, # – $p < 0.2$, ## – $p < 0.1$, ### – $p < 0.05$ – in comparison with overcrowded "vehicle" group (Mann-Whitney U-test for independent samples).

Thus, intranasal introduction of IA in the dose of 8,000 IU/kg to rats housed in standard conditions led to decrease of locomotor activity and time spent in the center of the maze, which characterized increase of anxiety level. In contrast, introduction of IA in the dose of 50 IU/kg led to decrease in anxiety level, which has been confirmed by some behavioral parameters (freezing, time of being into the open arm, latency of the first entrance into the close arm).

Overcrowding changed the behavior of control rats in the same manner as administration of low dose of IA (50 IU/kg) to rats housed in standard conditions.

Small dose of IA (50 IU/kg) normalized anxiety level of the overcrowded rats, whereas large dose did not change some behavioral parameters (locomotor activity, freezing) but increased duration of staying in the open arm of the maze.

Forced Swimming Test

In the control rats, intranasal administration of IA in dose of 50 IU/kg and 8,000 IU/kg induced increases in the time of passive swimming (immobility). This parameter in the group "IA, 50 IU/kg" (191.5 ± 3.8 s) and in the group "IA, 8,000 IU/kg" (189.2 ± 6.2 s) was longer than in the group "Vehicle" (164.8 ± 7.9 s, p < 0.01 and p < 0.05 respectively) (Figure 3(A, 1)). Time of swimming decreased in these groups in comparison with control rats (Figure 3(A, 2)).

Overcrowding induced increases in the time of passive swimming (210.5 ± 5.9 s) in comparison with control rats (164.8 ± 7.9 s, p < 0.01) (Figure 3(B, 1)), and decreases in the time of the first episode of active swimming (33.5 ± 3.6 s) compared with the respective control (65.5 ± 3.1 s, p < 0.001) (Figure 3(B, 3)). In the overcrowded conditions, IA treatment decreased the time of passive swimming (142.3 ± 16.2 s in the "IA, 50 IU/kg" group and 171.5 ± 10 s in the "IA, 8,000 IU/kg" group) in comparison with "vehicle" group (210.5 ± 5.9 s, p < 0.01). Time of the first episode of active swimming increased in the groups "IA, 50 IU/kg" (84.5 ± 13.4 s) and "IA, 8,000 IU/kg" (61.0 ± 5.8 s) in comparison with control group (33.5 ± 3.6 s, p < 0.001 and p < 0.01 respectively).

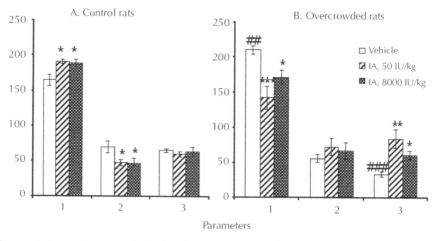

Figure 3. Behavioral measures in the forced swimming test in the control (A) and overcrowded (B) rats.

Values are the mean ± SEM 1 – time of passive swimming or immobility (s), 2 – time of swimming (s), 3 – time of the first episode of active swimming or 'climbing' (s) * – p < 0.05, ** – p < 0.01, *** – p < 0.001 – in comparison with the "vehicle" group, ## – p < 0.01, ### – p < 0.001 – in comparison with the corresponding control group housed in standard conditions (Stident's t-test for independent samples). Other designations as in Figure 1.

Thus, both doses of IA in standard conditions led to increases in depressive-like behavior. The same effect produced overcrowding in vehicle-treated rats. Both doses on IA, normalized behavior of overcrowded rats, but the effect of low dose was greater.

CONCLUSION

Low dose of IA did not change (open field) or decreased (light-dark choice, elevated plus maze), whereas high dose of IA increased (elevated plus maze) or did not change baseline level of anxiety in rats kept in standard conditions.

Overcrowding increased anxiety level. Low dose of IA normalized the behavior in all tests, but high dose of IA either did not exert influence on behavior (open field, light-dark test) or this influence was mixed in rats kept in overcrowded condition.

Both low and high doses of IA increased depressive-like behavior (forced swim test) in rats, kept in standard conditions.

Results suggest that long-term intranasal administration of high as well as low doses of IA to healthy (unstressed) individuals can exert negative effect on the baseline anxiety level and provoke depressive-like state. At the same time, the administration of low (but not high) doses of IA in stressful conditions might be useful, because it can prevent the development and/or normalize anxiety and depressive-like behavior that emerge in response to stressors.

KEYWORDS

- **Corticotropin-releasing hormone**
- **Interferon-alpha**
- **Interferon-alpha receptors**
- **Intranasal administration**
- **Social stresses**

ACKNOWLEDGMENT

The work was supported by RFH (grant № 07-06-00282a).

We are grateful to T. Alekseeva for help with english text correction.

Chapter 14

Neurotransplantation of Neural and Mesenchymal Stem Cells for Correction of Posthypoxic Disorders

Loseva E. V., Podgornyi O. V., Poltavtseva R. A., Marey M. V., Loginova N. A.,Kurskaya O. V., Sukhikh G. T., Chilachyan R. K., and Aleksandrova M. A.

INTRODUCTION

Brain hypoxia is widespread in clinical picture of neuropsychic deceases and is a typical post-resuscitation complication. Effects of the hypoxia include diffuse degeneration and death of the neurons, leading to learning, and memory disturbances (Boksa et al., 1995; Hymel et al., 2007; Jellinger, 2008; Voronina, 2000). Hypoxic hypoxia (HH) is one of the well studied animal (rat) models of diffuse brain degeneration. Therefore, HH is a very suitable model for study of similar deceases (Polezhaev and Aleksandrova, 1983). Neurotransplantation of few differentiated brain tissues contained stem cells is a new and promising strategy for treatment of neurogenerative diseases, including brain hypoxia (Aleksandrova, 2001; Loseva, 2001; Polezhaev and Aleksandrova, 1983; Polezhaev et al., 1993). The ability of stem cells to express wide spectrum of active molecules (growth factors, neurotrophic factors, cytokines etc.) underlies their action. These active molecules are *per se* the natural nanostructures that are necessary for activation of reparative processes in damaged brain (Bath and Lee, 2010).

At the present time, scientists concentrate on the neurotransplantation of fetal neural stem cells (NSC)—precursors of neurons and glia that are present in the nervous system in all life (Armstrong and Svendsen, 2000; Burns et al., 2009). Transplantation of NSC from embryonic and adult tissues give possibility to create new neurogenic zones in the brain that may be beneficial for treatment of wide spectrum of human neurodegenerative deceases (Chu et al., 2008; Kim, 2007; Pessina and Gribaldo, 2006; Podgornyi et al., 2004). However, use of human embryonic donor tissue creates numerous ethical problems. Besides, one of the unsolved problems is the problem of allogenic NSC immunological compatibility. So, the investigation of alternative sources of stem cells with neurogenic potential from adult human tissues is very important (Kurozumi et al., 2005; Moore et al., 2006; Smith et al., 2007). The cells of the bone-marrow are researched most extensively. One of the known alternatives for NSC is human bone-marrow derived multipotent mesenchymal stromal cells (MSC), which apparently have the maximal flexibility. The data about differentiation of MSC *in vitro* and *in vivo* are very conflicting. It is reputed that in the native population of MSC, part of the cells express neural markers (Minguell et al., 2005), and during the cultivation, MSC can give rise to the neuroglial and similar with neurons cells, which according to immunohistochemical and molecular analysis express specific markers (Magaki et al., 2005; Minguell et al., 2005). In neurotransplantation conditions, MSC can answer to signals of the brain microenvironment and differentiate into glia and neurons (Muñoz-Elias et al., 2004) and promote the regeneration of CNS tissue, but mechanisms of their action are practically unknown (Dezawa et al., 2004; Zhao et al., 2002). However, there are studies that disagree with the possibility of MSCs' neural differentiation (Jin and Schuchman, 2003; Neuhuber et al., 2004). Meanwhile, it is known that MSC express numerous growth factors and cytokines, which can keep up regeneration of brain tissue after hypoxia even without differentiation of MSC in neural phenotypes (Cipriani et al., 2007; Mayer et al., 2005).

The aim of the present study was to compare the effects of neurotransplantation of human NSC and MSC on the rat behavior and brain state after acute hypoxia. Our objectives were (1) to compare development of defensive conditioned reflex in rats under hypoxia and transplantation of NSC or MSC in striatum in comparison with control rats with hypoxia only, with hypoxia and shame operation and without hypoxia; (2) to compare the morpho-functional state of neurons in the neocortex of contralateral nonoperated brain hemisphere in the same groups, and (3) to examine changes in cell population (NSC and MSC) in the neurotransplants (*in vivo*) compared to cells cultured *in vitro* using immunohistochemical analysis.

MATERIALS AND METHODS

Cultivation of NSC

As a donor, material unviable human fetuses obtained from healthy women after medical abortion (9.5 weeks' gestation) were used in compliance with guidelines of World Health Organization (WHO), accepted by Public Health Ministry of Russian Federation. Tissue fragments were isolated from periventricular area of fetal brain, put into F12 medium, and cell suspension prepared by repeated pipetting was then cultured in DMEM/F12 growth medium with N2 supplement containing epidermal growth factor (EGF), basal fibroblast growth factor (bFGF), and leukemia-inhibiting factor (LIF). Neurospheres formed in this culture were examined by immunohistochemical method at day 65 after the start of culturing. Neurospheres were mechanically dissociated to single stem/progenitor cells suspension which was used for transplantation.

Cultivation of MSC

Adult human bone-marrow derived multipotent mesenchymal stromal stem cells (MSC) were obtained from the hip bone crest of adult human. Cell suspension was dissociated and plated in concentration of 5×10^4 cells on 1 ml of medium. Cells were cultured in the α-MEM medium with 10% autologous serum and 10% veal serum. At days 10-12 of culture cells were removed from plastic with help of 0.25% solution of tripsin and subcultured in new tissue culture flask with change of medium. Cells cultured for 30 days were used for transplantation (3 passages).

Hypoxic Hhypoxia (HH) and Neurotransplantation

Female Wistar rats weighting 250-300 g were exposed to 3 min HH in a special altitude chamber (180 mm Hg) (Polezhaev and Aleksandrova, 1983). Rats were anesthetized with 300 mg/kg chloral hydrate on day 1 after hypoxia before transplantation. The suspension of human neural stem/progenitor cells (NSC) (3 μl, 1.5×10^5 cells per rat) or adult human bone-marrow derived multipotent mesenchymal stromal and stem cells (MSC) were stereotactically transplanted into striatum area of the rat brain (A 0–0,5 mm; L, 2, 5 mm; V, 4 mm) from groups HH + TNSC and HH + TMSC (see below), respectively. Transplantation of both NSC and MSC was not followed by immunosuppression.

Behavioral Experiments

Behavioral experiments were performed on 45 female Wistar rats weighting 250-300 g. All animals (except group Norm, n = 16) were exposed to 3 min HH in a special altitude chamber (180 mm Hg) (Polezhaev and Aleksandrova, 1983). Rats were divided into four groups: with HH only (group HH, n = 11), with HH and saline introduction into the brain (group HH + S, n = 9), with HH and transplantation of NSC (group HH + TNSC, n = 6), with HH and transplantation of MSC (group HH + TMSC, n = 5).

All rats were trained to a defensive conditioned two-way avoidance reflex (CTAR) (shuttle-box test) using an electric shock (20–25 V) as the unconditioned stimulus in a shuttle box with presentation of a tone (60 dB, 300 Hz) for 5 sec; training was performed on two occasions. Rats from groups with HH were trained in three learning sessions (4th, 9th, and 19th day after operation). In group Norm, reflex was developed in two learning sessions with time interval 5 day. The development of defensive conditioned reflex was assessed using an 8-point scale (Loseva and Alekseeva, 2007). Rats were presented with no more than 60 combinations of the sound and electrocutaneous stimuli in each training session. The interstimulus interval was 30 sec. Assessments of the behavior of each animal were made on a points scale, according to the experimental protocols. Rats which did not avoid or escape the electric shock but sat in the chamber and squeaked or jumped were assigned one point. These animals received no more than 10 electric shocks after the sound signal. A total of 20 such combinations were presented. Rats only escaping from electrocutaneous stimulation throughout the experiment were given two points. Animals which not only escaped but also avoided the electric shock on 3–4 occasions in a row were given three points; those avoiding the shock 5–9 times were assigned four points. Rats performing 10 correct avoidance responses in a row were regarded as having acquired the reflex. Four rates of acquisition of the reflex were used: slow (> 55 combinations), intermediate (40–55 combinations), rapid (39–20 combinations) and over rapid (less then 20 combinations). In terms of the rate of acquisition of the CTAR, animals were assigned five, six, seven, and eight points respectively.

The mean scores and their standard errors were calculated for the each training sessions for each group, using the assessment method described above, in accordance with the CTAR training protocols. Data were analyzed statistically using the non-parametric Mann–Whitney test (for comparison of different groups) and the Wilcoxon test for differences between pairs (intragroup comparisons), run on Statistica.

Histological and Immunohistochemical Studies

On a day after last CTAR learning session part of the rats from control groups and all rats with transplants were narcotized, the brain was perfused with 4% paraformaldehyde in PBS (pH 7.2–7.4) and treated with 30% sucrose. Coronal 20 µm brain sections were cut, using a freezing microtome, and mounted on slides covered with gelatin. Brain slices from all groups were used for histological study. Sections from brains with transplants were assessed immunohistochemically.

For histological analysis, the Nissle staining of frozen section of rat brain from all groups (Norm, n = 4; HH, n = 5; HH + S, n = 6; HH + TNSC, n = 6; HH + TMSC, n = 5) was used. From each rat, four brain sections were analyzed. It is known that hypoxia leads to focal or diffusion degeneration in brain. Such degeneration leads to wrinkling or edema of cells. Therefore the percentage ratio of normal, wrinkled and edematic neurons (25 cells per each section, 100 cells per rat) was determined in the neocortex (V layer) of contralateral nonoperated brain hemisphere. These types of neurons reflect their structure-functional state. Calculation of neurons were performed in random field of view with magnification 800, using microscope Axioplan 2 (Zeiss, Germany). Data were analyzed statistically using the non-parametric Kholmogorov-Smirnov test (for comparison of different groups) run on Statistica.

For immunohistochemical analysis, brain sections from groups with transplants (HH + TNSC, n = 6; HH + TMSC, n = 5) were used. However, as was shown by us earlier, MSC were eliminated by day 20 after transplantation. Therefore, it was decided to do immunohistochemical analysis of the MSC transplants from group (HH + TMSC, n = 5) at day 10 after transplantation.

The brain sections for immunohistochemical study were assayed using primary antibodies against next proteins-markers: human nestin (Abcam, 1:100 and Chemicon, 1:200), vimentin (Chemicon, without dilution), β-tubulin III (Abcam, 1:100), glio fibrillary acid protein (GFAP) (Chemicon, 1:200), Ki61 (Abcam, 1:50), fibronectine (Santa Crus, 1:100), neurofilaments (ICN, 1:10) and human cell nuclei (hNuc, 1:50, Chemicon). For staining, the tissue specimens were incubated over night (4°C) in solution of primary antibodies. After washing in PBS, material was treated for 2 hr at room t° in solution of secondary goat anti rabbit antibodies (Jackson, 1:100, conjugated with fluorescence dye Texas Red) and mouse (Jackson, 1:100, conjugated with fluorescence dye Cy-2). Double immunocytochemical staining was performed by simultaneous incubation with primary antibodies of different host animals and secondary antibodies labeled with different fluorescence dyes. When needed, sections were stained with nuclear fluorescence dye Hoechst 33342, in concentration of 5 µg/kg (Sigma). All specimens were mounted in glycerol, covered with cover slide and examined in luminescent or combined light. Photographs were made using digital camera Nikon CoolPix 4500.

DISCUSSION

According to the results of present work, all groups of rats after hypoxia failed to develop defensive reflex worth than group Norm, which agrees with literature data (Girman and Golovina, 1989). At the same time among rat groups with hypoxia, the group with NSC transplants demonstrated best results. Group with MSK transplants was in a level with group with HH showing tendency to improve compared with sham operated group.

Analysis of morpho-functional state of neurons in the neocortex of contralateral nonoperated brain hemisphere showed that there was no difference in this respect between groups with transplants of both NSC and MSC. Ratio of cell types in these groups was worse than in group Norm, but better, than in control groups with hypoxia without transplantation. So, in the latest period after transplantation in rat brain after hypoxia the neuroprotective influence of both human NSC and MSC was observed.

To determine the effects of the human NSC and MSC transplantation on learning and state of brain of rat-recipients, cells of these transplants were analyzed. As was shown by us earlier, cultured human NSC contain all cell types capable of neuronal differentiations, including stem cells, committed cells, early neuroblasts and astrocytes (Aleksandrova et al., 2002, 2005), that agrees with literature data (Wen et al., 2009). In present work, it was established that NSK transplanted in rat brain practically did not provoke the immune reaction, survived successfully and kept neurogenic potential. It is known, that factors of adult brain microenvironment maintain the differentiation of different types of neural cells from NSC, their migration, reciprocal growth of processes and generation of synaptic connections (Cummings et al., 2005). In turn, transplanted neural progenitors express fibroblast growth factor and other growth factors, which can promote formation of neuro-vascular clusters in host brain and improve regeneration of damaged tissue (Jenny et al., 2009).

According to literature data, MSC include the cells of neuronal pool initially (Minguell et al., 2005; Woodbury et al., 2000). But in our previous experiments in the MSC culture fibroblast-like prolonged and spread cells were dominant. They showed co-expression of fibronectin and vimentin (markers of stroma). Among these cells, very few expressed nestin, but there were no cells with markers of neuronal and glial differentiation (β-tubulin III and GFAP) (Aleksandrova et al., 2006). In present work human MSC, transplanted into the rat brain provoked strong gliosis, macrophage invasion and were resorbed very quickly, which contradict data of other authors (Azizi et al., 1998; Moore et al., 2006). Brain microenvironment did not stimulate neural differentiation in MSC, though it was shown in some investigations (Muñoz-Elias et al., 2004), and in our own experiments these cells saved expressions of vimetin and fibronectin, which are inherent to fibroblasts (Table 1).

Table 1. Comparative analysis of the NSC and MSC differentiation in culture and after transplantation in rat brain.

Types of stem cells	Markers of differentiation					
	Nestin	Vimentin	GFAP	β-III-Tubulin	Fibronectin	NF
NSC *in vitro*	+++	+++	++	++	-	+
NSC in brain	+++	+++	++	++	-	+
MSC *in vitro*	+/-	+++	-	-	+++	-
MSC in brain	-	+++	-	-	+++	-

Along with this, an interesting fact that neurofilaments of host neurons grow into transplant area was discovered. We suggest that active processes growth may be stimulated by local changes in soluble and insoluble components of territorial matrix in the MSC transplantation area. On the one hand, MSC release trophic factors, growth factors and cytokines (Kurozumi et al., 2005; Zhang et al., 2004); on the other hand they express fibronectin, which maintains axonal growth and stimulate vascularization (Pearlman and Sheppard, 1996; Wang and Milner, 2006). Similar data about vessel growth were obtained with transplantation of human MSC in the region of spinal cord trauma; meanwhile authors underscored significant individual variability of MSC cultures (Neuhuber et al., 2005).

Obtained results indicate unquestionable advantage of NSC in comparison with MSC regarding possibility to differentiate in representative types of neural cells and duration of survival in recipient brain. Where transplants of NSK after 20 days were viable and did not provoke the immune reaction, the transplants of MSC provoked inflammation, which was expressed in strong reactive gliosis and macrophage reaction in recipient brain and these transplants were completely eliminated to 20 days. These results partially explain the fact that rats with NSC transplants developed defensive reflex, better than rats with transplants of MSC.

At the same time, on the morphological level in contralateral hemisphere, neuroprotective effect of MSC transplants was similar with the effect of NSC transplants. Since there are fibroblasts in MSC transplants (not less than 10 days), so probably growth factors and cytokines released by them lead to neuroprotective effect, which agrees with results of other investigations (Sarnowska et al., 2009).

RESULTS

Conditioned Two-way Avoidance Reflex (CTAR) Training

In group Norm, all rats developed CTAR by second learning session, so third learning session was not done. In other rat groups, CTAR training was performed in 3 learning sessions in 4–5, 9 and 19 days after operation. The results of CTAR training of all rat groups in 3 learning sessions are present in Figure 1.

It was shown (Wilcoxon test) that the only group Norm, studied better in second learning session in comparison with first one ($p < 0,001$), groups HH, HH + S ($p = 0,1$) and HH + TMSC ($p < 0,1$) studied better in third leaning session when compared to first one. In the same time group, HH + TNSC studied better, both in second and third learning session, in comparison with first one (p = 0,1; tendency).

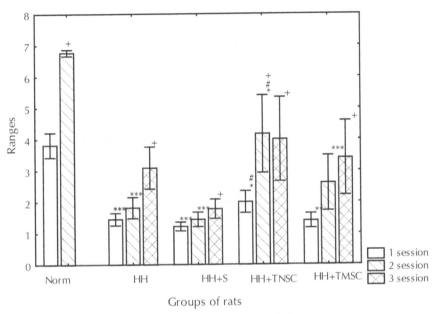

Figure 1. Two-way avoidance defensive conditioning in a shuttle box test.

Values are the mean ± SEM. Mann-Whitney test: * $p < 0,05$, **$p < 0,01$, ***$p < 0,001$ in comparison with appropriate learning session in group Norm; # $p < 0,1$ in comparison with appropriate learning session in group HH + S. Wilcoxon test: + $p < 0,05$ in comparison with first learning session inside groups. Three columns in each group –3 learning sessions. The names of groups are shown in text.

All groups with HH without transplantation and group HH + NMSC studied worse than group Norm in first and second learning session with high significance level ($p < 0,01$–$0,001$). Only in group HH + TNSC, the differences were less significant (first session, $p < 0,05$; second session, $p < 0,1$).

There was no difference (Mann-Whitney test) among groups HH, HH + S. and HH + TMSC in three learning sessions. In the same time group, HH + TNSC studied better in first and second sessions than group HH + S ($p < 0,1$).

The estimation of mean ranges (8-point scale), for 1 learning session (Mann-Whitney test) in all groups of rats with HH showed that in group HH + TNSK, development of conditioning was better than in groups HH and HH + S ($p = 0,1$ and $p < 0,05$ accordingly), and in group HH + TMSC, this index was higher, than in group HH + S ($p = 0,1$). So, between groups with HH, the best learning was in group with TNSC, which was evident by second learning session already. Group with TMSC did not differ from groups HH and HH + TNSC, but learned better, than group HH + S. Group HH + S demonstrated the worst ability to learn.

State of Neocortical Neurons in All Rat Groups

For histological analysis, the Nissle staining of frozen section of rat brain from all groups was used. Quantitative analysis of morpho-functional state of neurons in the neocortex of contralateral nonoperated brain hemisphere from all rat groups is presented in Figure 2. It was shown, that in all groups with HH, there were less normal and more wrinkled edematic neurons in comparison with group Norm. Only in groups with transplants (HH + TNSC and HH + TMSC), the number of edematic neurons did not differ from norm.

Group HH did not differ from group HH + S in the number of normal and edematic neurons, but in group HH + S there were more wrinkled neurons. It was found that in both groups with HH and transplants, there were more normal and less edematic neurons in comparison with groups with HH without transplantation (HH and HH + S), and the number of wrinkled neurons was less than in group HH + S. So, the state of pyramid neurons in neocortex was close to Norm only in groups with transplants of NSC and MSC, the worse state of neurons was in group HH + S.

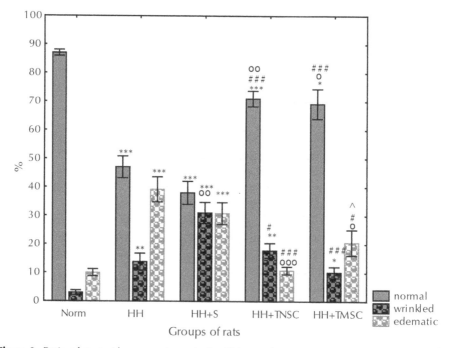

Figure 2. Ratio of pyramid neurons types in the V layer of neocortex somatosensory region of contralateral nonoperated brain hemisphere of rats from different groups (mean ± SEM).

Values are the mean ± SEM. Types of neurons: first bars—normal, second bars – wrinkled, third bars—edematic. Kholmogorov-Smirnov criterion: * $p < 0.05$, **$p < 0.01$, ***$p < 0.001$ in comparison with appropriate type of cells in group Norm; o–p

< 0.05, oo – p < 0.01, ooo – p < 0.001 in comparison with appropriate type of cells in group HH; # – p < 0.05, ## – p < 0.01, ### – p < 0.001 in comparison with appropriate type of cells in group HH + S; ^-p < 0.05 in comparison with appropriate type of cells in group HH + TNSC.

State of Embryonic NSC Transplants in Rat Brain after Hypoxia

Results of histological study of rat brain after hypoxia and transplantation of cultured embryonic NSC showed that after 20 days there were transplants in striatum of all rat brains. Non-scarred zones and regions with moderate glial scars and almost no macrophages were revealed at the boundary between the transplants and host brain tissue. Transplants were vascularized with vessels from the host brain.

Immunogistochemical analysis showed that transplanted cells visualized by staining with antibodies to human cell nuclei were present in the brain of all recipients. Transplants were vascularized with vessels from the host brain (Figure 3a).

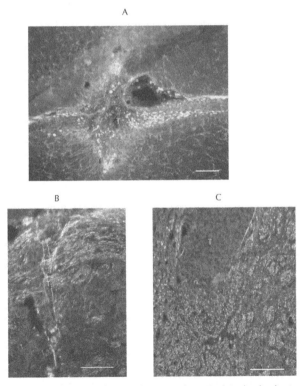

Figure 3. Transplants of NCK culture (day 20 after transplantation) in the forebrain of adult hypoxic rats (A) Transplant (T) of NSC culture led to mild gliosis without formation of glial barrier in recipient brain. Staining with antibodies against human cell nuclei and gliofibrillar acid protein, bar 100 µm, (B) Transplant (T) of NSC culture contained filaments, stained for nestin (vertical filaments). Filaments, stained with antibodies against neurofilament protein, are in the recipient brain tissue. Bar 100 µm, and (C) Transplant (T) of NSC culture contained cells, stained with antibodies against nestin, and filaments in recipient brain striatum, stained with antibodies against neurofilaments. Bar 100 µm.

Most transplanted cells were aggregated in compact clusters, though part of them migrated to different distances. Immunohistochemical staining for nestin showed that transplants consisted of a considerable number of cells that expressed nestin, a marker for stem cells. These cells had small round bodies and long oppositely directed processes. Some processes were directed along the long axis of the transplant or ingrown in brain tissue of recipient (Figure 3b). Immunocytochemical staining with antibodies to vimentin (marker of astrocytic precursors and neurons) showed that there are many vimentin-positive cells in transplants. Neuroblasts, stained by antibodies to β-tubulin III, were evenly distributed in transplants and had, as a rule, bipolar form with processes.

Double staining with antibodies against GFAP showed reaction of host glial cells and differentiation of astrocytes in the transplants. Rat brain astrocytes were slightly activated in response to xenotransplanted human cells. No continuous glial scars were revealed at the host-transplant boundary. Only in some regions, glial fibers lay along the boundary (Figure 3a). Only a small number of transplanted cells underwent differentiation into astrocytes. Double immunocytochemical staining with antibodies to human nuclei and glial protein identified several groups of 5–10 cells expressing both markers. Astroblasts were morphologically similar to nestin-positive cells in the transplants.

Staining with antibodies to neurofilaments showed absence of expression of this protein in transplanted cells. But axons of recipients were stained by these antibodies that allowed determining their growth in transplants of NSC (Figure 3b).

So cultured embryonic human NSC survive, retain multipotent activity, and migrate in the rat brain with extensive neuronal degeneration in xenotransplantation conditions. Cells from all periods of neural differentiation from stem cells to neurons and glia were present in transplants. Reciprocal innervation was observed between transplants and recipient brain.

State of MSC Transplants in Rat Brain after Hypoxia

Histological analysis of recipient brain after hypoxia and transplantation of cultured human MSC showed that in all cases track from entry needle went through the neocortex, white matter and ended in striatum. Both in 10 and 20 days, the similar collagen scar developed in transplant area, leading to strong morphological changes in surrounding tissues (Figure 4a). Evident glial reaction was observed around all transplants. The processes of reactive astrocytes were orientated radially to the transplants with evidence of extended gliosis.

In 10 days after transplantation, MSC were present in brain of all rats (n = 5) after hypoxia, visualized using antibodies anti-human cell nuclei protein (Figure 4a). Bulk of the transplanted cells was in striatum. There was no cell migration in recipient brain. At all preparations, transplanted cells were surrounded with bulk of macrophages that were observed as auto fluorescent macrophages (Figure 4a, 4b). In 20 days after transplantation, into rat brain after hypoxia alone, cells positive for human cell nuclei staining were visualized in track region in two rats out of 5. There was significant macrophage agglomeration in area of transplantation. So, practically complete elimination of transplanted MSC took place by day 20.

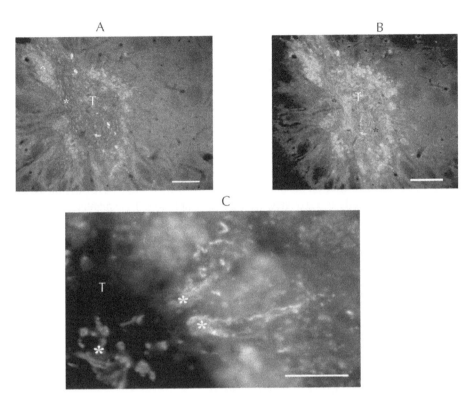

Figure 4. Transplants of human MSC culture (day 10 after transplantation) in the forebrain of adult hypoxic rats. Transplant (T) is separated by macrophage bank (^) from recipient brain tissue. Note presence of the fibroblasts in this T., secreting fibronectin. (A) Staining with antibodies against human cell nuclei (*), (B) Staining with antibodies against fibronectin (*). Bar 100 μm, and (C) Growth of recipient axons (*) into the transplant (T), stained with antibodies against neurofilaments. Bar 50 μm.

According to immunohistochemical analysis, in 10 days cells stained positive against vimentin were present in transplants. This showed that fibroblast-like MSC continue expression of this protein after transplantation. Also vimentin-positive cells were observed around transplants which indicated reactive gliosis development in recipient brain tissue. Besides, vimentin transplanted cells produced fibronectin visualized by staining against human cell nuclei and fibronectin (Figure 4a, 4b). The whole transplant area was immuno-positive to fibronectin, which indicated formation of separate matrix territory by fibroblast-like cells. Interestingly, transplanted cells failed to differentiate down neuronal lineage. However, ingrowth of hosts' neuronal processes deep into transplant area was evident (Figure 4c). Possibly fibronectin depositions in the transplant have attracted murine neurons ingrowth.

Thus, by day 10 after transplantation of human MSC in hypoxic rat brain, only fibroblast-like cells were present in transplants, and by day 20 even these were practically eliminated. At both time-points, gliosis and clusters of macrophages appeared in the area of transplants.

CONCLUSION

It was shown that development of two-way avoidance defensive conditioning in a shuttle box improved in rats-recipients with NSC, but not MSC transplants compared to control. Both transplants exerted neuroprotective influence on the rat brain. The NSC both *in vitro* (before transplantation) and *in vivo* (at day 20 after transplantation) gave rise to all neural cell types: stem cells, precursors of neurons and glia, neurons and glial cells. The MSC population *in vitro* and *in vivo* (at day 10 after transplantation) consisted of the fibroblast-like cells, which were eliminated by day 20 after transplantation and were surrounded by reactive glia. We suggested that effects of NSC may be connected with their good survival and potential to differentiate into neurons and with trophic influence on the brain of recipient, whereas MSC have possible positive trophic effect only at early stages after transplantation. Transplanted NSC hold much promise for replacement therapy of neurodegenerative brain diseases associated with hypoxia/ischemia.

KEYWORDS

- **Behavioral experiments**
- **Brain hypoxia**
- **Conditioned two-way avoidance reflex**
- **Hypoxic hypoxia**
- **Immunohistochemical study**
- **Neural stem cells**
- **Neurotransplantation**

ACKNOWLEDGMENT

This work was supported by the grants of the Russian Foundation for Basic Research (№ 08-04-00081-a, № 11-04-00338-a and № 11-04-00510-a).

We are grateful to T. Alekseeva for help with English text correction.

Chapter 15

Spray Drying in Pharmaceutical Manufacturing an Overview

Prathima Srinivas

INTRODUCTION

Spray drying is presently one of the most widely used and promising technologies in the pharmaceutical industry. It is an ideal process where the end product would comply with precise quality standards regarding particle size distribution, residual moisture/ solvent content, bulk density and morphology. Spray drying uses the aerosol phase to dry the particles. In this process, an atomized stream to be dried is made to come in contact with a gas stream that is at a higher temperature than the liquid stream. Higher temperature of the gas stream causes evaporation of the liquid from the droplets, thus forming particles. One advantage of spray drying is the remarkable versatility of the technology, evident when analyzing the multiple applications and the wide range of products that can be obtained. From very fine particles for pulmonary delivery to big agglomerated powders for oral dosages, from amorphous to crystalline products and the potential for one-step formulations.

Spray drying is being used for various applications, the mechanisms of spray drying to form particles is however still not completely understood. One of the reasons for this is that the spray drying process, characterized by rapid and simultaneous heat and mass transfer between the droplets of the feed solution and the heating gas, is complex to describe in a mathematical model as many of the model parameters are not readily measurable. The feed can be a solution, suspension, dispersion or emulsion. The dried product can be in the form of powders, granules or agglomerates depending upon the physical and chemical properties of the feed, the dryer design and final powder properties desired (Michael, 1993). Benefits of spray drying include (i) high precision control over particle size, bulk density, degree of crystallinity, residual solvents, (ii) Typical application in pre-formulated products, microencapsulations, solid solutions, (iii) improved bioavailability, improved product stability for products with unusual or difficult characteristics, sticky or hygroscopic products, slowly crystallizing products, difficult to isolate products, (iv) Rapid drying for temperature sensitive materials.

PRINCIPLE

When a solution or slurry is poured in the center of the rotating disk, a very high quantity of mist is produced in its surrounding and results in a spray. When a spray droplet comes in contact with hot air, the water in droplet evaporates and vaporizes instantly, and only the solid of feed liquid is left resulting in a dried product.

COMPONENTS

The spray drying system consists of the following:

(i) A spray drying chamber with a cylinder-on-cone geometry, (ii) The atomizer which feeds to the top of the vessel and the heating gas feeds to the side wall near the top, (iii) Thermocouples are set along the wall of the vessel to measure the temperature of the heating gas, and (iv) conical section has an opening at the bottom to remove the spent gas and particles.

A cyclone is used to separate the gas from the particles. The atomizer is used to introduce the liquid feed to the spray drying chamber. The atomizer used in this work can be set to produce 10–100 micron sized droplets. Heaters are provided to heat the heating gas before it enters the spray drying chamber. The heaters are used to generate temperatures as high as 1,000°F. A peristaltic pump is used to meter the feed solution to the atomizer.

PROCESS

The spray drying process is a well-established unit operation in the pharmaceutical industry (Vehring, 2007). To manufacture spray dried dispersion (SDD), a spray solution which consists of API and polymer is dissolved in a common solvent delivered to an atomizer inside a spray drying chamber concurrently with a hot drying gas. Organic solvents are typically used to produce SDDs because the API tends to be poorly water-soluble. Nitrogen drying gas is employed to provide an inert processing atmosphere when processing organic solvents. The spray solution is atomized into droplets using a spray nozzle. Many different types of spray nozzles can be used including two-fluid, ultrasonic, rotary, and pressure (or hydraulic) nozzles (Masters, 1991). When the spray-solution droplets contact the hot drying gas, the solvent in the droplets evaporates, leaving dried SDD particles entrained in the drying gas that exits the drying chamber. These particles are collected and then separated from the gas stream, usually by a cyclone separator. Most laboratory-scale spray dryers operate in a single pass mode where the drying gas is passed through the chamber only one time before it is vented to the appropriate waste stream. Many large pilot-scale and production-scale spray dryers operate in closed-loop or recycle mode where the solvent-laden drying gas is passed through a condenser, reheated, and introduced back into the drying chamber. The optimum process conditions for spray dryers operated in a recycle mode differ from those operated in a single-pass mode due to the influence of the solvent vapor in the inlet drying gas (Dan et al., 2009).

Spray drying is a very fast method of drying due to the very large surface area created by the atomization of the liquid feed. As a consequence, high heat transfer coefficients are generated and the fast stabilization of the feed at moderate temperatures makes this method very attractive for heat sensitive materials.

The spray drying technique involves five stages namely:

1. **Feed preparation**: This can be a homogenous solution, suspension or paste, which is free from impurities and can be properly pumped.

2. **Atomization**: It is the most critical step in the process. A liquid feed stock is atomized into droplets via either a nozzle or a rotary atomizer. Nozzles use pressure or compressed gas to atomize the feed while a rotary atomizer uses a wheel rotating at high speed. The degree of atomization controls the drying rate and therefore the dryer size. The most commonly used atomization techniques are:

   i. Pressure nozzle atomization: Spray created by forcing the fluid through an orifice. This is an energy efficient method which also offers the narrowest particle size distribution. Pressure nozzles are often preferred due to their simplicity, scalability, and ease of droplet-size tuning (Khavkin, 2004).

   ii. Two-fluid nozzle atomization: Spray created by mixing the feed with a compressed gas. It is the least energy efficient method; useful for making extremely fine particles.

   iii. Centrifugal atomization: Spray created by passing the feed through or across a rotating disk. Most resistant to wear and can generally be run for longer periods of time.

3. **Drying**: Heated process gas (air or nitrogen) is brought into contact with the atomized feed using a gas disperser leading to evaporation. A constant rate phase ensures that moisture evaporates rapidly from the surface of the particle. This is followed by a falling rate period where the drying is controlled by diffusion of water to the surface of the particle.

4. **Particle formation**: As the liquid rapidly evaporates from the droplet, a particle forms and falls to the bottom of the chamber.

5. **Recovery and Separation of powder from moist gas**: The powder is recovered from the exhaust gases using a cyclone or bag filter. The whole process generally takes no more than a few seconds. It is carried out in an economical (e.g., recycling the drying medium) and pollutant-free manner.

Critical Parameters in Design

Atomizers: The heart of any spray dryer is the atomizer, small in size, big in importance, installing the right atomizer is essential to spray drying success. The atomizer must fulfill several important functions which are summarized below:

   (i) It must disperse the feed material into small droplets, which should be well distributed within the dryer and mixed thoroughly with the hot gas.

   (ii) The droplets produced must not be so large that they are incompletely dried, nor so small that product recovery is difficult. Small particles may also overheat and become scorched.

   (iii) The atomizer must also act as a metering device, controlling the rate at which the material is fed into the dryer using different types of atomization nozzles like air atomization or two fluid nozzles, airless atomization nozzles, pressure nozzles, rotary or disk nozzles, and ultrasonic nozzles (Patel et al., 2009).

Critical parameters of spray drying include:

(a) *Inlet temperature of air*: Higher the temperature of inlet air, faster is the moisture evaporation. However, this method is not suitable for heat sensitive product (Michael, 1993).

(b) *Outlet temperature of air*: It governs the sizing of powder recovery equipment, higher is the outlet air temperature larger will be the size of powder recovery equipment and conveying ducts and plenums. Outlet air temperatures control final moisture content of powder (Maury et al., 2005).

(c) *Viscosity*: High viscosity hinders correct drop formation. As the viscosity is lowered, less energy or pressure is required to form a particular spray pattern (Patel et al., 2009).

(d) *Solid content*: Care must be taken with high solid loads (above 30%) to maintain proper atomization and to ensure correct droplet formation.

(e) *Surface tension*: Addition of a small amount of surfactant can significantly lower the surface tension. This can result in a wider spray pattern, smaller droplet size, and higher drop velocity.

(f) *Feed temperature*: As the temperature of a solution to be sprayed is increased, the solution may easily dry as it brings more energy to the system.

(g) *Volatility of solvent*: A high volatility is desirable in any drying process. Unfortunately, choices are limited today. In many cases, these restrict the solvent choice to water.

(h) *Nozzle material*: most pharmaceutical applications use stainless steel inserts. However, tungsten carbide nozzles are often available and have excellent resistance to abrasion and good corrosion resistance. (Patel et al., 2009).

Air Flow and Types of Spray Dryer

Co-current Flow

In a co-current dryer, the spray is directed into the hot air entering the dryer and both pass through the chamber in the same direction. Where smaller average particle sizes are desired, this typical configuration of co-current flow is used with a rotary atomizer. Finer powders are normally required for pressing very small pieces or for applications such as plasma sprays. For this configuration, the typical average particle size is 25–100 microns, depending on the capacity of the spray drying system. When using the co-current drying configuration, all of the spray dried powder is often conveyed with the spent drying air to the cyclone collector, eliminating the need to externally mix the two fractions. By using this concept, the yield is normally 95–98%, with the remaining small fraction collected in the bag filter (Ove, 2002).

Counter-current Flow Dryer

In this dryer design, spray and air are introduced at opposite ends of the dryer, with the atomizer positioned at the top and the air entering at the bottom. A counter-current dryer offers more rapid evaporation and higher energy efficiency than a concurrent design. Because the driest particles are in contact with hottest air, this design is not suitable for heat-sensitive products. Counter-current dryers normally use nozzles for atomization because theenergy of the spray can be directed against the air movement. Soaps and detergents are commonly dried in counter-current dryers.

Mixed Flow Dryer

Dryers of this type combine both concurrent and counter current flow. The most common configuration for producing press powders is mixed flow drying with a fountain nozzle. Like the counter-current design, a mixed flow dryer exposes the driest particles to the hottest air, so this design is not used with heat-sensitive products. The air is introduced through the top of the drying chamber, and the ceramic slurry is atomized by a nozzle that sprays upward from the base of the drying chamber. The maximum average particle size of the product discharged from the drying chamber is 75–150 microns, depending on the size of the drying chamber. Using a pressure nozzle, a very narrow particle size distribution can be obtained with a typical yield of 85–95%, depending on the specific gravity of the spray dried ceramic. However, if the feed rate to the spray dryer is low (< 100 lbs/hr), the orifice in the pressure nozzle becomes so small that plugging is inevitable. In such cases, a two-fluid nozzle is used, and the expected yield is reduced to 75–85% (Ove, 2002).

Open Cycle Dryer

In an open cycle dryer, drying air is drawn from the atmosphere, heated, conveyed through the chamber and then exhausted to the atmosphere. This is by far the most commonly used design.

Closed Cycle Dryer

Some ceramic slurry has to be prepared in organic solvents rather than water to prevent oxidation of one or more of the ceramic ingredients. In these applications, a closed-cycle spray drying system using an inert gas, such as nitrogen, is typically used. This concept has successfully been used to process tungsten carbide (hard metals) since the late 1960s. In closed-cycle spray drying plants, the atomized slurry is contacted by hot nitrogen in the spray drying chamber and processed into a free flowing powder like any other ceramic formulation. Dried product is discharged from the drying chamber and the cyclone, and the spent drying gas is introduced into a condenser system. The solvent evaporated in the drying chamber is condensed and recovered. The off-gases from the condenser are then reheated in an indirect heater for reuse in the drying chamber. Due to the flammability of the solvents, the equipment in the spray drying system has to be explosion-proof, and the drying system itself has to be gas-tight to prevent leakage of solvent vapor into the operating area. This type of spray drying system typically operates under a slight positive pressure to ensure that no explosive mixture of in-leaking ambient air and solvent vapor can be created. Additionally, the instrumentation and control system usually includes oxygen monitors and other safety controls (Ove, 2002).

Semi-closed Cycle Dryer

This design is a cross between open and closed cycle dryers and it is not gas tight. There are many variations on this design, with the most important being the "direct heated" or "self-inertizing" system. In the self-inertizing design, a direct-fired heater is used and the air entering the system is limited to that required for combustion. An amount of air equal to the combustion air is bled from the system at the other end of the process. The gas (mainly products of combustion) is recycled through the dryer. The recycled gas has very low oxygen content, making it suitable for materials that cannot be exposed to oxygen, due to explosive hazard or product degradation.

Single Stage Dryer

In a single stage dryer, the moisture is reduced to the target (typically 2–5% by weight) in one pass through the dryer. The single stage dryer is used in the majority of designs.

Two Stage Dryer

In a two stage dryer, the moisture content of product leaving the chamber is higher (typically 5–10%) than for the final product. After leaving the chamber, the moisture content is further reduced during a second stage. Second stage drying may be done in a fluidized bed dryer or a vibrating bed dryer. Two stage dryers allow the use of lower temperatures in the dryer, making the design a good choice for products that are particularly heat sensitive.

Horizontal Dryer

The chamber of a horizontal dryer has the form of a rectangular box with either a flat or a "V" shaped bottom. Nozzles in a box dryer normally spray horizontally, with the dried particles falling to the floor, where they are removed to a bagging area by a sweep conveyor or screw conveyor. Box dryers are usually small and the particle residence timerelatively short, requiring the use of low flow nozzles such as the low flow version of the BETE Twist & Dry, which produce relatively small particles. Manufacturers of flat-bottom box dryers include: CERogers, Marriott Walker, Henningsen Foods, Food Engineering Co. and Henszey Co. manufacturers of "V" bottom dryers include: Blaw-Knox, Bufflovak and Mora Industries.

Vertical Dryer

The chamber of a vertical (tower) dryer has the form of a tall cylinder with a cone-shaped bottom. Spray nozzles may be located at the top (co-current flow) or bottom (counter-current flow or mixed flow) of the Chamber BETE Twist & nozzles are commonly used in vertical dryers. Inlets for the drying air may be located at the top, bottom or side of the chamber. Vertical spray dryers are usually large and the residence time of sprayed particles is relatively long, allowing the use of higher flow nozzles such as the TD, which produce relativelylarge particles. Manufacturers of vertical spray dryers include Stork, Niro, and APV Anhydro Dobry et al. (2009).

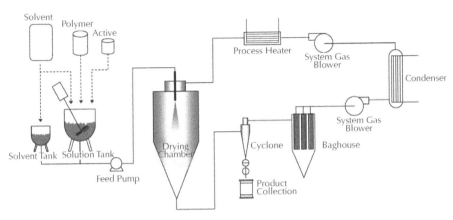

Figure 1. General spray drying equipment configuration.

ADVANTAGES

Spray drying offers several advantages over existing technologies.

Particle size and Stability

In the pharmaceutical industry, spray drying is used to manufacture particles that form the basis for dry dosage forms for parenteral, nasal, or pulmonary delivery, and are administered as suspensions, powders, or aerosols. These particles must be able to stabilize the active pharmaceutical ingredient and provide physical stability for the dosage form on storage. They must have adequate powder flow properties and dispensability, and, in the case of respiratory delivery, suitable aerodynamic properties. In recent years, particle engineering has been used to design complex particles which meet these demands (Reinhard et al., 2008). Hollow, low density particles with controlled surface morphology, particles with functional layers, or particles comprising smaller subunits such as nanoparticles or defined voids, have been introduced (Edwards et al., 2002; Kuo and Lechuga-Ballesteros, 2003; Platz et al., 2002; Weers et al., 2001).

An overview of studies on droplets suspended from thin filaments can be found in recent reports. Lin and Gentry (2002) observed the particle formation process of millimeter-sized droplet suspended from a filament, and investigated particle density and morphology as a function of latent heat of crystallization, solubility, and drying rate. The technique was further refined by Lin and Chen (2002, 2004), which was used to monitor the drying process of milk droplets. Drops suspended from filaments have been used frequently to study the morphology of dried particles (El-Sayed et al., 2002; Sunkel and King, 1993; Walton and Mumford, 1999), beginning with Charles worth and and Marshall (1960), who studied crust formation in evaporating drops. However, the use of a filament to suspend droplets has limitations. Most frequently mentioned are the need to work with relatively large droplets in the millimeter diameter range, and deviation from normal heat transfer because of heat conduction between droplet and filament.

Bioavailability

Since many modern therapeutic compounds are most stable in a crystalline form they often display poor aqueous solubility and low dissolution rates—reducing the bioavailability of the API and slowing absorption. With spray drying co-precipitation of API can be done with a polymer in a stable amorphous solid dispersion (SD), thereby greatly improving the dissolution rate. Spray drying has the potential to open doors for new, important treatments that are currently used to increase the bioavailabity of the drugs.

Dong et al. (2008) encapsulated a poorly water-soluble ibuprofen and ethanol in gelatin microcapsule by spray drying technique and found that the gelatin microcapsule dramatically increased the initial dissolution rate of ibuprofen compared to ibuprofen powder in pH 1.2 simulated gastric fluids. Moreover, it gives significantly higher initial plasma concentrations, C_{max} and AUC of ibuprofen in rats than did ibuprofen powder, indicating that the drug from gelatin microcapsule could be more orally absorbed in rats.

Encapsulation

Encapsulation offers drug developers a number of commercial and medial advantages. Spray drying, as well as spray congealing, makes it possible to create particles in order to fashion specific controlled release patterns and other properties. Sustained release of some antibiotics allows for a reduction in dosage, a reduction of concentration peaks and offers an effective way of treatment for chronic illnesses. In addition to reducing side effects, on a more practical level, enhanced taste masking can be achieved as can physical protection of the API. Encapsulation with a concurrent drier, heat exposure is minimized. The product is usually recovered about 15°C below the outlet temperature (Wan et al., 1992). This has been applied to microencapsulation of products such as antibiotics, vaccines, peptides and proteins. The application of the spray drying encapsulation technique is used to prepare "dehydrated" powders of substances which do not have any water to dehydrate. For example, instant drink mixes are spray dries of the various chemicals which make up the beverage. The technique was once used to remove water from food products; for instance, in the preparation of dehydrated milk. Because the milk was not being encapsulated and because spray drying causes thermal HYPERLINK "http://en.wikipedia.org/wiki/Thermal_degradation"HYPERLINK "http://en.wikipedia.org/wiki/Thermal_degradation" degradation, milk dehydration and similar processes have been replaced by other dehydration techniques. Skimmed milk powders are still widely produced using spray drying technology around the world, typically at high solids concentration for maximum drying efficiency.

Aseptic Production

Spray drying offers a number of advantages over other aseptic drying methods such as freeze drying. By precisely controlling the drying process, spray drying gives far greater command over the shape, density and morphology of the final product.

Inhalation

Pain-free and self-administered delivery systems are preferred by patients and medical professions whenever possible. This expanding field of drug delivery has, until now, been difficult to develop from small-scale to commercial levels of production. There is a rapid development of highly specialized spray drying nozzles that give increased particle engineering capabilities, even on large-scale—making it possible to accurately manipulate aerodynamic particle size and properties. Many spray drying technologies make it easier than ever to efficiently produce therapies in the form of free-flowing particles that are ideally suited for inhalation (Seville et al., 2007).

Compressibility

Solid dosage pharmaceuticals have often required a separate granulation step to produce a powder that has the correct flow properties to accommodate a high-speed tablet press. By using spray drying, granulation can now be an integrated part of a continuous process. This produces a more efficient, streamlined production system and reduces costs too.

Control Release Products

Creating a shell-like structure around the granular allows spray drying to be used for the manufacture of controlled-release products.

Granulation

In general, a spray dried granulation has improved flow, better distribution of drug, colors, and so on requires less lubricant than wet massed products (Michael, 1993). Spray drying results in a shell of concentrated binder at the surface of the granular material, providing strong tablets and maximum use of binder.

Others

Spray drying is used to get concentrated form, high retention of nutritive value, relatively good for heat sensitive products, protects, and retains aroma, availability of seasonal products, needs less space in storage, offers option of a one-step continuous process away from the two-step micronisation and blending phases, they are readily scalable for clinical and commercial manufacturing.

APPLICATIONS

Low Density Particles

A new approach to prepare low density drug particles is done by spray drying. Hartwig and Heike (2004) used a new particle engineering technology with the aim to design low density and aerodynamically suitable particles for inhalation. An oil-in-water emulsion consisting of an aqueous phase containing the dissolved model drug salbutamol sulphate, suitable surfactants, such as poloxamer or phosphatidylcholine, a bulking agent like lactose or a cyclodextrin derivative, and a lipid-phase that essentially consists of a liquefied propellant is spray dried. By means of this process particles of very low density (0.02 g/cm^3) and a drug load of 40% were prepared. The particles exhibited a porous to hollow structure, are thin-walled and of irregular shape. Depending on the composition of the aqueous phase, mean geometric particle sizes of less than 5 μm were obtained. It could be shown that a higher amount of poloxamer in the feed emulsion resulted in particles with improved dispensability. Reducing the vapor pressure of the inner propellant phase by addition of dichloromethane decreased the agglomeration tendency of the powders as a result of the irregular particle morphology and hence resulted in higher fine particle fractions.

Also, micronized but spherical particles can be prepared by spray drying. The amorphous particles are characterized by a low area of contact and a smaller and more homogeneous particle size distribution resulting in a higher respirable fraction than mechanically micronized drugs (Chawla et al., 1994; Dellamary et al., 2000; Vidgrén et al., 1987). Spray drying also allows a control over particle shape, morphology and density dependent on the spray drying conditions (Hickey et al., 1996).

Solid Dispersions

The SDs technology, where the API is dispersed at the molecular or nanoparticle level as an amorphous material within a solid matrix, is a proven, effective technique for improving drug solubility. The SDs can be produced practically at the lab and can be scaled at a commercial level, *via* spray drying or melt extrusion technology. Both processes have advantages and limitations. The advantages of spray drying technology are tremendous formulation flexibility from the wide variety of solvents, polymers and adjuvant that can be employed, the ability to work with temperature sensitive APIs and the enhancement in performance that can be obtained by mixing the API and polymer at the molecular level in solution and then freezing this morphology in place through rapid solvent removal (Serajuddin, 1999). Bhaskar Chauhan et al. (2005) prepared SDs of glibenclamide (GBM); a poorly water-soluble drug and polyglycolized glycerides (Gelucire®) with the aid of silicon dioxide (Aerosil® 200); as an adsorbent by spray drying technique. The SDs and spray dried GBM in comparison with pure GBM and corresponding physical mixtures (PMs) were initially characterized and then subjected to ageing study up to 3 months. Initial characterization of SDs and spray dried GBM by DSC showed that GBM was present in its amorphous form (AGBM). Improvement in the solubility and dissolution rate was observed for all samples.

Nano Spray drying

There has been an increasing interest in the development of protein nanotherapeutics for diseases such as cancer, diabetes and asthma (Larry, 2005). Spray drying with prior micro mixing is commonly used to obtain these powders. However, the separation and collection of protein nanoparticles with conventional spray dryer setups has been known to be extremely challenging due to its typical low collection efficiency for fine particles less than 2 μm. To date, there has been no feasible approach to produce these protein nanoparticles in a single step and with high yield (>70%).

In a study, Sie et al. (2011) explored the feasibility of the novel Nano Spray Dryer B-90 (equipped with a vibrating mesh spray technology and an electrostatic particle collector) for the production of bovine serum albumin (BSA) nanoparticles. A statistical experimental design method (Taguchi method based on three levels, five variables L18 orthogonal array robust design) was implemented to study the effect of and optimize the experimental conditions of spray mesh size, BSA solution concentration, surfactant concentration, drying air flow rate and inlet temperature on size and morphology (axial ratio). Particle size and morphology were predominantly influenced by the spray mesh size and surfactant concentration, respectively. The drying air flow rate and inlet temperature had minimal impact. Optimized production of smooth spherical nanoparticles (median size: 460 ± 10 nm, axial ratio: 1.03 ± 0.00, span 1.03 ± 0.03, yield: $72 \pm 4\%$) was achieved using the 4 μm spray mesh at BSA concentration of 0.1% (w/v), surfactant concentration of 0.05% (w/v), drying flow rate of 150 l/min and inlet temperature of 120°C. The Nano Spray Dryer B-90 was thus found to offer a new, simple and alternative approach for the production of protein nanoparticles suited for a variety of drug delivery applications.

Nano sized hydroxyapatite (HA) particles were prepared (Laurence and Limin, 2004) by sol gel or precipitation methods, in which the products were washed by aqueous or non-aqueous liquids to remove impurities or undesired components. This study evaluated properties of nano HA materials prepared by a spray drying method in which the HA product was not exposed to any liquid after its formation. Powder X-ray diffraction patterns suggested the material was amorphous, exhibiting a single broad peak at 30.5° (2θ). High resolution transmission electron microscopic analysis showed that the particles, some of which were 5 nm in size exhibited well-ordered HA lattice fringes. Small area diffraction patterns were indicative of HA. These results showed that a spray drying technique can be used to prepare nanometer sized crystalline HA that have significantly different physicochemical properties than those of its bulk-scale count.

Nanoparticle suspensions very often present a physicochemical instability during their storage. In order to overcome this lack of stability and facilitate the handling of these colloidal systems, the water elimination from the aqueous dispersions to obtain a dry solid form appears as the most promising strategy. Some studies (Patrice et al., 2007) report the use of the spray drying technique for the nanocapsules (NC) suspensions conversion into redispersible dried solid particles in presence of different water-soluble excipients as drying auxiliaries. Following the combination of additives solutions with NC suspension, the final dispersion homogeneity was favored, avoiding phase separations. According to the size measurement after a simple atomization experiment, the NC which has a thin and fragile shell structure can withstand the shear forces developed for the feed disintegration in droplets. During drying, certain additives molecules are able to act as NC protectors. The physicochemical characterization of the spray dried powders included an investigation of their properties, such as residual moisture content, particulate density, morphology and redispersion in water. Using a NC concentration of 1% (w/v), the best result was obtained with the preparation containing 10% (w/v) of lactose which led to more desirable powder morphology and favoring NC suspension reconstitution with only $\approx 2\%$ of the size distribution in the micrometer range. The spray drying technique is thus found to be an attractive method to improve the NC conservation and facilitate future handling.

Dry Elixir

Dry elixir is a solid form of microcapsules simultaneously containing ethanol and drug in water-soluble polymer shell. The poorly water-soluble drugs encapsulated in the drug elixir are readily dispersed and dissolved in aqueous media as a result of the cosolvent effect of ethanol, resulting in enhanced bioavailability. A dry elixir containing drug elixir in wall-forming materials as a novel oral dosage form was developed using the spray drying technique using a poorly water-soluble flubriprofen (FP) drug (Choong-Koook et al., 1995). The dry elixir was produced when a solution of water-soluble dextrin and drug dissolved in an ethanol water cosolvent system was spray dried. The resulting dry elixir was spherical in shape with a geometric mean diameter of about 13 μm and small pieces of broken shells adhered to large spherical particles. The dissolution rate of FP in the dry elixir within the first 5 min increased markedly compared to FP fine powder and appeared to be proportional to the ethanol content in the dry elixirs. The C max and absolute bioavailability of FP powder, well dispersed FP suspension and FP dry elixir were found to be 14.6, 17.2, and 31.3 μg/ml.

Cyclodextrins

Cyclodextrins have been reported in a number of studies in the pharmaceutical field to interact with many drug molecules to form inclusion complexes. These inclusion complexes have been extensively used to improve the solubility, stability and bioavailability of various drugs (Szejtli, 1982; Uekama, 1981). The preparation method of cyclodextrin inclusion complexes includes kneading, grinding, freeze drying, slow evaporation and co precipitation (Czugler et al., 1981; Kikuchi et al., 1987; Kurozumi et al., 1975; Uekama et al., 1983). Shan-Yang Lin et al. (1989) preparedthe freeze-dried warfarin-cyclodextrin inclusion complex not only to improve the dissolution rate of warfarin (> 1,000-fold) but also to prolong the prothrombin time of Warfarin. They also found that acetaminophen was included in the cavity of cyclodextrinwhen prepared by the grindingmethod and formed an inclusion complex (Lin and Yang, 1986). However, these procedures weretime-consuming and required multistage processing including initial reaction, recrystallization, filtration and drying. Some preparation methods use organic solvents as media. The residual organic solvent in the inclusion complexes, however, could be difficult to eliminate completely from the products.

Spray drying offers significant versatility over other means of drying. One of the advantages of the spray drying process is the direct formation of solid particulates from droplets undergoing chemical reaction during drying (Abdul-Rahman and Crosby, 1973). Aminophylline, pyrabital, and theophylline- phenobarbital complex have been directly prepared from aqueous droplets with the spray drying technique by Kawashima et al. (1984), which combined the synthesis, the drying and the agglomeration process into one process. This technique offers a one-step process with the advantage of reducing the preparation steps, saving time and cost, as well as better process control. Inclusion complexes of drugs (acetaminophen, indomethacin, piroxicam, and warfarin) with P-cyclodextrin were experimentally prepared by using a spray drying technique (Kata and Lukacs, 1986; Tokumura et al., 1985). The spray dried products were evaluated by X-ray diffractometry, differential scanning calorimetry (DSC) and IR spectroscopy. The micromeritic properties and dissolution behavior of spray dried products were examined. It was found that the spray drying technique could be used to prepare the amorphous state of drug inclusion complexes. The dissolution rates of drugs from tablets made by the spray dried products were faster than those of the pure drug and the PM of drug and β-cyclodextrin. The enhanced dissolution rate of spray dried products might be attributed to the decreased particle size, the high-energetic amorphous state and inclusion complex formation.

SMEDDS

In recent years, self-emulsifying and self-micro emulsifying drug delivery systems (SEDDS and SMEDDS) have shown a reasonable success in improving oral bioavailability of poorly water-soluble and lipophilic drugs (Holm et al., 2003; Humberstone and Charman, 1997; Kang et al., 2004; Lawrence and Rees, 2000). The SEDDS and SMEDDS are normally prepared either as liquids or encapsulated in soft gelatin capsules, which have some shortcomings especially in the manufacturing process, leading to high production costs (Franceschinis et al., 2005). Moreover, these dosage forms may be inconvenient to use and incompatibility problems with the shells of the soft gelatin are usual (Tuleu et al., 2004). Incorporation of a liquid self-emulsifying formulation into a solid dosage form may combine the advantages of SEDDS with those of a solid dosage form and overcome the disadvantages of liquid formulations described above (Nazzal and Khan, 2006). Recently, increasing research has focused on this area. A solid state microemulsion for the delivery of cyclosporine was prepared by coating a pre-microemulsion with enteric coating materials (Kim et al., 2001). A eutectic-based self-nanoemulsified drug delivery system of ubiquinone was incorporated into a tablet dosage form, using blends of maltodextrin, modified povidone and microcrystalline cellulose (MCC) (Nazzal et al., 2002). The release of lipid formulations from thistablet dosage form could be controlled by the addition of MCC of finer particle size and colloidal silicates. Pellets containing self-emulsifying mixtures were prepared by extrusion/spheronizationor wet granulation in high-shear mixer, with inclusion of MCC and lactose. The *in vitro* release of the drug from such pellets could be controlled by coating with a polymer film. However, these solid SEDDS were almost prepared by extrusion/spheronization, containing water-insoluble materials as solid carriers. Spray drying has been employed to prepare dry emulsions by removing water from an ordinary emulsion containing a water soluble solid carrier. The initial emulsion mostly consisted of oil, water and an ordinary emulsifying agent, and the droplet size of reconstituted emulsions from dry emulsions was usually more than 1µm.

Some studies (Tao et al., 2008) developed a new solid SMEDDS of nimodipine by spray drying, using Dextran 40 as water-soluble solid carrier. Reconstitution properties of the spray dried powders were investigated and correlated to solid state characterization of the powders performed by Scanning Electron Microscope (SEM), DSC, and X-ray powder diffraction; to determine whether the solid SMEDDS maintained the absorption characteristics of the liquid SMEDDS. A comparative bioavailability study was performed in fasted rabbits with the solid SMEDDS, the liquid SMEDDS and a conventional tablet of nimodipine. The liquid SMEDDS consisted of ethyl oleate, Labrasol, Cremophor_ RH 40 and nimodipine. The solid SMEDDS was prepared by spray drying the liquid SMEDDS in a laboratory spray dryer, using dextran as solid carrier. The imaging of TEM and photo correlation spectroscopy revealed no difference in the droplet size of reconstituted micro emulsion between both SMEDDS. Solid state characterization of the solid SMEDDS was performed by SEM, DSC, and X-ray powder diffraction. The same dose of nimodipine in the solid SMEDDS and in the liquid SMEDDS resulted in similar AUC and C_{max} values, but the maximum absorption was retarded by the solid SMEDDS. The AUC and C_{max} after oral administration of the solid SMEDDS were 2.6- and 6.6-fold higher, respectively, compared to those of the conventional tablet. These results demonstrate that the solid SMEDDS may preserve an improved bioavailability with releasing micro emulsion lipid droplets from the formulation *in vivo*. Thus, this solid self micro emulsifying system may provide a useful solid dosage form for oral poorly water-soluble drugs.

Microencapsulation

Microencapsulation is defined as a process in which tiny particles or droplets are surrounded by a coating, or embedded in a homogeneous or heterogeneous matrix, to give small capsules with many useful properties. It can provide a physical barrier between the core compound and the other components of the product. More especially, in the food field, microencapsulation is a technique by which liquid droplets, solid particles or gas compounds are entrapped into thin films of a food grade microencapsulating agent. The core may be composed of just one or several ingredients and the wall may be single or double-layered. a large number of different microencapsulation processes such as: spray drying, spray-cooling, spray-chilling, air suspension coating, extrusion, centrifugal extrusion, freeze-drying, coacervation, rotational suspension separation, co-crystallization, liposome entrapment, interfacial polymerization, molecular inclusion, and so on (Desai and Park, 2005; Gibbs et al., 1999; Gouin, 2004; King, 1995; Shahidi and Han, 1993).

Although most often considered as a dehydration process, spray drying can be used to encapsulate active material within a protective matrix formed from a polymer or melt (Dziezak, 1988). The application of spray drying process in microencapsulation involves three basic steps (Dziezak, 1988) namely, preparation of the dispersion or emulsion to be processed; homogenization of the dispersion; and atomization of the mass into the drying chamber.

In the spray drying process, the initial emulsion droplets are in the order of diameter 1–100 μm. Before the spray drying step, the formed emulsion must be stable over a certain period of time (Liu et al., 2001), oil droplets should be rather small and viscosity should be low enough to prevent air inclusion in the particle (Drusch, 2006). Emulsion viscosity and particle size distribution have significant effects on microencapsulation by spray drying. High viscosities interfere with the atomization process and lead to the formation of elongated and large droplets that adversely affect the drying rate (Rosenberg et al., 1990). The core material retention during microencapsulation by spray drying is affected by the composition and the properties of the emulsion and by the drying conditions. The obtained oil-in-water emulsion is then atomized into a heated air stream supplied to the drying chamber and the evaporation of the solvent, usually water, consequently leads to the formation of microcapsules. As the sprayed particles fall through the gaseous medium, they assume a spherical shape with the oil encased in the aqueous phase. The short time exposition and the rapid evaporation of water keep the core temperature below 40°C, in spite of the high temperatures generally used in the process.

Direct Compression

Direct compression is the preferred method for the preparation of tablets because of several advantages. However, as specific material properties are required to allow direct compression, materials have been co-processed via spray drying to obtain compounds having superior properties (hygroscopicity, flowability, and compactability) for direct compression compared to the individual excipients or their PMs (Gohel and Jogani, 2003). During co processing, no chemical changes occur and all the reflected changes show up in the physical properties of the particles (Gohel, 2005). Several coprocessed excipients for direct compression are commercially available: ludipress (a-lactose monohydrate, polyvinylpyrrolidone, and crospovidone), Cellactose and Microcelac (a-lactose monohydrate and cellulose), Cel–O–Cal (cellulose and calcium sulphate), Prosolv (microcrystalline cellulose and silicon dioxide), and F-Melt (mannitol, xylitol, inorganic excipient, and disintegrating agent, developed for fast dissolving dosage forms). (Tanaka et al., 2005) Hauschild and Picker (2004) evaluated a co-processed compound based on a lactose monohydrate and maize starch for tablet formulation. Compared to its PM the co-processed material had a better flow ability, a higher tablet tensile strength and faster tablet disintegration. Heckel analysis showed that the spray dried mixture deformed plastically with limited elasticity, whereas the PM exhibited a predominantly elastic behavior. Microcelac 100, a co-processed spray dried filler/binder for direct compression and composed of 25% w/w microcrystalline cellulose and 75%w/w α-lactose monohydrate, showed superior flow ability and binding properties compared to PMs of microcrystalline cellulose with different lactose grades for example α-lactose monohydrate (lactose 100 M), anhydric β-lactose (Pharmatose DCL21), and spray dried lactose (Pharmatose DCL11).

Synthesis of PMN (Pb Mn Nb) Samples

Lead magnesium niobate ceramics, Pb $(Mg1/3Nb2/3)O_3$ (PMN) and related compounds, are the most widely studied lead-based relaxor ferroelectric materials, because of their excellent dielectric and electrostrictive properties, making them very promising candidates for applications such as multilayer capacitors, sensors and actuators(Gupta and Kulakarni, 1994).The main problem in the fabrication of pure perovskite PMN samples is the formation of the unwanted pyrochlore phase that decreases the dielectric and electromechanical performances of the material (Costa et al., 2002). Several processes were investigated to eliminate or reduce the pyrochlore phase, including either the modification of the mixed oxide procedure, such as the "columbite" method, or wet chemical processes, such as chemical precipitation (co-precipitation, stepwise precipitation, partial oxalate route), sol-gel and citrate routes, freeze-drying, and spray-pyrolysis methods (Costa et al., 2002). The main feature of the wet chemical processes is the mixing of the reagents at a molecular level that leads to a strong improvement of reactivity of the precursor powders. The enhancement of reactivity is particularly important for the PMN system where incomplete reactions between components involve the formation of parasite secondary phases. Although the spray drying is commonly applied to water-based ceramic suspensions for the powders atomization (Lukasiewicz, 1989), its application to solutions is especially useful in the preparation of multi component ceramic powders whose properties are strongly dependent on chemical homogeneity (Johnson, 1987). Unlike spray-pyrolysis, where the solution is dried and precursor directly pyrolized inside the reaction chamber, the spray drying process atomizes the solution producing an amorphous powder which is calcined in a further step. The spray drying of solutions is a direct synthesis from solution (DSS) method never used before to obtain PMN powders. In comparison to other solution techniques, the spray drying process is quite simple and permits a good theoretical simulation of experimental parameters to optimize the process.

Vaccines

Some of the key considerations involved in preparing a dry vaccine formulation include: (1) the exposure of virus particles to various thermal and mechanical stresses during processing, (2) the selection of excipients which confer protection against a variety of degradation mechanisms. Furthermore, the formulation components must be compatible with the processing method chosen, for example avoidance of crystallization and collapse of glassy matrix during a freeze drying process. Depending on the freezing rate and the buffer component(s) chosen, the occurrence of salt crystallization (and its rate of formation) is affected, potentially leading to pH change that may affect the stability of the labile biomolecules (Pikal-Cleland et al., 2000). In addition, with selective crystallization, the effectiveness of excipients as stabilizers may decrease and the concentration of the remaining unfrozen formulation increases, potentially leading to aggregation (Izutsu et al., 1993, Randolph, 1997). With spray drying, the extent of virus enrichment on the surface of the spray dried particles is expected to have a strong influence on its storage stability (Abdul-Fattah et al., 2007). Spray drying provides advantages of offering high volume product throughput (>5000 lb/hr) and reduced manufacturing times over other protein preservation/drying technologies such as freeze drying. While the spray dried powders could easily be reconstituted for injection, they could also be incorporated into a variety of other dosage formats, including, but not limited to, mucoadhesive thin films, transdermal skin patches, controlled release polymer matrices, enteric coated tablets, wafers, and aerosizable powders for inhalation, offering a multitude of options available for the route of vaccination as well as for the delivery device/vehicle (Satoshi et al., 2009). The aerosol route is particularly appropriate for pharmaceuticals and biotherapeutics that target the lungs, and some of the formulations described herein have aerosol properties that may allow for measles vaccination by the pulmonary route.

Satoshi et al., (2009) used a combination of unique stabilizers and mild spray drying process conditions to produce heat-stable measles vaccine powder. Live attenuated measles vaccine from Serum Institute of India was formulated with pharmaceutically approved stabilizers, including sugars, proteins, amino acids, polymers, surfactants, and plasticizers, as well as charged ions. In addition, the effects of buffer salt and pH on the storage stability of measles virus were examined. The potency of the dried vaccine stored at several temperatures was quantified by TCID50 assay on Vero cells. As a comparison to other process methods, lead formulations were also subjected to freeze drying and foam drying. The optimized measles vaccine formulation tested at 37°C was stable for approximately 8 weeks (i.e., time for 1 log TCID50 loss). The measles titer decreased in a bi-phasic manner, with initial rapid loss within the first week but relative stability thereafter. Key stabilizers identified during the formulation screening processes were L-arginine, human serum albumin, and a combination of divalent cations. Spray drying was identified as the optimal processing method for the preparation of dried vaccine, as it generally resulted in negligible process loss and comparable, if not better storage stability, with respect to the other processes. Processing methods and formulation components were developed that produced a measles vaccine stable for up to 8 weeks at 37°C, which surpassed the WHO requirement for heat stability of 1 week at that temperature.

Dry Powder Inhalers (DPI)

In the case of spray dried powders for inhalation, residual moisture can also have an effect on powder dispersion and powder flow characteristics. Efficient and reproducible particle disaggregation is essential for the generation of a respirable powder aerosol. The presence of moisture may influence the cohesive nature of the powder and lead to the formation of aggregates. For inhalation drug delivery applications, this task is especially challenging as the particles are designed to be aerodynamically light with small stokes number characteristics such as low terminal velocity and the ability to readily follow gas flow streams. Such particle performance attributes are highly desired for dry powder inhalation products which target the deep lung to enable efficient particle dispersion and drug transport past the upper airway constrictions. Small particles are cohesive in nature, which leads to agglomeration, poor flow ability and hygroscopicity, the latter owing to the fact that an amorphous solid phase is invariably produced as a result of a typical milling-based particle reduction method (Jeffery et al., 2004).

A clear advantage of spray drying process is that it is readily scalable for clinical and commercial manufacturing. Dry particles produced from spray drying are single particles comprised of drug alone or drug and excipients with low levels of residual solvent. Particle properties such as particle size, morphology and composition can be readily manipulated to obtain highly dispersible particles, avoiding the use of a secondary processing, such particle size as blending with a larger particle size carrier. It has been demonstrated that spray drying is suitable for the production of dry powders containing proteins and peptides since they can be processed from a stable solution and biological activity is kept intact upon reconstitution. Spray dried powders for inhalation aerosol particles can carry up to 100% drug (compared to only 1–2% carried by liquid aerosol particles). As a result, larger therapeutic doses can be delivered to the alveolar epithelium through dry powder system. An additional advantage of dry powder formulations is the low-microbial growth thereby minimizing the potential to cause serious lung infection. Some disadvantages of using spray drying to produce aerosol particles include the fact that yield is dependent on the formulation and that in the case of proteins heat inactivation and surface denaturation are possible. These issues can be addressed through both formulation and process design and reduce the effective shear and thermal exposure during processing. Some examples include nanoparticles used for aerosol delivery to the lung, amino acid modified spray dried powders with enhanced aerosolisation properties for pulmonary drug delivery. B-estradiol dry powder inhalers for aerosolisation properties (Helena ans Rita, 2009).

Protein Stabilization via Spray Drying

Therapeutic peptides and proteins are far more stable in the solid state compared to the liquid state. Delicate proteins often significantly degrade within hours when held at room temperature in the liquid state. A recent survey has shown that 12 of the 30 commercial products are available only as dry powder and 28 of the 30 require refrigeration. Improved chemical stability may be obtained by removing water from the formulations. Upon water removal, the protein or peptide is molecularly dispersed in non-crystalline solid, also known as glassy solid. The molecular mobility of the therapeutic protein or peptide is greatly reduced compared to the liquid state and thus chemical stability is improved. Extent of molecular mobility depends on the glass transition temperature which should be maintained well above storage temperature (Bodmeier and Chen, 1998).

CONCLUSION

The production of particles from the process of spraying has gained much attention in recent years. The basic theory of spray drying is now well understood and enables excellent control of the critical variables which affect product attributes. Multistage processes, new spray techniques, and temperature-gradient systems hold promise for future pharmaceutical application (Masters, 1991). One can conclude that spray drying is a process that meets the demand of sophisticated drug delivery systems through an efficient, one-step process capable of precise particle size and drug content control.

KEYWORDS

- **Bovine serum albumin**
- **Flubriprofen**
- **Glibenclamide**
- **Hydroxyapatite**
- **Nanocapsules**
- **Physical mixtures**
- **Solid dispersion**
- **Spray dried dispersion**
- **Spray drying**

ACKNOWLEDGMENT

The author wishes to acknowledge the support of her post graduate students Mrs. Preethi Mylavarapu and Ms. Mownika G in survey of literature.

Chapter 16

RNA nanotechnology in Nanomedicine

Wade W. Grabow, Kirill A. Afonin, Paul Zakrevsky, Faye M. Walker,
Erin R. Calkins, Cody Geary, Wojciech Kasprzak, Eckart Bindewald,
Bruce A. Shapiro, and Luc Jaeger

INTRODUCTION

The impact that ribonucleic acid (RNA) has had in the multi-disciplined field of nano-technology is evident by the emergence of the subfield known as RNA nanotechnology or ribo-nanotechnology (Guo, 2010). Ribo-nanotechnology has been able to establish itself and stand on its own due to the unique structural and chemical properties of RNA. In many ways, RNA constitutes a satisfying compromise between the relatively simple self-assembling principles associated with DNA and the diverse structural and functional attributes of proteins. The development of RNA as a viable building block for nano-scale self-assembly has been facilitated by the atomic scale solution structures associated with large naturally occurring RNAs like the ribosome and the group I intron (Ban et al., 2000; Cate et al., 1996; Yusupov et al., 2001). Recently, the rapid emergence of RNA as an important tool for applications in the more focused fields of nanomedicine, and synthetic biology results from an increased appreciation of non-coding RNA (ncRNA) and their assorted biological roles (Eddy, 2001). In the past several decades molecular biology has revealed that RNAs function as carriers of information messenger RNA (mRNA), informational translators transfer RNA (tRNAs), enzymatic catalysts (ribozymes) (Cech et al., 1981; Nissen et al., 2000), structural elements (DsrA and GcvB) (Busi et al., 2009; Cayrol et al., 2009a, 2009b), processing guides (snoRNAs) (Steitz and Tycowski, 1995), allosteric sensors (riboswitches) (Winkler et al., 2002), as well as gene regulators (siRNAs and miRNAs) (Tuschl, 2001).

Considering the vast set of cellular responsibilities, RNA molecules constitute key cellular biopolymers having incredible potential as therapeutics drugs. The rational development of scaffolds that allow precise positioning of different therapeutic agents or biosensors in three-dimensional (3D) space is an important goal in nanomedicine. In this manner, nanoscaffolds offer the ability to simultaneously deliver specific therapeutics and control their respective composition and stoichiometry. Because of their inherent self-assembly and therapeutic properties, RNA nanostructures offer unique scaffolds that can potentially be used as functional structures to offer new applications in nanomedicine and synthetic biology.

THE PRESENT STATE OF RIBO-NANOTECHNOLOGY

The remarkable potential of RNA for nanomedicine applications (Davis et al., 2010; Grabow et al., 2011; Guo et al., 2010; Heidel and Davis, 2011; Shukla et al., 2011; Tarapore et al., 2011; Venkataraman et al., 2010), in many ways, depends upon the development of design strategies aimed at controlling the synthesis and folding of artificial RNA architectures for assembling multifunctional RNA components inside and outside cellular systems. Tremendous progress has been achieved towards this end in the past few years. For example, previous work in RNA nanotechnology (Guo, 2010) has demonstrated the design of modular RNA units forming dimers (Afonin et al., 2008; Jaeger et al., 2001), functionalized closed trimers (Khaled et al., 2005), hexamers (Grabow et al., 2011; Guo, 2002), 1D and 2D arrays (Nasalean et al., 2006; Severcan et al., 2010). The use of tertiary assemblies of RNA that have been rationally engineered to assemble into thermostable nanoparticles garnering increased resistance to nuclease cleavage (Grabow et al., 2011; Severcan et al., 2010). The discovery and redesign of the packaging RNA (pRNA), part of the DNA-packaging motor of Bacteriophage Phi29, has been used to demonstrate many of the advantages associated with RNA nanotechnology (Guo et al., 2005; Shu et al., 2011a; Tarapore et al., 2011). Furthermore, extensive studies of RNA assemblies that assemble via kissing-loop interactions (Chworos et al., 2004; Grabow et al., 2011; Severcan et al., 2009a, 2010) and are stabilized by the tertiary folding multi-helix junctions (Geary et al., 2011) have provided valuable experimental insight into some of the thermodynamic constraints that dominate RNA folding.

Clearly, the current state of the art in RNA nanotechnology pales in comparison to natural cellular machineries like the ribosome (Figure 1(A)) (Ramakrishnan, 2010; Steitz, 2010; Yonath, 2010), spliceosome (Ohi et al., 2007; Sander et al., 2006) or the pRNA motor of bacteriophage Phi29 (Morais, Koti et al. 2008; Simpson et al., 2000) which exemplify the ability of RNA both to self-assemble into highly complex nanoparticles and to carry out highly sophisticated functions. It is apparent that even larger RNA architectures based on ncRNA might be able to form naturally in cells (Busi et al., 2009; Cayrol et al., 2009a, 2009b). However, most of these types of cellular RNA nanostructures also rely on proteins to fold and assemble into functional RNA-based complexes. One key issue that remains for the development of more complex architectures pertains to the advancement of efficient strategies for designing and producing 3D multifunctional RNA architectures that fold under isothermal conditions within real cellular contexts. The kinetic control of RNA folding and assembly during transcription in a cell is a far more challenging task than its thermodynamic control in a test tube (e.g., Feng et al., 2011; Jomaa et al., 2011).

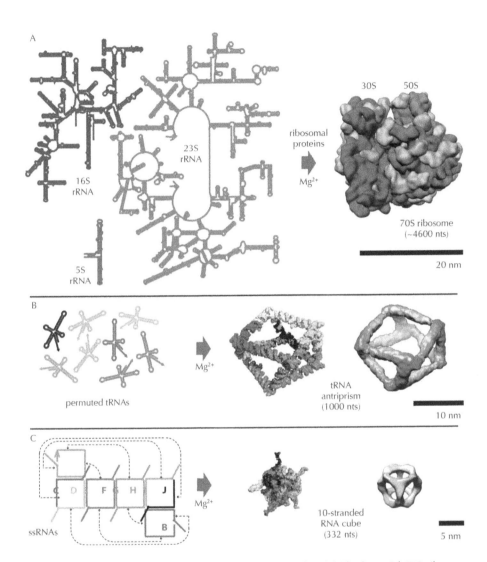

Figure 1. Examples of natural and artificial RNA nanoparticles. (A) The bacterial 70S ribosome includes at least three rRNAs totaling 4,600 nucleotides (nts), which represent two third of the total mass of the ribosome, (B) The tRNA antiprism is formed by thermodynamic control of the self-assembly of eight RNA units based on the tRNA fold. This polyhedral structure was solved at 24.5 E resolution by single particle reconstruction cryo-EM (Severcan et al., 2010), and (C) The 10-stranded cube is formed by isothermal self-assembly of ten RNA strands during *in vitro* transcription. This polyhedral structure was solved at 11.7 E resolution by single particle reconstruction cryo-EM (Afonin et al., 2010).

RNA-based nano-scaffols

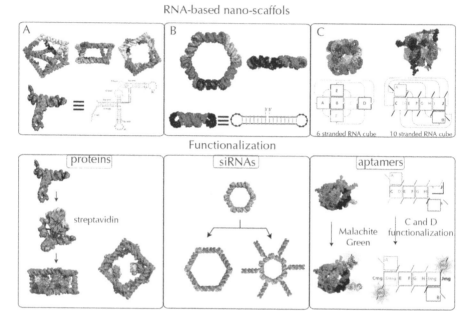

Figure 2. RNA nano-scaffolds assembled through the RNA architectonics strategy relying on pre-folded RNA structural motifs (A, B) forming (A) RNA antiprism, (B) RNA nanorings, and (C) single stranded RNAs forming hexameric cubes based on single-stranded tile design strategy. Lower panels demonstrate ways in which the nanoparticles have been functionalized (Afonin et al., 2010; Grabow et al., 2011; Severcan et al., 2010)

RIBO-NANOTECHNOLOGY DESIGN STRATEGIES

Currently, two complementary approaches to engineer versatile, programmable, 3D RNA nano scaffolds have been employed to allow precise control over geometry, size, and stoichiometry and offer the potential for additional functionalization: one approach based on the tertiary self-assembly of multiple RNA units and the other based on the isothermal annealing of RNA strands. Both design strategies have demonstrated the ability to generate RNA scaffolds that have been functionalized with proteins (strepta-vidin for RNA antiprism, Figure 2(A)), short interfering RNAs (siRNAs) (RNA nanor-ings, Figure 2(B)), or RNA aptamers (Malachite Green aptamer for 3D RNA cubes, Figure 2(C)) (Afonin et al., 2010; Grabow et al., 2011; Severcan et al., 2010). In what follows we describe the current RNA self-assembly designs strategies as well as some of the challenges that will need to be addressed as ribo-nanotechnology advances.

The RNA Architectonics Strategy

The first design strategy, commonly referred to as RNA architectonics, regards RNA tertiary fragments (motifs) as independently stable structures which can be extracted from known X-ray and NMR solution structures of natural RNA molecules and re-combined into novel RNA supramolecular assemblies through 3D computer modeling (see section 4) (Bindewald et al., 2008a, 2008b; Chworos and Jaeger, 2007; Jaeger and Chworos, 2006; Severcan et al., 2009b). This strategy places a certain number of fixed constraints on a given sequence such that the 3D hydrogen bonding network associated with the desired tertiary motif remains uninterrupted. The first artificial RNA nanostructures were design using this strategy (Chworos et al., 2004; Jaeger and Leontis, 2000). More recently, octameric antiprism (Severcan et al., 2010) and hexameric nanorings (Grabow et al., 2011; Paliy et al., 2009; Yingling and Shapiro, 2007) have been designed and characterized extensively. In terms of the assembly protocols, the use of natural RNA tertiary fragments typically requires pre-folding of all individual monomer units prior to their assembly. Traditionally, the pre-folding step is thought to be essential to facilitate the correct folding and formation of tertiary interactions and structural motifs in each monomer unit.

In the case of the nanoring, we demonstrate that the particular geometry of the RNAI/IIi kissing-loop complex as originally proposed (Yingling and Shapiro, 2007) and the design and incorporation of six sequence specific kissing-loop complexes provides complete thermodynamic control over RNA self-assembly to form hexagonal RNA nanorings (Grabow et al., 2011). Because the nanoring's overall geometry is dictated solely by the geometry of the kissing-loop complexes at the interface of the individual subunits, the nanoring design leaves the interior stem available for encoding virtually any siRNA sequence. Two orthogonal approaches have been developed to allow the incorporation of up to six siRNA duplexes (Figure 2(B), bottom). The first encodes siRNA sequences directly within the helical stems of the nanoring units and has been shown to confer increased resistance toward ribonucleases (Figure 2(B), bottom left), while the second (Figure 2(B), bottom right, Figure 3(A), top) appends siRNA duplexes to the periphery of the nanoring by extension of the 3' ends of the strand and annealing the corresponding antisense strands (Grabow et al., 2011).

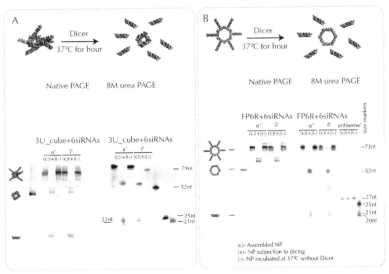

Figure 3. Demonstration of the two design strategies offering complementary scaffolds with the ability to package multiple siRNAs. Native and denaturing PAGE gels showing dicer processing of siRNAs appended to (A) RNA cubes and (B) nanorings (Adapted from Grabow, et al. *Nano Letters* (2011)).

Single-stranded Tile Strategy

The second design strategy used to generate RNA scaffolds having the ability to be functionalized with aptamers (Figure 2(C)) or siRNAs (Figure 3(A), bottom) is similar to well-established methods used in the design and construction of DNA "origami" nanomaterials (Chen and Seeman, 1991; Rothemund, 2006; Yin et al., 2008a, 2008b). However, the higher thermodynamic stability associated with an A-form helix and the increased stability of RNA non-canonical base pairs, presents additional challenges to minimize alternative folding traps and to ensure the successful formation of 3D RNA nano-objects. This approach employs a computer aided technique to engineer RNA cubes (see section 4) that are reported in this work as a second type of functionalized nano-scaffold. Typically, the second strategy utilizes relatively short (26–48 nt) single-stranded RNAs amenable to chemical synthesis and customized chemical modifications to build 3D scaffolds using canonical Watson–Crick interactions exclusively (Afonin et al., 2010) (Figure 2(C)). This strategy is, in many ways, reminiscent of the assembly strategy purportedly used by DsrA in bacteria (Cayrol et al., 2009b). While the potential use of functional RNA assemblies as packaging and delivery vehicles of therapeutic RNAs is presently in progress (Grabow et al., 2011; Khaled et al., 2005; Tarapore et al., 2011; Venkataraman et al., 2010), many challenges associated with producing more sophisticated RNA nano-architectures still need to be addressed.

COMPUTATIONAL TOOLS AND STRATEGIES FOR RNA NANO-DESIGN

The majority of the RNA nanostructures constructed and characterized to date have been designed using a significant amount of human effort. From the onset, various 3D computer interfaces programs like Swiss PDB viewer have been used to manually assemble RNA motifs into specific, preconceived nanoparticles. Manual approaches to RNA nanostructure design and characterization are time consuming and expensive. As a result, a number of computational approaches to RNA nanoparticle design have been developed to aid RNA nanoparticle design. As discussed in previous sections, one can view the design process as falling into at least two categories, corresponding to the RNA architectonics and single-stranded strategies respectively. Though the two design strategies are complementary to one another, because they approach the concept of nano design from different perspectives they require unique computational methods. A brief introduction to some of the current computational-based strategies and the ways in which they support the different nanodesign strategies are provided below. Finally, the role that RNA dynamics plays in computationally accommodating the proper assembly of particles will also be considered. Recently, several computational tools, which have greatly enhanced this design effort, have been developed and are discussed below.

RNA Motif Databases

The RNA architectonics design strategy is driven by the identification and characterization of stable tertiary RNA motifs. At a fundamental level, this requires categorizing the minimal set of nucleotides that are conserved or semi-conserved in a RNA sequence to make the characteristic motif of interest. The sequence parameters represent, as exemplified by the well characterized UA handle, the structural designability of a motif and constitute one type of database required for RNA nanostructure design (Geary et al., 2011; Jaeger et al., 2009). Several databases like Structural Classification of RNA (SCOR) and nucleic acid database (NDB) contain annotated RNA structures classified by either function, type of tertiary interaction, or 3D geometry from X-ray crystallography and NMR experimentation (Berman et al., 1996; Klosterman et al., 2002; Tamura et al., 2004). Similarly, the RNA Junction database, which is composed of over 13,000 junction motifs and kissing loops derived from the PDB database, catalogues structural RNA motifs that contain documented, reoccurring, base-interactions and tertiary contacts that may not necessarily adhere to standard Watson-Crick helical base pairs. The database currently consists of junctions that are defined from 2-way (bulge and internal loops) up to and including 9-way junctions. A key component of the database is its ability to search for junctions that have specified angle ranges between adjoined helices. The junction angle about which helices may be connected is often an important component of nanoparticle design. Similarly, kissing loop interactions, which make up an important motif for RNA assembly, are also incorporated.

3D Nano-construction Tools

A number of design tools have been developed that help arrange, join, and model RNA structural elements in a 3D workspace (Bindewald et al., 2008a; Jossinet et al.. 2010; Martinez et al., 2008; Xia et al., 2010). NanoTiler is a versatile computational design tool that is capable of utilizing motifs found in the RNAJunction database, in conjunction with "standard" A form RNA helical connectors of varying lengths to generate defined nanoparticles (Bindewald et al., 2008b). Besides generating the initial 3D atomic models of desired RNA nanostructures, algorithms associated with the program are capable of generating a set of sequences based on 3D models that have been shown experimentally to have a high probability to self-assemble into the desired constructs. This latter aspect requires a sequence generator to produce sequences that have both the proper intra-strand secondary structure interactions, as well as, the proper inter-strand interactions. NanoTiler not only permits the topological specification of the desired structure, but also the specification of constraints imposed by certain bases to conserve desired tertiary motifs. Examples, of some of these computationally designed and *in vitro* verified structures are shown in Figures 1(C) and 2(B–C). In the case of the cubes, NanoTiler was used to design the cube corner elements *de novo* when no natural motif with the desired property could be found. NanoTiler's sequence optimizer was then able to generate the sequences that were used in the self-assembly experiments. In the case of the hexagonal nanoring, which was initially constructed from six copies of the *ColE1* kissing-loop complex and six spacer helices, the Nano-Tiler's deformation scheme was used to apply translation, bending and twisting alterations to the connecting helices until a connectivity score representing the "goodness-of-fit" between the closing ends was minimized.

The RNA2D3D is another interactive modeling program developed to aid in modeling 3D RNA structures (Martinez et al., 2008). Given the secondary structure pairing information and the primary sequence, the program transforms the paired regions of a secondary structure into idealized helices, facilitates extending the helical geometry into single-stranded fragments (all types of loops), or extending the flanking helical regions into the loops, automates stacking of user-selected helices, and facilitates modeling of pseudoknots and arbitrary tertiary interactions. It also allows one to perform 3D transformations of user-selected structure fragments and to "clean-up" modeling results via molecular mechanics energy-minimization and short molecular dynamics (MD) runs. Some of its modeling features, such as the ability to incorporate fragments of experimentally determined structures into the full model, the ability to connect multiple RNA chains via kissing-loop interactions, or the option to dynamically add base-pairs to the selected helical regions are inherently useful in nanostructure modeling applications.

RNA Dynamics and Assembly

The RNA is a dynamic molecule. Initial computational modeling of the hexagonal nanoring and the RNA tectosquare showed that the 3D all atomic models, when treated as rigid objects, should not form closed rings. In the case of the tectosquare, built out of four monomers incorporating the so-called right angle motif and connected via re-programmed (mutated) HIV-1 kissing loops, exploratory modeling using the software package RNA2D3D showed that the incorporation of one extra base pair in the 5' stem of each L-shaped corner element caused the initially open ends to move (mostly rotated) past each other. More precise RNA2D3D modeling showed that a coaxial rotation of 22° in one stem in each of the four L-shaped corner elements comprising the square was needed to close the square (i.e. bring two halves of the initially open kissing loop together) (Figure 4(A–C)). These results provide information regarding the amount of perturbation that would be required in the rigid building block components to provide closure.

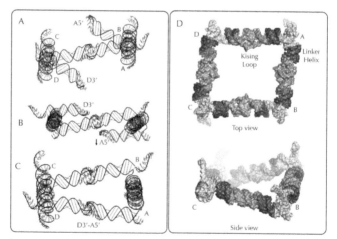

Figure 4. Exploration of the building block flexibilities required to close a tectosquare with the programs RNA2D3D (A–C) and NanoTiler (D). (A) Open structure based on ideal geometry building blocks, (B) Effects of adding one base pair to 5' arm of each building block, (C) Tectosquare closure resulting from coaxial rotation of one arm in each building block by 22°, and (D) NanoTiler-assembled tectosquare incorporating the kissing loop and the right angle corner dynamic states selected from molecular dynamics (MD) simulations and connected together with linker helices subject to controlled distortions within the observed MD limits (Kasprzak et al., 2011).

Ultimately MD studies of component building blocks and assembled structures showed that there was enough dynamic motion, including twisting, bending and stretching, in the building blocks to accomplish full structure closure (Kasprzak et al., 2011). While the survey of the dynamic states of tectosquare building blocks yielding a closed full nano-structure was a time-consuming method, the same conclusions were more rapidly indicated by the NanoTiler, which applied deformations required to produce closure to the helical connector elements, again involving twisting, bending and stretching (Figure 4(D)) (Kasprzak et al., 2011).

Future Challenges in Ribo-nanotechnology
Based on the current knowledge of RNA tertiary motif sequence signatures (e.g., Geary et al., 2011; Jaeger et al., 2009), researchers now have the toolkit to design and construct much larger and more complex RNA assemblies. Despite the fact that extensive studies on RNA assemblies have provided important experimental insight into some of the constraints that dominate RNA folding, more sophisticated strategies, eventually similar to those employed by nature, will be required.

Presently, researchers are far from being able to design multifunctional RNA particles structurally and functionally as complex as the ribosome (Figure 1(A)). Most rationally designed RNA particles to date are "opened" regular polygonal structures. In the future, it would be of interest to develop design strategies for "irregular" solid shapes that do not have internal molecular symmetry. These RNA particles are expected to be more dense and able to compact a larger number of nucleotides per volume than previous RNA particles (Afonin et al., 2010; Severcan et al., 2010). However, additional advancements are to be made that focus on characterizing RNA nanoparticles initially produced *in vivo*, inside the cell, and containing allosteric properties.

Increasing RNA Chemical Stability
The decreased chemical stability of RNA in comparison to DNA, while posing real challenges to certain biomedical applications, is a major source of its in cellular diversity. The RNA strands are continually made, broken down, and reused. Natural RNAs like introns take advantage of this chemical instability to generate the final mature RNA product of a gene. In any case, different strategies have been employed to increase the chemical stability of RNA. The most simple and often overlooked strategy to stabilize RNA can be achieved through its own folding and/or assembly. In the case of the nanoring, assembly of the individual RNA subunits through kissing-loop interactions provides increased ribonuclease resistance not afforded to the individual unassembled subunits (Grabow et al., 2011). Moreover, the use of tertiary assemblies rationally engineered to assemble into thermostable nanoparticles garnering increased resistance to nuclease cleavage while still allowing the incorporation of diceable siRNAs substrates to be embedded within the RNA nanoparticle itself (Grabow et al., 2011). A second strategy employed by the nanoring and others involves creating circularized RNAs devoid of 5'- and 3'- ends (Abe et al., 2007; Grabow et al., 2011). Circularization provides protection from the ubiquitous ribonucleases that attack the ends of RNA molecules. Chemical modification of individual nucleotides at the hydroxyl group in the 2' position of the pentose ring, which is responsible for phosphate backbone

cleavage, represents one of the most common stabilization strategies (Allerson et al., 2005; Chen et al., 2005). Importantly, the incorporation of chemically modified nucleotides produces RNA having similar properties to natural unmodified RNA. The ability to direct self-assembly and to retain functional activity has been shown in the case of the pRNA, while the biological efficacy of chemically modified RNA has been demonstrated in the case of siRNAs (Choung et al., 2006; Liu et al., 2011).

Isothermal Assembly: Kinetic Versus Thermodynamic Control

Requirements associated with controlling the kinetic influences related to dynamic assemblies are highlighted by comparison of the two design strategies detailed above. In contrast to the first design strategy, monomers associated with the second strategy are designed to avoid stable internal secondary structures and does not rely on structural or tertiary interactions. In this manner, the sequence constraints associated with the NP design do not fall on one particular sequence or region of a sequence, but they are spread over the purview of the entire system. As a result, the assembly protocol for the second strategy often involves one-pot isothermal incubation which has been found to be amenable to co-transcriptional assembly (Afonin et al., 2010). In the case of tRNA cubes associated with the first assembly strategy, attempts to assemble monomers co-transcriptionally at 37°C were unsuccessful (data not shown). These results highlight the fact that the design of RNA nanoparticles based on thermodynamic properties alone are susceptible to kinetic traps associated with the assembly process. *In vitro*, kinetic traps can be avoided by using traditional assembly protocols involving denaturation, snap-cool, and incubation at elevated temperatures (~ 50°C) to produce tRNA cubes with high yield (Severcan et al., 2010).

It is well-known that naturally occurring tRNAs contain numerous nucleotides that are post-transcriptionally modified (Limbach et al., 1994). Such chemical modifications are used to ensure proper folding as well as contribute to increased thermal stability. Interestingly, demonstrations that RNA nanorings, which are categorized by the first assembly strategy, are able to co-transcriptionally assemble under isothermal conditions *in vitro* show that the folding and assembly of relatively simple thermodynamically designed subunits can take place simultaneously (Figure 5). This suggests that the incorporation of simpler structural motifs like the kissing-loops and stems used in the nanoring mitigates the formation of kinetic traps, which are prone to dominate thermodynamically designed assemblies under isothermal conditions.

In the case of tRNA, post-transcriptional editing creates essential structural elements at the primary, secondary, and tertiary levels, involving both loop nucleotides and base-paired stems which ensure proper tRNA folding and functionality (Limbach et al., 1994). Furthermore, rRNA modifications have been shown to occur in nucleotides that participate in the formation of specific conserved helices (Mahendran et al., 1994). Using RNA editing to help direct folding invokes two basic requirements, namely the ability to recognize key nucleotides in a given sequence can direct one folding pathway over another and the ability to make modifications on these key nucleotides in a specific manner. Currently, several computational programs exist which are meant to identify pseudoknots (Bindewald et al., 2010; Reeder et al., 2007; Rivas and Eddy, 1999; Shapiro et al., 2007; Xayaphoummine et al., 2005), however, the requirement to find specific points in a folding process that may lead to kinetic traps or misfolded products demonstrates that more sophisticated kinetic folding algorithms are still required (Laing and Schlick, 2011). Algorithms are needed that are able to not only recognize alternative folding pathways, but also identify critical points of divergence so that specific nucleotides requiring modifications can be suggested. As the design of therapeutic RNAs becomes larger, alternative strategies may need to be modeled after larger ncRNAs that have the tendency to form compact yet disordered intermediates. In this manner, the formation of stable secondary structures is coupled to the emergence of a desired tertiary fold (Woodson, 2010).

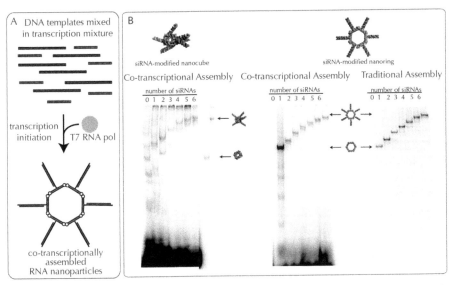

Figure 5. Co-transcriptional assembly of siRNA-functionalized nanoparticles (A) Self-assembly scheme involving simultaneous transcription of individual RNA monomers in one-pot and (B) Native PAGE experiments showing co-transcriptional assembly of RNA transcripts corresponding to cubes (left) and nanorings (right) (Afonin, et al. in preparation). The DNA templates corresponding to each RNA strand involved in the desired nanoparticle were added in equimolar concentrations in the presence of T7 polymerase, NTPs, and polymerization buffer at 37°C. Transcription mixture after ~ 3 hr was run on 7% native PAGE gel without prior purification.

Conditional Allosteric Response

Much progress has been made in the identification, characterization, and employment of natural occurring riboswitches for the control of gene expression (Breaker, 2008; Mandal and Breaker, 2004). Riboswitches can be characterized as RNA elements that undergo a structural shift of their expression platform in response to the binding of a regulatory molecule. Numerous aptamer elements have been both discovered or selected for in laboratories that possess high specificity for different small metabolites. Owing to their high degree of specificity, aptamers have gained routine employment in the quest to deliver drugs selectively to targeted cells (Levy-Nissenbaum et al., 2008). The high degree of specificity however comes at a cost when considering the synthetic design of nanoparticles that are able to switch between conformational states. Natural, coordinated switching between two biological conformations often comprises a delicate balance between two structures having very similar thermodynamic stabilities, which can be directed towards one conformation over the other based on environmental conditions including temperature, the concentration of a metabolite, or the concentration of the RNA species itself (Breaker, 2008; Flamm et al., 2001). Once again, advances in computational methods may provide additional tools to better understand and engineer structures with the ability to balance between two alternative conformations.

Further advancements in nanomedicine and synthetic biology will be made through design strategies involving functional RNA assemblies able to respond conditionally to particular environmental cellular cues (Venkataraman et al., 2010). Naturally occurring siRNAs, miRNAs, and snoRNAs functionally regulate protein translation by their association with corresponding mRNAs. Cancers are also susceptible to translational control and a number of ncRNAs have been identified as reliable biomarkers, used to distinguish cancer cells from normal cells as well as to identify different types of cancers (Mallardo et al., 2008). In this respect, RNAs engineered to interact with biomarkers which are conditionally present as the result of a particular cancer to serve key roles in cancer replication may be a novel strategy in RNA nanomedicine.

Nanoparticle Characterization *in vivo*

Ultimately, the advancements in RNA nanomedicine involving isothermal folding *in vivo* will require new methods for validating RNA self-assembling nanostructures directly within their respective cellular contexts. It is therefore essential to develop fast and efficient methods for characterizing their 3D architectures and structural features *in vivo*. While NMR, TEM, and AFM were initially successfully used to validate RNA nanostructures (e.g., Chworos et al., 2004; Davis et al., 2005; Severcan et al., 2009a), one of the most powerful approaches to elucidate the architectures of complex 3D RNA particles is single particle reconstruction cryo-EM (Frank, 2009). Recently, the first artificial 3D nanoparticles of RNA, a programmable RNA antiprism based on tRNAs (Severcan et al., 2010) (Figure 1(B)) and two RNA cubic scaffolds (Afonin et al., 2010) (Figure 1(C)) were captured *in vitro*.

Two of the more promising techniques for *in vivo* imaging of nanostructures involve fluorescent- and EM-based methods. Recently RNA aptamers coupled to autofluorescent protein complexes have been used in the detection and localization of RNA transcripts in living cells (Przybyla and Watts, 2010; Schifferer and Griesbeck, 2009; Valencia-Burton et al., 2007; Yiu et al., 2011). Similar strategies targeting protein localization have demonstrated the ability to multiplex various protein fluorophores (Przybyla and Watts 2010). Alternatively, recent progress in EM techniques associated with visualizing particular protein structures within cells using clonable EM tags constitutes a second method available for structural visualization of RNA *in vivo* (Diestra et al., 2009; Shu et al., 2011b).

CONCLUSION

The functional diversity of RNA molecules has allowed ribo-nanotechnology to make significant contributions to the greater field of nanotechnology over a relatively short time period. Likewise, the progression of ribo-nanotechnology, in many ways, has contributed to the advent of the subfields of nanomedicine and synthetic biology. The rather diverse biological roles and exquisite self-assembly characteristics or RNA make it a choice material for the design of biologically functional materials on the nano-scale. While significant progress has been made to understand the folding constraints associated with using naturally occurring and artificially designed RNAs for addressing novel biomedical applications *in vitro*, further advancements are required to in order to move toward the level of structures and functions found in naturally occurring RNA nanostructures.

KEYWORDS

- **Molecular dynamics**
- **NanoTiler**
- **Nucleic acid database**
- **Ribo-nanotechnology**
- **Ribonucleic acid**
- **Short interfering RNA**
- **Structural classification of RNA**

ACKNOWLEDGMENT

This research was supported by NIH R01GM-079604 (to Luc Jaeger). This research was supported [in part] by the Intramural Research Program of the NIH, National Cancer Institute, Center for Cancer Research (to Kirill A. Afonin and Bruce A. Shapiro). This publication has been funded in part with federal funds from the National Cancer Institute, National Institutes of Health, under Contract HHSN 261200800001E (to Wojciech Kasprzak and Eckart Bindewald). The content of this publication does not necessarily reflect the views or policies of the Department of Health and Human Services, nor does mention of trade names, commercial products, or organizations imply endorsement by the U.S. Government.

References

1

Barry, B. W. (2001). Novel Mechanism and devices to enable successful transdermal drug delivery. *European J. Pharm. Sci.* **14**(2), 101–114.

Bendas, E. R. and Tadros, M. I. (2007). Enhanced Transdermal Delivery of Salbutamol Sulfate via Ethosomes. *AAPS PharmSciTech.14* **8**(4), E107.

Bhalaria, M. K., Naik, S., and Mishra, A. N. (2009). Ethosomes: A novel system for antifungal drugs in the treatment of topical fungal disease. *Ind. J. Exp. Bio.* **47**, 368-375.

Bouwstra, J. A. and Honeywell-Nguyen, P. L. (2002). Skin structure and mode of action of vesicles. *Adv. Drug Deliv. Rev.* **54** Suppl 1, S41–S55.

Bouwstra, J. A., Honeywell-Nguyen, P. L., Gooris, G. S., and Ponec M., (2003). Structure of the skin barrier and its modulation by vesicular formulations. *Prog. Lipid Res.* **42**, 1–36.

Byung, S. J., Yong, M. H., Kwang, H. L., and Moon, J. C. (2004). Preparation and characterization of calcein Entrapped ethosome. J. Korean Ind. Eng. Chem. **15**(2), 205-210.

Cevc, G. (2004). Lipid vesicles and other colloids as drug carriers on the skin. *Adv. Drug Deliv. Rev.* **56**(5), 675–711.

Cevc, G. and Blume, G. (1992). Lipid vesicles penetrate into intact skin owing to the transdermal osmotic gradients and hydration force. *Biochimica et Biophysica Acta* **1104**, 226-232.

Cevc, G., Blume, G., Schatzlein, A., Gebauer, D., and Paul, A. (1996). The skin: A pathway for systemic treatment with patches and lipid-based agents carriers. *Adv. Drug Del. Rev.* **18**, 349-378.

Cevc, G., Blume, G., and Schatzlein, A., (1997). Transfersomes-mediated transepidermal delivery improves the region-specificity and biological activity of corticosteroids *in vivo. J. Control. Release* **45**, 211-226.

Chin, J. H. and Goldstein, D. B. (1997). Membrane disordering action of ethanol: Variation with membrane cholesterol content and depth of the spin label probe. *Mol. Pharmacol.* **13**, 435.

Choi, M. J. and Maibach, H. J. (2005). Liposomes and Niosomes as topical drud delivery systems. *Skin Pharmacol. Physiol.* **18**, 209-219.

Cortesi R., Ravani, L., Zaid A. N., Menegatti, E., Romagnoli, R., Drechsler, M., and Esposito, E. (2010). Ethosomes for the delivery of anti-HSV-1 molecules: Preparation, characterization and *in vitro* activity. *Pharmazie* **65**(10), 743-749.

Daniels, R. (2004). Strategies for skin Penetration Enhancement, Skin care Forum. *Cognis* **37**, 89-96.

Dayan, N. and Touitou, E. (2000). Carriers for skin delivery of trihexyphenidyl HCl: Ethosomes *vs* liposomes. *Biomaterials* **21**(18), 1879-1885.

David, C. P. (2001). *New drug delivery systems, in Handbook of modern pharmaceutical analysis.* S. Ahuja and S. Scypinski (Eds.), vol 3 Separation Science and technology. Academic Press, USA.

Dayan. N. and Touitou, E. (2002). Carrier for skin delivery of trihexyphenidyl HCl: Ethosomes *vs* liposomes. *Biomaterials* **21**, 1879-1885.

Deo, M. R., Sant, V. P., Prakash, S. R., Khopade, A. J., and Banakar, U. V. (1997). Proliposomes based transdermal delivery of levonorgestrel. *J. Biomaterials Appli.* **12**, 77-85.

Dubey, V., Mishra, D., Dutta, T., Nahar, M., Saraf, D. K., and Jain, N. K. (2007). Dermal and transdermal delivery of an anti-psoriatic agent via ethanolic liposomes. *J. Control Release* **123**, 148-154.

El Maghraby, G. M., Williams, A. C., and Barry, B. W. (2001). Skin delivery of 5-fluorouracil from ultradeformable and standard liposomes *in vitro. J. Pharm. Pharmacol.* **53**, 1069–1077.

El Maghraby, G. M., Williams, A. C., and Barry, B. W. (2006). Can drug-bearing liposomes penetrate intact skin? *J. Pharm. Pharmacol.* **58**, 415–429.

Elsayed, M. M., Abdallah, O. Y., Naggar, V. F., and Khalafallah, N. M. (2006). Deformable liposomes and ethosomes: Mechanism of enhanced skin delivery. *Int. J. Pharm.* **322**, 60–66.

Elsayed, M. M., Abdallah, O. Y., Naggar, V. F., and Khalafallah, N. M. (2007). Deformable liposomes and ethosomes as carriers for skin delivery of ketotifen. *Pharmazie* **62**, 133–137.

Esposito, E., Menegatti, E., and Cortesi, R. (2004). Ethosomes and liposomes as topical vehicles for azelaic acid: A preformulation study. *J. Cosmet. Sci.* **55**, 253-264.

Fang, Y. P., Tsai, Y. H., Wu, P. C., and Huang, Y. B. (2008). Comparison of 5-aminolevulinic acid- encapsulated liposome versus ethosome for skin delivery for photodynamic therapy. *Int. J. Pharm.* **356**, 144–152.

Godin, B. and Touitou, E. (2003). Ethosomes: New prospects in transdermal delivery. *Crit. Rev. Ther. Drug. Carrier Syst.* **20**, 63-102.

Godin, B. and Touitou, E. (2004). Mechanism of bacitracin permeation enhancement through the skin and cellular membrane from an ethosomal carrier. *J. Control. Release* **94**, 365-379.

Godin, B., Touitou, E., Rubinstein, E., Athamna, A., and Athamna, M. (2005a). A new approach for treatment of deep skin infections by an ethosomal antibiotic preparation: An *in vivo* study. *J. Antimicrob Chemother.* **55**(6), 989–994.

Godin, B. and Touitou E. (2005b). Erythromycin ethosomal systems: Physicochemical characterization and enhanced antibacterial activity. *Curr. Drug Deliv.* **2**(3), 269-725.

Gupta, P., Singh, P., Mishra, V., and Jain, S. (2004). Topical immunization: Mechanistic insight and novel delivery system. *Ind. J. Bio.* **3**, 9-21.

Hadgraft, J. (1996). Recent developments in topical and transdermal delivery. *European J. Drug Metab Pharmacokinet* 21, 165-173.

Hans Schreief and Joke Bouwstrab (1994). Liposomes and niosomes as topical drug carriers: Dermal and transdermal drug delivery. *Journal of Controlled Release* **30**, 1-15.

Harris, R. A. (1987). Effect of ethanol on membrane order: Fluorescence studies. *Ann. N.Y. Acad Sci.* **492**, 125.

He, R., Cui, D. X., and Gao, F. (2009). Preparation of fluorescence ethosomes based on quantum dots and their skin scar penetration properties. *Mater. Lett.* **63**, 1662–1664.

Hogaki, K., Ammuaikit, C., and Kimura, T. (2003). Strategies for overcoming the stratum corneum. *Am. J. Drug Deliv.* **1**(3), 187-214.

Honeywell-Nguyen, P. L. (200b). The effect of surfactant-based elastic and rigid vesicles on the penetration of lidocain across human skin. *STP Pharma. Sci.* **12**, 57–262.

Honeywell-Nguyen, P. L., De Graff, A. M., Wouter Groenink, H. W., and Bouwstra, J. A. (2002a). The *in vivo* and *in vitro* interactions of elastic and rigid vesicles with human skin. *Biochim. Biophys. Acta* **1573**, 130–140.

Honeywell-Nguyen, P. L. and Bouwstra, J. A. (2003). The *in vitro* transport of pergolide from surfactant-based elastic vesicles through human skin: A suggested mechanism of action. *J. Control. Release* **86**, 145–156.

http://www.ntt-inc.com/Opportunities/StategicPartnerships/tabid/75/Default.aspx

Hyo Jung Gwak and Byung Suk Jin (2007). Preparation and Characterization of EGCG Entrapped Ethosome. *J. Korean Ind. Eng. Chem.* **18**(2), 130-135.

Jacobs, M., Martin, G. P., and Marriott, C. (1988). Effects of phosphatidylcholine in the topical bioavailability of corticosteroids assessed by the human skin blanching assay. *J. Pharm. Pharmacol.* **40**, 829–833.

Jain, N., Talegankar, S., and Jam, N. K., (2004). New ways to enter the blood stream. Emerging Strategies in Transdermal drug delivery. *The Pharma Review:Sep–Oct*, 41–66.

Jain, S., Bhandra, D., and Jain, N. K. (1997). Transfersome –*A novel carrier for effective transdermal drug delivery*. Controlled and novel drug delivery 1st edition- CBS publishers and distributors, New Delhi, pp. 426–451.

Jain, S., Tiwary, A. K., Sapra, B., and Jain, N. K. (2007). Formulation and evaluation of ethosomes for transdermal delivery of lamivudine. *AAPS Pharm. Sci. Tech.* **8**(4).

Jakob, T. M., Stefan, V., Ann-Therese, K., Carl, S., Jeanne, D. J., and Klaus, E. Andersen (2010). Ethosome Formulations of Known Contact Allergens can Increase their Sensitizing Capacity. *Acta Derm Venereol.* **90**, 374–378.

John, D. and Mullins (1980). *Medicated Application, Remington Pharm Sci.* 16th edition,

Mack publishing Company Eastern, Pennsylvania. vol 87, 1518-1519.

Kikwai, L., Babu, R. J., Prado, R., Kolot, A., Armstrong, C. A., Ansel, J. C., and Singh, M. (2005). *In vitro* and *in vivo* Evaluation of Topical Formulations of Spantide II. *AAPS Pharm. Sci. Tech.* 6(4), 34–39.

Kirjavainen, M., Urtti, A., Valjakka-Koskela, R., Kiesvaara, J., and Monkkonen, J. (1999b). Liposome-skin interactions and their effects on the skin permeation of drugs. *Eur. J. Pharm. Sci.* 7, 279–286.

Koli, J. R. and Lin, S. (2009). Development of anti oxidant ethosomes for topical delivery utilizing the synergistic properties of Vit A palmitate, Vit E and Vit C. *AAPS Pharm. Sci. Tec.* 11, 1-8.

Kumar, R. and Katare, O. P. (2005). Lecithin Organogels as a Potential Phospholipid Structured for Topical Drug Delivery. A Review. *AAPS Pham. Sci. Tech.* 06(02), 56-61.

Lasch, J., Laub, R., and Wohlrab, W. (1992). How deep do intact liposomes penetrate into human skin? *J. Control. Rel.* 18(1), 55-58.

Liu, X., Liu, H., Liu, J., He, Z., Ding, C., Huang, G., Zhou, W., and Zhou, L. (2011). Preparation of a ligustrazine ethosome patch and its evaluation *in vitro* and *in vivo*. *Int. J. Nanomedicine* 6, 241-247.

Lodzki, M., Godin, B., Rakou, L., Mechoulam, R., Gallily, R., and Touitou, E. (2003). Cannabidiol—transdermal delivery and anti-inflammatory effect in a murine model. *J. Control Release* 93, 377–387.

Lopez-Pinto, J. M., Gonzalez-Rodriguez, M. L., and Rabasco, A. M. (2005). Effect of cholesterol and ethanol on dermal delivery from DPPC liposomes. *Int. J. Pharm.* 298(1), 1–12.

Merdan, V. M., Alhaique, F. E., Touitou, E. (1998). Vesicular carriers for Topical delivery. *Acta Technologiae et Legis Medicoment* 91, 1-6.

Mishra, D., Mishra, P. K., Dubey, V., Nahar, M., and Jain, N. K. (2007). Systemic and mucosal immune response induced by transcutaneous immunization using Hepatitis B surface antigen-loaded modified liposomes. *J. Control Release* 33, 424-433.

Paolino, D., Lucania, G., Mardente, D., Alhaique, F., and Fresta, M. (2005). Ethosomes for skin delivery of ammonium glycyrrhizinate: *In vitro* percutaneous permeation through human skin and *in vivo* anti-inflammatory activity on human volunteers. *J. Control Release* 106, 99–110.

Ranjit, S. and Vyas, S. P. (1996). Selective drug delivery through and within the skin using liposomes. *Indian J. Pharm. Sci.* 58(1), 9-17.

Rao, Y., Zheng, F., Zhang, X., Gao, J., and Liang, W. (2008). *In vitro* percutaneous permeation and skin accumulation of finasteride using vesicular ethosomal carriers. *AAPS Pharm. Sci. Tech.* 9(3), 860-865.

Sang, M. L. and Byung, S. J. (2005). Stability of ascorbyl palmitate entrapped in ethosome. *Applied Chemistry* 9(1), 145-148.

Schmid, M. H. and Korting, H. C. (1994). Liposomes: A drug carrier system for topical treatment in dermatology. *Crit. Rev. Ther. Drug carrier Syst.* 11, 97-118.

Shumilov, M., Bercovich, R., Duchi, S., Ainbinder, D., and Touitou, E. (2010). Ibuprofen transdermal ethosomal gel: Characterization and efficiency in animal models. *J. Biomed. Nanotechnol.* 6(5), 569-576.

Singh, H. P., Utreja, P., Tiwary, A. K., and Jain, S. (2008). Elastic liposomal formulations for sustained delivery of Colchicine: *In vitro* characterization and *In vivo* evaluation of anti gout activity. *AAPS Pharm. Sci. Tec.* 11, 54-64.

Touitou, E. (1996). Compositions for applying active substances to or through the skin. *US Patent* 5, 540, 934.

Touitou, E. (1998). Composition for applying active substances to or through the skin, *US Patent* 5, 716, 638.

Touitou, E. (2002). Drug delivery across the skin. *Expert Opin. Biol. Ther.* 2, 723-733.

Touitou, E., Alkabes, M., and Dayan, N. (1997). Ethosomes: Novel lipid vesicular system for enhanced delivery. *Pharm. Res.* S14, 305–306.

Touitou, E., Dayan, N., Bergelson, L., Godin, B., and Eliaz, M. (2000a). Ethosomes-novel vesicular carriers for enhanced delivery: Characterization and skin penetration properties. *J. Contr. Rel.* 65, 403-418.

Touitou, E., Godin, B., and Weiss, C. (2000b). Enhanced delivery into and across the skin by ethosomal carries. *Drug Dev. Research* 50, 406-445.

Touitou, E. and Godin, B. (2006). Vesicles for enhanced delivery into and through the skin. In *Enhancement in drug delivery*. E. Touitou and B. W. Barry (Eds.). CRC Press, Taylor & Francis Group, Boca Raton-London-New York, pp. 255-278.

Touitou, E and Godin, B. (2007). Dermal drug delivery with ethosomes: Therapeutic potential. *Future Medicine July* **4**(4), 465-472.

Trima Israel Pharmaceutical Products Maabarot Ltd., data on SupraVir cream file.

Verma, D. D., Verma, S., Blume, G., and Fahr, A. (2003). Liposomes increase skin penetration of entrapped and non-entrapped hydrophilic substances into human skin: A skin penetration and confocal laser scanning microscopy study. *Eur. J. Pharm. Biopharm.* **55**, 271–277.

Vora, B., Khopade, A. J, and Jain, N. K. (1998). Proniosome based transdermal delivery of levonorgestrel for effective contraception. *J. Control Release* **54**, 149-165.

William, A. B. (2007). Application of thermal analysis to the study of the dental materials. Handbook of Thermal Analysis and Calorimetry vol 5;.Recent Advances. *Techniques and Applications*. M. E. Brown and P. K. Gallagher (Eds.). Elsevier, pp. 670-677.

Yi-Ping Fang, Yaw-Bin Huang, Pao-Chu Wu, Yi-Hung Tsai (2009). Topical delivery of 5-aminolevulinic acid-encapsulated ethosomes in a hyperproliferative skin animal model using the CLSM technique to evaluate the penetration behaviour. *Eur. J. Pharm. Biopharm.* **73**(3), 391-398.

Zhaowu, Z., Xiaoli, W., Yangde, Z., and Nianfeng, L. (2009). Preparation of matrine ethosome, its percutaneous permeation *in vitro* and anti-inflammatory activity *in vivo* in rats. *J. Liposome Res.* **19**(2), 155-162.

Zhou, Yan, Wei, Yu-Hui, Zhang, Guo-Qiang, Wu, Xin-An (2010). Synergistic penetration of ethosomes and lipophilic prodrug on the transdermal delivery of acyclovir. *Archives of Pharmacal Research* **33**(4), 567-574.

Zhu, W. W., Zhai, G. X., and Zhao, J. (2007). Progress on ethosomes. *Food and Drug* **9**(01), 46–49.

2

Abdel, K., Maged, S., Alqasoumi, S. I., and Al-Taweel, A. M. (2009). Hepatoprotective constituents from cleome droserifolia. *Chem.Pharm. Bull.* **57**, 620–624.

Ahlemeyer, B. and Krieglstein, J. (2003). Neuroprotective effects of ginkgo biloba extract. *Cell Mol. Life Sci.* **60**, 1779–1792.

Ali, J., Akhtar, N., and Sultana, Y. (2008). Antipsoriatic microemulsion gel formulations for topical drug delivery of babchi oil (*Psoralea coryfolia*). *Methods Find Exp. Clin. Pharmacol.* **30**, 1–9.

Ali, M., Al-Qattan, K. K., Al-Enezi, F., Khanafer, R. M., and Mustafa, T. (2000). Effect of allicin from garlic powder on serum lipids and blood pressure in rats fed with a high cholesterol diet. Prostaglandins, Leukotrienes Essent. *Fatty Acids.* **62**, 253–259.

Anand, P., Kunnumakkara, A. B., Newman, R. A., and Aggarwal, B. B. (2007). Bioavailability of curcumin: Problems and promises. *Mol. Pharm.* **4**, 807–818.

Anand, R., Patnaik, G. K., Kulshreshtha, D. K., and Dhawan, B. N. (1994). Antiurolithiatic activity of lupeol, the active constituent from crateva nurvala. *Phyto. Res.* **8**, 417–421.

Arora, R. B., Singh, M., and Arora, C. K. (1962). Tranquillizing activity of jatamansone, a sesquiterpene from nardostachys jatamansi. *Life Sci.* **6**, 225–228.

Bagchi, M., Zafra-Stone, S., Sen, C. K., Roy, S., and Bagchi, D. (2006). DNA microarray technology in the evaluation of weight management potential of a novel calcium-potassium salt of (-)-hydroxycitric acid. *Toxicology Mechanisms and Methods*. **16**, 129–135.

Basu, S. P., Mandal, J. K., and Mehdi, N. S. (1994). Anticonvulsant effect of pongamol. *Ind. J. Pharm. Sci.* **56**, 163–167.

Bhattacharya, S. K., Reddy, P. K. S. P., Ghosal, S., Singh, A. K., and Sharma, P. V. (1976). Chemical constituents of Gentianaceae XIX: CNS-depressant effects of swertiamarin. *J. Pharm. Sci.* **65**, 1547–1549.

Boyd, B. J. (2008). Past and future evolution in colloidal drug delivery systems. *Exp. Opin. Drug Deliv.* **5**, 69–85.

Bradamante, S., Barenghi, L., and Villa, A. (2004). Cardiovascular protective effects of resveratrol. *Cardiovascular Drug Rev.* **22**, 169–188.

Burger, O., Ofek, I., Tabak, M., Weiss, E. I., Sharon, N., and Neeman, I. (2000). A high molecular mass constituent of cranberry juice inhibits Helicobacter pylori adhesion to human gastric mucus. *FEMS Immunol. and Med. Microbiol.* **29**, 295–301.

Caiolfa, V. R., Zamai, M., Fiorino, A., Frigerio, E., Pellizzoni, C., d'Argy, R., Ghiglieri, A., Castelli, M. G., Farao, M., Pesenti, E., Gigli, M., Angelucci, F., and Suarato, A. (2000). Polymerbound camptothecin: initial biodistribution and antitumour activity studies. *J .Control .Rel.* **65**, 105–119.

Catherine, C. N. (2007). Cranberry and blueberry: Evidence for protective effects against cancer and vascular diseases. *Mol. Nutri .Food Res.* **51**, 652–664.

Chen, H., Chang, X., Du, D., Liu, W., Liu, J., Weng, T., Yang, Y., Xu, H., and Yang,T. X. (2006). Podophyllotoxin-loaded solid lipid nanoparticles for epidermal targeting. *J. Control. Rel.* **110**, 296–306.

Chen, H., Chang, X., Weng, T., Zhao, X., Gao, H., Yang, Y., Xu, H., and Yang, X. (2004). A study on microemulsions systems for transdermal delivery of triptolide. *J.Control. Rel.* **98**, 427–436.

Constantides, P. P., Lambert, K. J., Tustian, A. K., Schneider, B., Lalji, S., Ma, W., Wentzel, B., Kessler, D., Worah, D., and Quay, S. C. (2000). Formulation development and antitumour activity of a filter steralizable emulsion of paclitaxel. *Pharm. Res.* **17**, 175–182.

Cozier, A., Jaganath, I. B., and Clifford, M. N. (2009). Dietary phenolics: chemistry, bioavailability and effects on health. *Nat. Prod. Rep.* **26**, 1001–1043.

Cruz, C., Correa-Rotter, R., Sanchez-Gonzalez, D. J., Hernandez-Pando, R., Maldonado, P. D., and Martínez-Martínez, C. M. (2007). Renoprotective and antihypertensive effects of S-allylcysteine in 5/6 nephrectomized rats. *Am. J.Physiol. Renal Physiol.* **293**, F1691–1698.

Cui., S., Zhao, C., Chen, D., and He, Z. (2005). Self-Microemulsifying Drug Delivery Systems (SMEDDS) for improving *in vitro* dissolution and oral absorption of Pueraria Lobata isoflavone. *Drug Dev. Ind. Pharm.* **31**, 349–356.

Ding,Y. L., Ma, S. X., Lu, X. R., and Wang, H. B. (1995). Ginseng saponin liposome. *Chin. Pharm. J.* **30**, 414–417.

Drewnowski, A. and Carmen Gomez-Carneros (2000). Bitter taste, phytonutrients, and the consumer: A review. *Am. J. Clin. Nutr.* **93**, 1424–1435.

Duarte, J., Perez-Palencia, R., Vargas, F., Ocete, M. A., Perez-Vizcaino, F., Zarzuelo, A., and Tamargo, J. (2001). Antihypertensive effects of the flavanoid quercetin in spontaneously hypertensive rats. *Br. J. Pharmacol.* **133**, 117–124.

El-Samaligy, M. S., Afifi, N. N., and Mahmoud, E. A. (2006). Increasing bioavailability of silymarin using a buccal liposomal delivery system: Preparation and experimental design investigation. *Int. J. Pharm.* **308**, 140–148.

Fang, J. Y., Hwang, T. L., Huanga, Y. L., and Fang, C. L. (2006). Enhancement of the transdermal delivery of catechins by liposomes incorporating anionic surfactants and ethanol. *Int. J. Pharm.* **310**, 131–138.

Fu, R. Q., He, F. C., Meng, D. S., and Chen, L. (2006). Preparation of paclitaxel-loaded poly (d,l-lactic acid) nanoparticles. *Acta Academiae Medicinae Militaris Tertiae.* **28**, 1573–1577.

Gautam, M., Diwanay, S., Gairola, S., Shinde, Y., Patki, P., and Patwardhan, B. (2004). Immunoadjuvant potential of asparagus racemosus in experimental system. *Ethnopharmacol.* **91**, 251–255.

Gelperina, S., Kisich, K., Iseman, M. D., and Heifets, L. (2005). The potential advantages of nanoparticle drug delivery systems in chemotherapy of tuberculosis. *Amer. J. Resp. Cric.Care Med.* **172**, 1487–1490.

Goel, R. K., Maiti, R. N., Manickam, M., and Ray, A. B. (1997). Antiulcer activity of naturally occurring pyrano-coumarin and iso-coumarins and their effect on prostanoid synthesis using human colonic mucosa. *Ind. J. Exp. Biol.* **35**, 1080–1083.

Greenwald, R. B., Conover, C. D., Pendri, A., Choe, Y. H., Martinez, A., Wu, D., Guan, S., Yao, Z., and Shum, K. L. (1999). Drug delivery of anti cancer agents: water soluble 4-poly (ethylene glycol) derivatives of the lignan, podophyllotoxin. *J. Control. Rel.* **61**, 281–294.

Gupta, P. A., Siripurapu, K. B., Ahmad, A., Palit, G., Arora, A., and Maurya, R. (2007). Anti-stress constituents of evolvulus alsinoides: An Ayurvedic crude drug. *Chem. Pharm. Bull.* **55**, 771–775.

Gurib-Fakim, A. (2006). Medicinal plants: Traditions of yesterday and drugs of tomorrow. *Molecular Aspects of Medicine.* **27**, 1–93.

Hong, W., Chen, D. W., Zhao, X. L., Qiao, M. X., and Hu, H. Y. (2008). Preparation and study *in vitro* of long-circulating nanoliposomes of curcumin. *Chin. J. Chinese Materia Medica.* **33**, 889–892.

Hou, J. and Zhou, S. W. (2008). Formulation and preparation of glycyrrhizic acid solid lipid nanoparticles. *ACTA Academiae Medicinae Militaris Tertiae.* **30**, 1043–1045.

Huffman, M. A. (2003). Animal self medication and ethno-medicine:Exploration and exploitation of the medicinal properties of plants. *Proc. Nutri. Soc.* **62**, 371–381.

Iriti, M. and Faoro, F. (2009). Bioactivity of grape chemicals for human health. *Nat. Prod. Comm.* **4**, 611–634.

Ji, D. Y., Wu, Q. Z., and Ping, Q. N. (2008). Synthesis of PLA-m PEG and preparation of docataxel polymer micelles. *J. China Pharm.Univ.* **39**, 223–227.

Joussen, A. M., Rohrschneider, K., Reichling, J., Kirchhof, B., and Kruse, F. E. (2008). Treatment of corneal neovascularisation dietary isoflavonoids and flavonoids. *Exp. Eye Res.* **71**, 483–487.

Kulkarni, S. K. and Dhir, A. (2008). *Withania somnifera*: An Indian ginseng. *Prog. Neuro-Psychopharm. Bio. Psych.* **32**, 1093–1105.

Kumar, S., Sahai, M., and Ray, A. B. (1985). Chemical constituents of the leaves of fluggea micrcarpa. *Planta Med.* **51**, 466.

Kurowska, E. M., Borradaile, N. M., Spence, J. D., and Carroll, K. K. (2000). Hypocholesterolemic effects of dietary citrus juices in rabbits. *Nutr. Res.* **20**, 121–129.

Laura R., Seijen ten Hoorn J., Melnikov S. M., and Velikov. K. P. (2010). Colloidal phytosterols: synthesis, characterization and bioaccessibility. *Soft Matter.* **6**, 928–936.

Lawes, C. M. M., Horrn, S. V., and Rodgers, A. (2008). Global burden of blood-pressure-related disease. *Lancet.* **371**, 1513–1518.

Lewis, Y. S. and Neelakantan, S. (1965). (-)-Hydroxycitric acid-the principal acid in the fruits of Garcinia cambogia desr. *Phytochemistry.* **4**, 619–625.

Li, H. L., Zhai, G. X., Zhu, W. W., Li, L. B., and Ma, Y. K. (2008). Studies on quercetin solid lipid nanoparticles and oral absorption in mice. *China Pharmacy Journal.* **43**, 435–438.

Li, L., Wang, D. K., Li, L. S., Jia, J., Chang, D., and Ali, L. (2007). Preparation of docetaxel sub micron emulsion for intravenous administration. *J. Shenyang Pharm. Univ.* **12**, 736–739.

Li, Y. C., Dong, L., Jia, K., Chang, X. M., and Xue, H. (2007). Preparation and anti-fibrotic effects of solid lipid nanoparticles loaded with silibinin. *Journal of Xian Jiaotong Univ. (Medical Sciences).* **28**, 517–520.

Lin, A. H., Li, H. Y., Liu, Y. M., and Qiu, X. H. (2007). Preparation and release characteristics of berberine chitosan nanoparticles *in vitro*. *China Pharmacy.* **18**, 755–757.

Liu, M., Dong, J., Yang, Y., Yang, X., and Xu, H. (2005). Anti-inflammatory effects of triptolide loaded poly (d,l-lactic acid) nanoparticles on adjuvant-induced arthritis in rats. *J. Ethnopharmacol.* **97**, 219–225.

Liversidge, G., Liversidge, E. M., Ruddy, S. B., and Callanan, F. (2009). Will nanoparticles deliver? *Drug Disc. Dev. Magazine.* **12**, 30–34.

Lu, M. F., Cheng, Y. Q., Li, L. J., and Wu, J. J. (2005). Progress of study on passive targeting of drug delivery system. *Mater. Rev.* **19**, 108–110.

Malfertheiner, P., Sipponen, P., Naumann, M., Moayyedi, P., Megraud, F., Xiao, S. D., Sugano, K., and Nyren, O. (2005). Helicobacter pylori eradication has the potential to prevent gastric cancer: a state-of-the-art critique. *Am. J.Gastroenterol.* **100**, 2100–2115.

Mandal, B. and Maity, C. R. (1986). Hypoglycemic action of Karanjin. *Acta Physiol. Pharmacol. Bulg.* **12**, 42–46.

Manickam, M., Ramanathan, M., Jahromi, M. A., Chansouria, J. P., and Ray, A. B. (1997). Antihyperglycemic activity of phenolics from pterocarpus marsupium. *J. Nat. Prod.* **60**, 609–610.

Markesbery, W. (1997). Oxidative stress hypothesis in alzheimer's disease. *Free Radic. Biol. Med.* **23**, 134–147.

Mehnert, W. and Mader, K. (2001). Solid lipid nanoparticles- production, characterization and applications. *Adv. Drug Deliv. Rev.* **47**, 165–196.

Mei, Z., Chen, H., Weng, T., Yang, Y., and Yang, X. (2003). Solid lipid nanoparticle and microemulsion for topical delivery of triptolide. *Eur. J. Pharm. Biopharm.* **56**, 189–196.

Mei, Z., Li, X., Wu, Q., Hu, S., and Yang, X. (2005). The research on the anti-inflammatory activity and hepatotoxicity of triptolide-loaded solid lipid nanoparticle. *Pharmacol. Res.* **51**, 345–351.

Min, K. H., Park, K., Kim, Y., Bae, S. M., Lee, S., Jo, H. G., Park, R., Kim, I., Jeong, S. Y., Kim, K., and Kwon, I. C. (2008). Hydrophobically modified glycol chitosan nanoparticles-encapsulated campthothecin enhance the drug stability and tumor targeting in cancer therapy. *J. Control. Rel.* **127**, 208–218.

Mukherjee, P. K., Sahoo, A. K., Narayanan, N., Kumar, S. N., and Ponnusankar, S. (2009). Lead finding from medicinal plants with hepatoprotective potentials. *Expert Opinion on Drug Discovery.* **4**, 545–576.

Mur, E., Hartig, F., Eibl, G., and Schirmer, M. (2002). Randomized double-blind trial of an extract from the pentacyclic alkaloidchemotype of uncaria tomentosa for the treatment of rheumatoid arthritis. *J. Rheumatol.* **29**, 678–681.

Musthaba, S. M., Ahmed, S., Ahuja, A., Ali, J., and Baboota, S. (2009a). Nano approaches to enhance pharmacokinetic and pharmacodynamic activity of plant origin drugs. *Curr. Nanoscience.* **5**, 344–352.

Musthaba, S. M., Baboota, S., Ahmed, S., Ahuja, A., and Ali, J. (2009b). Status of novel drug delivery technology for phytotherpeutics. *Expert Opin. Drug Deliv.* **6**, 625–637.

Negishi, H., Xu, J. W., Ikeda, K., Njelekela, M., Nara, Y., and Yamori, Y. (2004). Black and green tea polyphenols attenuate blood pressure increases in stroke-prone spontaneously hypertensive rats. *J. Nutr.* **134**, 38–42.

Nityanand, S., Srivastava, J. S., and Asthana, O. P. (1989). Clinical trials with gugulipid. A new hypolipidaemic agent. *J. Assoc. Physicians India.* **37**, 323–328.

Owens, D. E. and Peppas, N. A. (2006). Opsonization, biodistribution, and pharmcokinetics of polymeric nanoparticles. *Int. J. Pharm.* **307**, 93–102.

Pappas, E. and Schaich, K. M. (2009). Phytochemicals of cranberries and cranberry products: Characterization, potential health effects, and processing stability. *Cri. Rev. Food Sci. Nutri.* **49**, 741–781.

Pardieke, J., Hommoss, A., and Muller, R. H. (2009). Lipid nanoparticles (SLN, NLC) in cosmetic and pharmaceutical dermal products. *Int. J. Pharm.* **366**, 170–184.

Patel, A. R. and Joshi, V. J. (2008a). Evaluation of SLS: APG mixed surfactant systems as carrier for solid dispersion. *AAPS Pharm Sci Tech.* **9**, 583–590.

Patel, A. R., Kulkarni, S., Nandedkar, T. D., and Vavia, P. R. (2008b). Evaluation of alkylpolyglucoside as an alternative surfactant in preparation of peptide loaded nanoparticles. *J. Microencapsulation.* **25**, 531–540.

Patel, A. R., Bouwens, E. C. B. and Velikov, K. P. (2010a). Sodium caseinate stabilized zein colloidal particles. *J. Agri. Food Chem.* **58**, 12497–12503.

Patel, A. R., Hu, Y., Tiwari, J. K. and Velikov, K. P. (2010b). Synthesis and characterisation of zein-curcumin composite colloidal particles. *Soft Matter.* **6**, 6192–6199.

Patel, A. R., Nisjje, J. and Velikov, K. P. (2011). Novel polymer-polyphenol beads for encapsulation and delivery applications. *Soft Matter.* **7**, 4294–4301.

Patel, A. R. and Vavia, P. R. (2007). Preparation and *in vivo* evaluation of SMEDDS (Self-Microemulsifying Drug Delivery System) containing fenofibrate. *The AAPS Journal.* **9**, E344–352.

Patel, A. R. and Velikov, K. P. (2011). Colloidal delivery systems in foods: A general comparison with oral drug delivery. *LWT Food Sci. and Tech.* (in press), doi:10.1016/j.lwt.2011.04.005.

Peeyush, K. T., Gireesh, G., Jobin, M., and Paulose, C. S. (2009). Neuroprotective role of curcumin in the cerebellum of streptozotocin-induced diabetic rats. *Life Sciences.* **85**, 704–710.

Perez-Vizcaino, F., Duarte, J., and Andriantsitohaina, R. (2006). Endothelial function and cardiovascular disease: Effects of quercetin and wine polyphenols. *Free Radical Research.* **40**, 1054–1065.

Prabhakar, P. K. and Doble, M. (2009). Synergistic effect of phytochemicals in combination with hypoglycemic drugs on glucose uptake in myotubes. *Phytomedicine.* **16**, 1119–1126.

Riccioni, G. (2009). Carotenoids and cardiovascular disease. *Current Atherosclerosis Reports.* **11**, 434–439.

Roby, A., Erdogan, S., and Torchillin, V. P. (2006). Solubilization of poorly soluble PDT agent, meso-tetraphenylporphine in plain or immuno targeted PEG-PE results in dramatically improved cancer cell killing *in-vitro. Eur. J. Pharm. Biopharm.* **62**, 235–240.

Sahu, A., Bora, U., Kasoju, N., and Goswami, P. (2008a). Synthesis of novel biodegradable and self assembling methoxy poly (ethylene glycol)-palmitate nanocarrier for curcumin delivery to cancer cells. *Acta Biomater.* **4**, 1752–1761.

Sahu, A., Kasoju, N., and Bora, U. (2008b). Fluorescence study of the curcumin-casein micelle complexation and its application as a drug nanocarrier to cancer cells. *Biomacromol.* **9**, 2905–2912.

Samaligy, M. S., Afifi, N. N., and Mahmoud, E. A. (2006). Increasing bioavailability of silymarin using a buccal liposomal delivery system: preparation and experimental design investigation. *Int. J. Pharm.* **308**, 140–148.

Saraswat, B., Visen, P. K., Patnaik, G. K., and Dhawan, B. N. (1997). Protective effect of picroliv, active constituent of *Picrorhiza kurrooa*, against oxytetracycline induced hepatic damage. *Ind. J. Exp. Biol.* **35**, 1302–1305.

Saxena, A. K., Singh, B., and Anand, K. K. (1993). Hepatoprotective effects of eclipta alba on sub cellular levels in rats. *J. Ethnopharmacol.* **40**, 155–161.

Saxena, A. M., Murthy, P. S., and Mukherjee, S. K. (1996). Mode of action of three structurally different hypoglycemic agents: a comparative study. *Ind. J. Exp. Biol.* **34**, 406–409.

Sekizawa, T., Yanagi, K., and Itoyama, Y. (2001). Glycyrrhizin increases survival of mice with herpes simplex encephalitis. *Acta Virol.* **45**, 51–54.

Sharifi, A. M., Darabi, R., and Akbarloo, N. (2003). Investigation of antihypertensive mechanism of garlic in 2K1C hypertensive rat. *J. Ethnopharmacol.* **86**, 219–224.

Sharma, R. D., Sarkar, A., Hazra, D. K., Misra, B., Singh, J. B., Maheshwari, B. B., and Sharma, S. K. (1996). Hypolipidaemic effect of fenugreek seeds: A chronic study in noninsulin dependent diabetic patients. *Phytother. Res.* **10**, 332–334.

Shutenko, Z., Henry, Y., Pinard, E., Seylaz, J., Potier, P., Berthet, F., Girard, P., and Sercombe, R. (1999). Influence of the antioxidant quercetin *in vivo* on the level of nitric oxide determined by electron paramagnetic resonance in rat brain during global ischemia and reperfusion. *Biochem. Pharmacol.* **57**, 199–208.

Soler, C., Soriano, J. M., and Manes, J. (2009). Apple-products phytochemicals and processing: A review. *Nat. Prod. Comm.* **4**, 659–670.

Sonaje, K., Italia, J. L., Sharma, G., Bhardwaj, V., Tikoo, K., and Ravi Kumar, M. N. V. (2007). Development of biodegradable nanoparticles for oral delivery of ellagic acid and evaluation of their antioxidant efficacy against cyclosporine α-induced nephrotoxicity in rats. *Pharm. Res.* **24**, 899–908.

Song, Y. M., Ping, Q. N., and Wu, Z. H. (2005). Preparation of silybin nanoemulsion and its pharmacokinetics in rabbits. *J. China Pharm. Univ.* **5**, 427–431.

Soppimath, K. S., Aminabhavi, T. M., Kulkarni, A. R., and Rudzinski, W. E. (2001). Biodegradable polymeric nanoparticles as drug delivery devices. *J. Control. Rel.* **70**, 1–20.

Sreedevi, C. D., Latha, P. G., Ancy, P., Suja, S. R., Shyamal, S., Shine, V. J., Sini, S., Anuja,G. I., and Rajasekharan, S. (2009). Hepatoprotective studies on sida acuta burm. f. *J. Ethnopharmacol.* **124**, 171–175.

Stickel, F. and Schuppan, D. (2007). Herbal medicine in the treatment of liver diseases. *Digestive and Liver Disease.* **39**, 293–304.

Stinchcombe, T. E. (2007). Nanoparticle albumin-bound paclitaxel: A cremophor-EL-free formulation. *Nanomedicine.* **2**, 415–423.

Sugawara, T., Kushiro, M., Zhang, H., Nara, E., Ono, H., and Nagao, A. (2001). Lysophosphatidylcholine enhances carotenoid uptake from mixed micelles by caco-2 human intestinal cells. *J. Nutr.* **131**, 2921–2927.

Sun, H. W. and Quyang, W. Q. (2007). Preparation, quality and safety evaluation of berberine nanoemulsion for oral application. *J. Shanghai Jiaotong Univ. (Agri.Sci.).* **1**, 60–65.

Tiwari, A. K., Gode, J. D., and Dubey, G. P. (1990). Effect of terminalia arjuna on lipid profiles of rabbit fed hypercholesterolaemic diet. *Int. J. Crude Drug Res.* **28**, 48–51.

Tiyaboonchai, W., Tungpradit, W., and Plianbangchang, P. (2007). Formulation and characterization of curcuminoids loaded solid lipid nanoparticles. *Int. J. Pharm.* **337**, 299–306.

Tokudome, Y., Oku, N., Doi, K., Namba, Y., and Okada, S. (1996). Antitumor activity of vincristine encapsulated in glucuronide-modified long-circulating liposomes in mice bearing Meth A sarcoma. *Biochimica et Biophysica Acta (BBA) – Biomembranes.* **1279**, 70–74.

Torchillin, V. P. (2007). Micellar nanocarriers: Pharmaceutical perspectives. *Pharm. Res.* **24**, 1–16.

Tuteja, N., Singh, M. B., Misra, M. K., Bhalla, P. L., and Tuteja, R. (2001). Molecular mechanisms of DNA damage and repair: Progress in Plants. *Critical Reviews in Biochemistry and Molecular Biology.* **36**, 337–397.

Utsunomiya, T., Kobayashia, M., Itob, M., Pollarda, R. M., and Suzuki, F. (2000). Glycyrrhizin improves the resistance of MAIDS mice to opportunistic infection of *Candida albicans* through the modulation of MAIDS-associated type 2 T cell responses. *Clin. Immunol.* **95**, 145–155.

Van, D. E., Beukelman, C. J., Van den Berg, A. J. J., Kroes, B. H., Labadie, R. P., and Van Dijk, H. (2001). Effects of methoxylation of apocynin and analogs on the inhibition of reactive oxygen species production by stimulated human neutrophils. *Eur. J. Pharm.* **433**, 225-230.

Velikov, K. P. and Pelan, E. (2008). Colloidal delivery systems for micronutrients and nutraceuticals. *Soft Matter.* **4**, 1964-

Wang, Q. W., Liu, H., Lv, H. L., Zhang, X. F., and Chen, X. G. (2006). Enhancement of radiosensitivity by immunoliposomal docetaxel in human colon adenocarcinoma Lovo cell. *Chin. J. Exp. Surgery.* **23**, 795–797.

Winkler, C., Wirleitner, B., Schroecksnadel, K., Schennach, H., Mur, E., and Fuchs, D. (2004). *In vitro* effects of two extracts and two pure alkaloid preparations of uncaria tomentosa on peripheral blood mononuclear cells. *Planta Med.* **70**, 205–210.

Wissing, S. A., Kayser, O., and Muller, R. H. (2004). Solid lipid nanoparticles for parenteral drug delivery. *Adv. Drug Deliv. Rev.* **56**, 1257–1272.

Wnag, X., Jiang, Y., and Wang, Y. W. (2008). Enhancing anti-inflammation activity of curcumin through O/W nanoemulsions. *Food Chem.* **108**, 419–424.

Wu, W., Wang, Y., and Que, Li. (2006). Enhanced bioavailability of silymarin by self microemulsifying drug delivery system. *Eur. J. Pharm. Biopharm.* **63**, 288–294.

Xi., N., Hou, L. B., Wang, C. X., Yan, X. Q., Jiang, Q. F., and Guo, D. (2007). Preparation and *in vitro* drug release behaviour of hydroxycamptothecin semisolid lipid nanoparticles. *China Hospital Pharmacy Journal.* **27**, 139–142.

Yadav, R. S., Sankhwar, M. L., Shukla, R. K., Chandra, R., Pant, A. B., Islam, F., and Khanna, V. K. (2009). Attenuation of arsenic neurotoxicity by curcumin in rats. *Toxicol. Appl. Pharmacol.* **240**, 367–376.

Yajun, C., Jie, L., Xiangliang, Y., Xiaoling, Z., and Huibi, X. (2005). Preparation, in-vitro characterization and enhanced hepatoprotective effect. *J. Pharm. Pharmacol.* **57**, 259–264.

Yang, J. (2009). Brazil nuts and associated health benefits: A review. *LWT-Food Sci. Tech.* **42**, 1573–1580.

Yoshikawa, K., Amimotoa, K., Ariharaa, S., and Matsuura, K. (1989). Structure studies of new antisweet constituents from Gymnema sylvestre. *Tetrahedron Letters* **30**, 1103–1106.

Yoshikawa, M., Matsui, Y., Kawamoto, H., Umemoto, N., Oku, K., Koizumi, M., Yamao, J., Kuriyama, S., Nakano, H., Hozumi, N., Ishizaka, S., and Fukui, H. (1997). Effects of glycyrrhizin on immune-mediated cytotoxicity. *J. Gastroenterol. Hepatol.* **12**, 243–248.

Youdim, K. A. and Joseph, J. A. (2001). A possible emerging role of phytochemicals in improving age-related neurological dysfunctions: A multiplicity of effects. *Free Radical Biology and Medicine.* **30**, 583–594.

Zeisser-Labouebe, M., Lange, N., Gurny, R., and Delie, F. (2006). Hypericin-loaded nanopartilcles for the photodynamic treatment of ovarian cancer. *Int. J. Pharm.* **326**, 174–181.

Zhang, L. and Kosaraju, S. L. (2007). Biopolymeric delivery system for controlled release of polyphenolic antioxidants. *Eur. Poly. J.* **43**, 2956–2966.

Zhang, L. H., Huang, Y., Wang, L. W., and Xiao, P. G. (1995). Several compounds from Chinese traditional and herbal medicine as immunomodulators. *Phytotherapy Res.* **9**, 315–322.

Zhu, Y. X., Fan, J., Zhou, W., and Miao, Y. S. (2007). Preparation and characterization of paclitaxel magnetic liposomes. *J. Clin. Med. Practice.* **11**, 12–23.

3

Carlisle, R. C., Benjamin, R., Briggs, S. S., Sumner-Jones, S., McIntosh, J., Gill, D., Hyde, S., Nathwani, A., Šubr, V., Ulbrich, K., Seymour, L. W., and Fisher, K. D. (2008). Coating of adeno-associated virus with reactive polymers can ablate virus tropsim, enable retargeting and provide resistance to neutralising antisera. *J. Gene Med.* **10**, 400–411.

Carlisle, R. C., Di, Y., Cerny, A. M., Sonnen, A. F. P., Sim, R. B., Green, N. K., Šubr, V., Ulbrich, K., Gilbert, R. J. C., Fisher, K. D., Finberg, R. W., and Seymour, L. W. (2009). Human erythrocytes bind and inactivate type 5 adenovirus by presenting Coxsackie virus-adenovirus receptor and complement receptor 1. *Blood* **113**, 1909–1918.

Duncan, R. and Vicent, M. J. (2010). Do HPMA copolymer conjugates have a future as clinically useful nanomedicines? A critical overview of current status and future opportunities. *Adv. Drug Delivery Rev.* **62**, 272–282.

Eto, Y., Yoshioka, Y., Mukai, Y., Okada, N., and Nakagawa, S. (2008). Development of PEGylated adenovirus vector with targeting ligand. *Int. J. Pharm.* **354**, 3–8.

Fisher, K. D., Green, N. K., Hale, A., Šubr, V., Ulbrich, K., and Seymour, L. W. (2007). Passive tumour targeting of polymer-coated adenovirus for cancer gene therapy. *J. Drug Targeting* **15**, 546–551.

Katchalski-Katzir, E., Kasher, R., Balass, M., Scherf, T., Harel, M., Fridkin, M., Sussman, J. L., and Fuchs, S. (2003). Design and synthesis of peptides that bind alpha-bungarotoxin with high affinity and mimic the three-dimensional structure of the binding-site of acetylcholine receptor. *Biophys. Chem.* **100**, 293–305.

Kreppel, F. and Kochanek, S. (2008). Modification of adenovirus gene transfer vectors with synthetic polymers: A scientific review and technical guide. *Mol. Ther.* **16**, 16–29.

Morrison, J., Briggs, S. S., Green, N., Fisher, K., Šubr, V., Ulbrich, K., Kehoe, S., and Seymour, L. W. (2008). Virotherapy of ovarian cancer with polymer-cloaked adenovirus retargeted to the epidermal growth factor receptor. *Mol. Ther.* **16**, 244–251.

Oh, I. K., Mok, H., and Park, T. G. (2006). Folate immobilized and PEGylated adenovirus for retargeting to tumor cells. *Bioconjugate Chem.* **17**, 721–727.

Říhová, B. (2002). Immunomodulating activities of soluble synthetic polymer-bound drugs. *Adv. Drug Delivery Rev.* **54**, 653–674.

Stevenson, M., Hale, A. B. H., Hale, S. J., Green, N. K., Black, G., Fisher, K. D., Ulbrich, K., Fabra, A., and Seymour, L. W. (2007). Incorporation of a laminin-derived peptide (SIKVAV) on polymer-modified adenovirus permits tumor-specific targeting via alpha 6-integrins. *Cancer Gene Ther.* **14**, 335–345.

Šubr, V., Etrych, T., Ulbrich, K., Hirano T., Kondo, T., Todoroki, T., Jelínková, M., and Říhová, B. (2002). Synthesis and properties of poly[N-(2-hydroxypropyl)methacrylamide] conjugates of superoxide dismutase. *J. Bioactive Compat. Polym.* **17**, 105–122.

Šubr, V. and Ulbrich, K. (2006). Synthesis and properties of new N-(2-hydroxypropyl) methacrylamide copolymers containing thiazolidine-2-thione reactive groups. *React. Funct. Polym.* **66**, 1525–1538.

Ulbrich, K., Šubr, V., Strohalm, J., Plocová, D., Jelínková, M., and Říhová, B. (2000). Polymeric drugs based on conjugates of synthetic and natural macromolecules I. Synthesis and physicochemical characterisation. *J. Controlled Release* **64**, 63–79.

Willemsen, R. A., Pechar, M., Carlisle, R. C., Schooten, E., Pola, R., Thompson, A. J., Seymour, L. W., and Ulbrich, K. (2010). Multicomponent Polymeric System for Tumour Cell-Specific Gene Delivery Using a Universal Bungarotoxin Linker. *Pharm. Res.* **27**, 2274–2282.

4

Adegbite, A. E. and Olorode, O. (2002). Karyotype studies of three species of *Aspilia* Thouar (Heliantheae—Asteraceae) in Nigeria. *Plant Science Res. Comm.* **3**, 11–26.

Bean, C. P. and Livingston, J. D. (1959). Superparamagnetism. *Journal Applied Physics*, **30**, 120S–129.

Brice, M. R. Appenzeller, C. Y., Frederic, J., and Jean-Claude, B. (2005). *Applied and Environmental Microbiology*, **71**(9), 5621–5623.

Ferrer, G. G., Sanchez, M. S., Ribelles, J. L. G., Colomer, F. J., and Pradas, M. M. (2007). Nanodomains in a hydrophilic-hydrophobic IPN based on poly(2-hydroxyethyl acrylate) and poly(ethyl acrylate). *European Polymer Journal* **43**, 3136–3145.

Frutos, P., Pena, E. D., Frutos, G., and Barrales, R. J. M. (2002). Release of gentamicinsulphate from modified commercial bone cement .Effect of (2-hydroxyethyl ethylacrylate) *co*-monomer and poly(N-vinyl-2-pyrrilidone) additive on release mechanism and kinetics. *Biomaterials*, **23**, 3787–3797.

Goswami, S., Kiran, K., Panda, A. B., Sharma, P. P., Mahapatra, S. K., Bhoraskar, S. V., and Banerjee, I. (2011). *Int. J. Nano Dimn.* **2**(1), 37–48.

Goswami, S., Nad, S., and Chakrabarty, D. (2005). Modification of novolac resin by interpenetrating network formation with poly(butyl acrylate). *Journal of Applied Polymer Science.* **97**, 2407–2417.

Gupta P. K., and Hung C. T. (1989). *J. Pharm. Sci*, **78**, p. 745.

Kaul, V., Changez, M., and Dinda, A. K. (2005). Efficacy of antibiotics-loaded interpenetrating network (IPNs) hydrogel based on poly(acrylic acid) and gelatine for treatment of experimental osteomyelitis: *In vivo* study. *Biomaterials* **26**, 2095–2104.

Liu, L. S., Marshall, C. F, Kost, J., and Kevin, B. H. (2003). Pectin based systems for colon-specific drug delivery via oral route. *Biomaterials.* **24**, 3333–3349.

Majid, S. A., Lindberg, L. T., Gunterberg, B., and Siddiki, M. S. (1985). Gentamicin PMMA beads in the treatment of chronic osteomyelitis. *Acta Orthoedic Scand.* **56**, 265–268.

Nelson, C. L. (1987). Infected joint implants,principles of treatment. *Orthop Rev,* **16**, 215–223.

Nelson C. L., Evans, R. P., Blaha, J. D., Calhoun, J., Henry, S. L., and Patzakis, M. J. (1993). A comparison of gentamicin-impregnated poly(methylmethacrylate) bead implantation to conventional parenteral antibiotic therapy in infected total hip and knee arthoplasty. *Clin Orthop.* **295**, 96–101.

Neuberger, T., Schöpf, B., and Hofmann, H. (2005). Superparamagnetic nanoparticles for biomedical applications: Possibilities and limitations of a new drug delivery system. *J. Magn. Magn. Mater*. **293**, 483–496.

Madhukumar, P., Borse, P., Rohatgi, V. K., Bhoraskar, S. V., Singh, P., and Sastry M. (1994). *Mater. Chem. Phys.* **36**, 3–4, 354.

Ravishankar, H., Patil, P., Samel, A., Petreit, H. U., Lizio, R., and Iyer, J. (2011). *Int. J. Pharceutics* **411**, 05-21.

Sato, S. and Kim, S .W. (1984). Macromolecular diffusion through polymer membranes. *Int. J. Pharrn.*, **22**, 229–255.

Shantha, K. L. and Harding, D. R. K. (2003). Synthesis, characterization and evaluation of poly[lactose acrylate-*N*-vinyl-2 pyrrolidone] hydrogels for drug delivery. *European Polymer Journal* **39**, 63–73.

Sumathi, S. and Ray, A. R., (2002). Release behavior of drugs from Tamarind Seed Polysaccharides. *Journal of Pharmacy and Pharmaceutical Science*, **5**, 12–20.

Varshosaz, J. and Koopaie, N. (2002). *Iranian Polymer Journal* **11**, 123.

Vays, S. P. and Khar, R. K. (2004). *Targeted & controlled Drug Delivery.* CBC Publisher & Distributors, New Delhi, 459–463.

Widder, K. J., Senyei, A. E., and Scarpelli, D. G. (1978). *Proc. Soc. Exp. Biol. Med.* **58**, 141

Zhou, Z. H., Wang, J., Liu, X., and Chan, H. S. O., (2001). *J. Mater. Chem.* **11**, 1704.

5

Arpicco, S., Dosio, F., Brusa, P., Crosasso, P., and Cattel, L. (1997). New coupling reagents for the preparation of disulfide cross-linked conjugates with increased stability, *Bioconjugate Chemistry*, **8**, 327–337.

Bignotti, F., Sozzani, P., Ranucci, E., and Ferruti, P. (1994). NMR studies, molecular characterization, and degradation behavior of poly(amido amine)s. 1. Poly(amido amine) deriving from the polyaddition of 2-methylpiperazine to 1,4-bis(acryloyl) piperazine. *Macromolecules*, **27**, 7171–7178.

Casali, M., Riva, S., and Ferruti, P. (2001). Use of new aminosugar derivatives as comonomers for the synthesis of glycosylated poly(amido-amines). *Journal of Bioactive and Compatible Polymers*, **16**(6), 479–491.

Danusso, F. and Ferruti, P. (1970). Synthesis of tertiary amine polymers. *Polymer*, **11**(2), 88–113.

Devalapally, H., Chakilam, A., and Amiji, M. M. (2007). Role of nanotechnology in pharmaceutical product development. *Journal of Pharmaceutical Sciences*, **96**, 2547–2565.

Duncan R. (2003). The dawning era of polymer therapeutics. *Nature*, **2**, 347–360.

Duncan, R. (2006). Polymer conjugates as anticancer nanomedicines. *Nature*, **6**, 688–701.

Ferruti, P., Marchisio, M. A., and Barbucci, R. (1985). Synthesis, physico-chemical properties and biomedical applications of poly(amidoamine)s. *Polymer*, **26**(9), 1336–1348.

Ferruti, P., Ranucci, E., Bignotti, F., Sartore, L., Bianciardi, P., and Marchisio, M. A. (1994). Degradation behaviour of ionic stepwise polyaddition polymers of medical interest. *Journal of Biomaterials Science Polymer Edition*, **6**, 833–844.

Ferruti, P. (1996). Ion-chelating Polymers (Medical Applications). In *Polymeric Materials Encyclopedia*. J. C. Salamone (Ed.). CRC Press Inc, Boca Raton, Florida, pp. 3334–3359.

Ferruti, P., Manzoni, S., Richardson, S. C. W., Duncan, R., Pattrick, N. G., Mendichi, R., and Casolaro, M. (2000). Amphoteric linear poly(amido-amine)s as endosomolytic polymers: correlation between physico-chemical and biological properties. *Macromolecules*, **33**(21), 7793–7800.

Ferruti, P., Marchisio, M. A., and Duncan, R. (2002). Poly(amido-amine)s: Biomedical applications. *Macromolecular Rapid Communications*, **23**(5–6), 332–355.

Flory, P. J. (1953). Principles of polymer chemistry.

Franchini, J., and Ferruti, F. (2005). Poly(amidoamine)s for gene delivery. In *Polymeric gene delivery: Principles and Applications*. Mansoor M. Amiji (Ed.). CRC Press Inc, Boca Raton, Florida, pp. 255–278.

Lavignac, N., Lazenby, M., Foka, P., Malgesini, B., Verpilio, I., Ferruti, P., and Duncan, R. (2004). Synthesis and endosomolytic properties of poly(amidoamine) block copolymers. *Macromolecular Bioscience*, **4**, 922–929.

Manfredi, A., Suardi, M. A., Ranucci, E., and Ferruti, P. (2007). Polymerization kinetics of poly(amidoamine)s in different solvents. *Journal of Bioactive and Compatible Polymers*, **22**(2), 219–231.

Pattrick, N. G., Richardson, S. C. W., Casolaro, M., Ferruti, P., and Duncan, R. (2001). Poly(amidoamine)-mediated intracytoplasmic delivery of ricin A-chain and gelonin. *Journal of Controlled Release*, **77**(3), 225–232.

Ranucci, E., Ferruti, P., Lattanzio, E., Manfredi, A., Rossi, M., Mussini, P. R., Chiellini, F., and Bartoli, C. (2009). Acid-base properties of poly(amidoamine)s. *Journal of Polymer Science: Part A: Polymer Chemistry*, **4**, 69-77.

Ranucci, E., Sartore, L., Bignotti, F., Marchisio, M. A., Bianciardi, P., and Veronese, F. M. (1994). Recent results on functional polymers and macromonomers of interest as biomaterials or for biomaterial modification. *Biomaterials*, **15**, 1235–1241.

Ranucci, E., Spagnoli, G., Ferruti, P., Sgouras, D., and Duncan, R. (1991). Poly(amidoamine)s with potential as drug carriers: Degradation and cellular toxicity. *Journal of Biomaterial Science Polymer Edition*, **2**, 303–315.

Ranucci, E., Suardi, M., Annunziata, R., Ferruti, P., Chiellini, F., and Bartoli, C. (2008). Poly(amidoamine) Conjugates with Disulfide-Linked Cholesterol Pendants Self-Assembling into Redox-Sensitive Nanoparticles. *Biomacromolecules*, **9**, 2693–2704.

Richardson, S. C. W., Ferruti, P., and Duncan, R. (1999). Poly(amidoamine)s as potential endosomolytic polymers: Evaluation *in vitro* and body distribution in normal and tumour-bearing animals. *Journal of Drug Targeting*, **6**, 391–404.

Richardson, S. C. W., Pattrick, N. G., Lavignac, N., Ferruti, P., and Duncan, R. (2010). Intracellular fate of bioresponsive poly(amidoamine)s *in vitro* and *in vivo*. *Journal of Controlled Release*, **142**(1), 78–88.

Szejtli, J. (2004). Cyclodextrin and molecular encapsulation. *Encyclopedia of Nanoscience and Nanotechnology*, **2**, 283–304.

6

Aguila, A., Donachie, A. M., Peyre, M., McSharry, C. P., Sesardic, D., and Mowat, A. M. (2006). Induction of protective and mucosal immunity against diphtheria by an immune stimulating complex (ISCOMS) based vaccine. *Vaccine*, **24**, 5201–5210.

Akdis, C. A., Barlan, I. B., Bahceciler, N., and Akdis, M. (2006). Immunological mechanisms of sublingual immunotherapy. *Allergy*, **61**, 11–14.

Andrianov, A. K. and Payne, L. G. (1998). Polymeric carriers for oral uptake of microparticulates. *Adv. Drug Del. Rev.*, **34**, 155–170.

Banerjee, S., Medina-Fatimi, A., and Nichols, R. (2002). Safety and efficacy of low-dose *Escherichia coli* enterotoxin adjuvant for urease-based oral immunization against *Helicobacter pylori* in healthy volunteers. *Gut*, 51, 634–640.

Bergmeier, L. A., Tao L., Gearing, A. J. M., Adams, S., and Lehner, T. (1992). Comparison of IgA antibodies in vaginal and rectal fluids, serum and saliva following immunization of genital and gut-associated lymphoid tissue. In: *Proc. 7th Int. Cong. Mucosal Immunol. Excerpta Medica*, Amsterdam, The Netherlands, pp. 23–39.

Brayden, D. J., Jepson, M. A., and Baird, A. W. (2005). Keynote review: Intestinal Peyer's patch

M cells and oral vaccine targeting. *Drug Discov Today*, **10**, 1145–1157.

Carreno-Gomez, B., Woodley, J. F., and Florence, A. T. (1999). Studies on the uptake of tomato lectin nanoparticles in everted gut sacs. *Int. J. Pharm.*, **183**, 7–11.

Chen, H. (2000). Recent advances in mucosal vaccine development. *J. Control. Rel.*, **67**, 117–128.

Chen, H., Torchilin, V., and Langer, R. (1996). Lectin-bearing polymerized liposomes as potential oral vaccine carriers. *Pharm. Res.*, **13**, 1378–1383.

Clark, M. A., Blair, H., Liang, L., Brey, R. N., Brayden, D., and Hirst, B. (2002). Targeting polymerized liposome vaccine carrier to intestinal M cells. *Vaccine*, 20, 208–271.

Clark, M. A., Hirst, B. H., and Jepson, M. A. (2000). Lectin-mediated mucosal delivery of drugs and microparticles. *Adv. Drug Del. Rev.*, **43**, 207–223.

Clark, M. A., Jepson, M. A., Simmons, N. L., and Hirst, B. H. (1995). Selective binding and transcytosis of Ulex europaeus 1 lectin by mouse Peyer's patch M-cells *in vivo*. *Cell Tissue Res.*, **282**, 455–461.

Cleek, R. L., Ting, K. C., Eskin, S. G., and Mikos, A. G. (1997). Microparticles of poly (DL-lactic-co-glycolic acid)/poly (ethylene glycol) blends for controlled drug delivery. *J. Control. Rel.*, **48**, 259–268.

Coffin, S. E. and Offit, P. A. (1998).Induction of mucosal B-cell memory by intramuscular inoculation of mice with rotavirus. *J. Virol.*, **72**, 3479–3483.

Davis, S. S. (2001). Nasal vaccines. *Adv. Drug Del. Rev.*, **51**, 21–42.

Dea-Ayuela, M. A., Rama-Iniguez, S., Torrado-Santiago, S., and Bolas-Fernandez, F. (2006). Microcapsules formulated in the enteric coating copolymer Eudragit L100 as delivery systems for oral vaccination against infections by gastrointestinal nematode parasites. *J. Drug Target.*, **14**, 567–575.

Del Giudice, G., Covacci, A., Telford, J. L., Montecucco, C., and Rappuole R. (2001).The design of vaccine against *Helicobacter pylori* and their development. *Annu. Rev. Immunol.*, **19**, 523–563.

Desai, M. A., Mutlu, M., and Vadgama, P. (1992).A study of macro-molecular diffusion through native porcine mucus. *Experientia.* **48**, 22–26.

Dietrich, G., Griot-Wenk, M., Metcalfe, I.C., Lang, A. B., and Viret J-F. (2003). Experience with registered mucosal vaccines. *Vaccine*, **21**, 678–683.

Dilraj, A., Cutts, F. T., and de Castro, J. F. (2000). Response to different measles vaccine strains given by aerosol and subcutaneous routes to schoolchildren: a randomized trial. *Lancet,* **355**, 798–803.

Durrer, C., Irache, J. M., Duchene, D., and Ponchel, G. (1994).Study of the interactions between nanoparticles and intestinal mucosal. *Prog. Colloid Polym. Sci.*, **97**, 275–280.

Durrer, P., Gluck, U., and Spyr, C. (2003).Mucosal antibody response induced with a nasal virosome-based influenza vaccine. *Vaccine*, 21, 4328–4334.

Eriksson, K., Kilander, A., Hagberg, L., Norkrans, G., Holmgren, J., and Czerkinsky, C. (1998). Induction and expression of intestinal homoral immunity in HIV-infected individuals: prospects for vaccination against secondary enteric infections. *Pathobiology,* 66, 176–182.

Eyles, J., Alpar, H. O., Field, W.N., Lewis, D. A.,and Keswick, M. (1995). The transfer of polystyrene microspheres from the gastrointestinal tract to the circulation after oral administration in the rat. *J. Pharm. Pharmacol.* 47, 561–565.

Florence, A. T. (2005). Nanoparticle uptake by oral route: Fulfilling its potential? Drug Dis. *Today*, 2, 75-81.

Foster, N., Clark, M. A., Jepson, M. A., and Hirst, B. H. (1998). *Ulex europaeus 1* lectin targets microspheres to mouse Peyer's patch M-cells *in vivo. Vaccine*, 16, 536–541.

Giannasca, P. J., Boden, J. A., and Monath, T. P. (1997). Targeted delivery of antigen to hamster nasal lymphoid tissue with M-cell-directed lectins. *Infect. Immun.* 65, 4288–4298.

Giannasca, P. J., Giannasca, K. T., Leichtner, A. M., and Neutra M. R. (1999). Human Intestinal M Cells Display the Sialyl Lewis A Antigen. *Infect. Immun.*, 67, 946–953.

Gupta, P. N., Mahor, S., Rawat, A., Khatri, K., Goyal, A., and Vyas, S. P. (2006). Lectin anchored stabilized biodegradable nanoparticles for oral immunization: 1. Development and *in vitro* evaluation. *Int. J. Pharm.*, **318**, 163–173.

Gupta, P. N. and Vyas, S. P. (2011). Investigation of lectinized liposomes as M-cell targeted carrier-adjuvant for mucosal immunization. *Colloids & surfaces B: Biointerfaces*, **82**, 118–125.

Haining, W. N., Anderson, D. G., and Little S. R. (2004). pH-triggered microparticles for peptide vaccination. *J. Immunol.*, **173**, 2578–2585.

Henderson, B., Poole, S., and Wilson, M. (1996). Bacterial modulins: novel class of virulence factors which cause host tissue pathology by inducing cytokine synthesis. *Microbiol. Rev.*, **60**, 316–341.

Holmgren, J., Czerkinsky, C., Eriksson, K., and Mharandi A. (2003). Mucosal immunization and adjuvants: a brief overview of recent advances and challenges. *Vaccine*, 21, S2/89–S2/95.

Holmgren, J. and Czerkinsky C. (2005).Mucosal immunity and vaccines. *Nat. Med.*, **11** (Suppl. 4), S45–S53.

Hussain, N. and Florence, A. T. (1998). Utilizing bacterial mechanisms of epithelial cell entry: Invasin-induced oral uptake of latex nanoparticles. *Pharm. Res.*, **15**, 153–156.

Jaganathan, K. S., Singh, P., Prabakaran, D., Mishra, V., and Vyas, S. P. (2004). Development of a single-dose stabilized poly (D, L-lactic-co-glycolic acid) microsphere-based vaccine against hepatitis B. *J. Pharm. Pharmacol.*, **56**, 1243–1250.

Jaganathan, K. S. and Vyas, S. P. (2006). Strong systemic and mucosal immune responses to surface-modified PLGA microspheres containing recombinant Hepatitis B antigen administered intranasally. *Vaccine*, 24(19), 4201–4211.

Jain, S., Singh, P., Mishra, V., and Vyas, S. P. (2005). Mannosylated niosomes as adjuvant–carrier system for oral genetic immunization against Hepatitis B. *Immunol. Lettrs.*, 101, 41–49.

Jain, S. and Vyas, S. P. (2006). Mannosylated niosomes as adjuvant-carrier system for oral mucosal immunization. *J. Lipo. Res.*, 16, 331–345.

Jani P., McCarthy D. E., and Florence A. T. (1992). Nanosphere and microsphere uptake via Peyer's patches: observation of the rate of uptake in the rat after a single oral dose. *Int. J. Pharm.*, **86**, 239–246.

Jepson, M. A. and Clark, M. A. (1998). Studying M cells and their role in infection. *Trends Microbiol.*, **6**, 359–365.

Jung, T., Kamm, W., Breitenbach, A., Kaiserling, E., Xiao, J.X., and Kissel T. (2000). Biodegradable nanoparticles for oral delivery of peptides: is there is a role for polymers to affect mucosal uptake? *Eur. J. Pharm. Biopharm.*, **50**, 147–160.

Kabok, Z., Ermak, T. H., and Pappo, J. (1994). Microheterogeneity of follicle epithelium and M cells in rabbit gut-associated lymphoid tissues defined by monoclonal antibodies. *FASEB J.*, **8**, A1008.

Kozlowski, P. A., Cu-Uvin, S., Neutra, M. R., and Flanigan, T. P. (1997). Comparison of the oral, rectal, and vaginal immunization routes for induction of antibodies in rectal and genital tract secretions of women. *Infect. Immun.*, **65**, 1387–1394.

Le Fever, M. E., Boccio, A. M., and Jeol, D. D. (1989). Intestinal uptake of fluorescent microsphere in young and aged mice. *Proc. Soc. Exp. Biol. Med.*, **190**, 23–27.

Le Ray, A. M., Vert, M., Gautier, J. C., Benoit, J. P. (1994). Fate of poly (DL-lactide-co-glycolide) nanoparticles after intravenous and oral administration to mice. *Int. J. Pharm.*, **106**, 201–211.

Levine, M. M. (2003). Can needle-free administration of vaccines become the norm in global immunization? *Nat. Med.*, **9**, 99–103.

Litwin, A., Flanagan, M., and Entis, G. (1996). Immunologic effects of encapsulated short ragweed extract: a potent new agent for oral immunotherapy. *Ann. Allergy Asthma Immunol.*, **77**, 132–138.

Lo, D., Tynan, W., and Dickerson, J. (2003). Peptidoglycan recognition protein expression in mouse Peyer's patch follicle associated epithelium suggests functional specialization. *Cell Immunol.*, **224**, 8–16.

Lo, D., Tynan, W., and Dickerson, J. (2004). Cell culture modeling of specialized tissue: identification of genes expressed specifically by follicle associated epithelium of Peyer's patch by expression profiling of caco-2/Raji co-cultures. *Int. Immunol.*, **16**, 91–99.

Macian, F. (2005). NFAT proteins: key regulators of T-cell development and function. *Nat. Rev. Immunol.*, **5**(6), 472–484.

Magistris, M. T. D. (2006). Mucosal delivery of vaccine antigens and its advantages in pediatrics. *Adv. Drug Del. Rev.*, **58**, 52–67.

Migliaresi, C., Fambri L., and Cohn, D. (1994). A study on the *in-vitro* degradation of poly (lactic acid). *J. Biomat. Sci. Poly Ed.*, **5**, 591–606.

Moghimi, S. M., Hawley, A. E., Christy, N. M., Gray, T., Illum, L., and Davis, S. S. (1994). Surface engineered nanospheres with enhanced drainage into lymphatics and uptake by macrophages of the regional lymph nodes. *FEBS Lett.*, **344**, 25–30.

Nesburn, A. B., Burke, R. L., Ghiasi, H., Slanina, S. M., and Wechsler, S. L. (1998). Therapeutic periocular vaccination with a subunit vaccine induces higher levels of herpes simplex virus specific tear secretory immunoglobulin A than systemic vaccination and provide protection against recurrent spontaneous ocular shedding of virus in latently infected rabbits. *Virology*, **252**, 200–209.

Neutra, M. R., and Kozlowski, P. A. (2006). Mucosal vaccines: the promise and the challenge. *Nat Rev Immunol.*, **6**, 148–158.

Norris, D. A., Puri, N., and Sinko, P. J. (1998). The effect of physical barriers and properties on the oral absorption of particulates. *Adv. Drug Del. Rev.*, **34**, 135–154.

Nugent, J., Po, A. L., and Scott, E. M. (1998). Design and delivery of non-parenteral vaccines. *J. Clin. Pharm. Ther.*, **23**(4), 257–285.

O'Hagan, D. T., Rafferty, D., Wharton, S., and Illum, L. (1993). Intravaginal immunization in sheep using a bioadhesive microsphere antigen delivery system. *Vaccine*, **11**, 660–664.

O'Hagan, D. T. (1996). The intestinal uptake of particles and the implications for drug and antigen delivery. *J. Anat.*, **189**, 477–482.

Ogra, P. L., Faden, H., and Welliver, R. C. (2001). Vaccination strategies for mucosal immune responses. *Clin. Microbiol. Rev.*, **14**, 430–445.

Olaguibel, J. M., and Alvarez Puebla, M. J. (2005). Efficacy of sublingual allergen vaccination for respiratory allergy in children: Conclusions from one meta-analysis. *J. Investig. Allergol. Clin. Immunol.*, **15**, 9–16.

Pappo, J., and Ermak, T. H. (1989). Uptake and translocation of fluorescent latex particle by rabbit Peyer's patch follicle epithalium: a quantitative model for M cell uptake. *Clin. Exp. Immunol.*, **76**, 227–280.

Partidos, C. D. (2000). Intranasal vaccines: forthcoming challenges. Pharm. Sci. Tech. Today, 3(8), 273–281.

Payne, L. G., Jenkins, S. A., and Woods A. L. (1998). Poly[di(carboxylatophenoxy)phospha-zene] (PCPP) is a potent immunoadjuvant for an influenza vaccine. *Vaccine*, **16**, 92–98.

Perez O., Bracho G. and Lastre M. (2006). Proteoliposome-derived Cochleate as an immunomodulator for nasal vaccine. Vaccine, 24, S2 /52-S2/53.

Rescigno, M., Urbano M., and Valzasina B. (2001). Dendritic cells express tight junction proteins and penetrate gut epithelial monolayers to sample bacteria. *Nat. Immunol.* **2**, 361–367.

Ryan, E. J., Daly, L. M., and Mills, K. H. G. (2001). Immunomodulators and delivery systems for vaccination by mucosal routes. *TRENDS in Biotech.*, 19(8), 293–304.

Sahoo, S. K., Panyam, J., Prabha, S., and Lab-hasetwar, V. (2002). Residual polyvinyl alcohol associated with poly (D,L-lactide-*co*-glycolide) nanoparticles affects their physical properties and cellular uptake. *J. Control. Rel.*, **82**, 105–114.

Shakweh, M., Besnard, M., Nicolas, V., and Fattal, E. (2005). Poly (lactide-co-glycolide) particles of different physicochemical properties and their uptake by Peyer's paches in mice. *Eur. J. Pharm. Biopharm.*, **61**, 1–13.

Simon, L., Shine, G., and Dayan, A.D. (1994). Effect of animal age on the uptake of large particulates across the epithelium of rat small intestine. *Int. J. Exp. Pathology.*, **75**, 369–373.

Singh, P., Prabakaran, D., Jain, S., Mishra, V., Jaganathan, K. S., and Vyas, S. P. (2004). Cholera toxin B subunit conjugated bile salt stabilized vesicles (bilosomes) for oral immunization. *Int. J. Pharm.*, **278**, 379–390.

Sminia, T., and Kraal, G. (1999). Nasal-associated lymphoid tissue. In: *Mucosal Immunology*, P. L. Ogra, J. Mestecky, M. E. Lamm, W. Strober, J. Bienenstock and J. R. McGhee (eds.), 2nd ed. Academic Press, New York. pp. 357–379.

Smythies, L. E., Novak, M. J., Waites, K. B., Lindsey, J. R., Morrow, C. D., and Smith, P. D. (2005). Poliovirus replicons encoding the B subunit of *Helicobacter pylori* urease protect mice against H. pylori infection. *Vaccine*, 23, 901–909.

Strous, G. J., and Dekker, J. (1992). Mucin-type glycoproteins. *Crit. Rev. Biochem. Mol. Biol.*, **27**, 57–92.

Sturesson, C. and Degling, W. L. (2000). Comparison of poly (acryl starch) and poly (lactide-*co*-glycolide) microspheres as drug delivery system for a rotavirus vaccine. *J. Control. Rel.*, **68**, 441–450.

Tafaghodi, M., Sajadi, Tabasi, S. A., and Jaafari, M. R. (2006). Formulation, characterization and release studies of alginate microspheres encapsulated with tetanus toxoid. *J. Biomater. Sci. Polym.* Ed., **17**, 909–924.

Thanavala, Y., Mahoney, M., and Pal, S. (2005). Immunogenicity in humans of an edible vaccine for hepatitis B. *Proc. Natl. Acad. Sci. USA*, **102**, 3378–3382.

Tommaso, A. D., Saletti, G., and Pizza, M. (1996). Induction of antigen-specific antibodies in vaginal secretions by using a nontoxic mutant of heal labile enterotoxin as mucosal adjuvant. *Infect. Immun.*, **64**, 974–979.

Uchida, T., Martin, S., Foster, T. P., Wardley, R. C. and Grimm, S. (1994). Dose and load studies for subcutaneous and oral delivery of poly (lactide-*co*-glycolide) microspheres containing ovalbumin. *Pharm. Res.*, **11**, 1009–1015.

Van Overtvelt, L., Razafindratsita, A., and St-Lu, N. (2006). Sublingual vaccines based on wild-type recombinant allergens. *Allerg Immunol* (Paris), **38**, 247–249.

Vyas, S. P., Singh, A., and Sihorkar, V. (2001). Ligand-receptor-mediated drug delivery: an emerging paradigm in cellular drug targeting. *Crit. Rev. Ther. Drug Carrier Syst.*, **18**, 1–76.

Wheeler, A.W. and Sharif, S. (1996). Sublingual delivery of vaccines: can we enhance the immune response induced via this route? *Eur. J. Pharm. Sci.*, **4**, S39.

Wu, H. Y. and Russell, M. W. (1997). Nasal lymphoid tissue, intranasal immunization, and compartmentalization of the common mucosal immune system. *Immunol. Res.*, **16**, 187–201.

Yanagita, M., Hiroi, T., and Kitagaki, N. (1999). Nasopharyngeal-associated lymphoreticular tissue (NALT) immunity: fimbriae-specific Th1 and Th2 cell-regulated IgA responses for the inhibition of bacterial attachment to epithelial cells and subsequent inflammatory cytokine production. *J. Immunol.*, **162**, 3559–3565.

Young, V. B., Falkow, S., and Schoolnik, G. K. (1992). The invasin proteinof *Yersinia enterocolitica*: internalization of invasin bearing bacteria by eukaryotic cells is associated with reorganization of the cytoskeleton. *J. Cell Biol.*, **116**, 197–207.

Zhou, F., Kraehenbuhl, J.-P., and Neutra, M. R. (1995). Mucosal IgA response to rectally administered antigen formulated in IgA-coated liposomes. *Vaccine*, 13, 637–644.

7

Bhumakar, D. R., Joshi, H. M., Sastry, M., and Pokharkar, V. B. (2007). Chitosan Reduced Gold Nanoparticles as Novel Carriers for Transmucosal Delivery of Insulin Pharm. *Res* **24**, 1415–1426.

Crooks, R. M., Lemon, B. I., Sun, L., Yeung, L. K., and Zhao, M. (2001). Dendrimer – encapsulated metals and semiconductors: Synthesis, characterization and applications. *Top. Curr. Chem* **212**, 81–135.

Dai, J., and Bruening, M. L. (2002). Catalytic nanoparticles formed by reduction of metal Ions in multilayered polyelectrolyte films. *Nano Lett.* **2**, 497501.

Davendra, J., Hemant Kumar, D., Sumita, K., and Kothari, S. L. (2009). Synthesis of plant mediated silver nanoparticles using papaya fruit extract and evalution of their antimicrobial activities. *Digest Journal of Nanomaterials and Biostructures* 4(4), 723–727.

Dubey, S. P., Lahtinen, M., Sarkka, H., and Sillanpaa, M. (2010). Bioprospective of *Sorbusaucuparia* leaf extract in development of silver and gold nanocolloids. *Colloids Surfaces B* **80**, 26–33.

Dwivedi, A. D., and Gopal, K. (2010). Biosynthesis of silver and gold nanoparticles using *Chenopodium album* leaf extract. *Colloids Surfaces A* **369**, 27–33.

Gittins, D. I., Bethell, D., Nichols, R. J., and Schiffrin, D. J. (2000).Diode-like electron transfer across nanostructured films containing a redox ligand. *J. Mater. Chem* **10**, 79–83.

Jaidev, L. R., and Narasimha, G. (2010). Fungal mediated biosynthesis of silver nanoparticles, characterization and antimicrobial activity. *Colloids Surfaces B* **81**, 430–433.

Konwarh, R., Gogoia, B., Philip, R, Laskarb, M. A., and Karak, N. (2011). Biomimetic synthesis of silver nanoparticles by Citrus limon (lemon) aqueous extract and theoretical prediction of particle size. *Colloids Surfaces B* **82**(1), 152–159.

Lok, C. N., Ho, C. M., Chen, R., He, Q. Y., Yu, W. Y., Sun, H., Tam, P. K., Chiu, J. F., and Che C. M. (2006). Proteomic Analysis of the Mode of Antibacterial Action of Silver Nanoparticles. *J. Proteome Res* **5**, 916–924.

Hayat, M. A. (Ed.) (1989). *Colloidal Gold: Principles, Methods and Applications*, Vol. 1, Academic Press, San Diego, CA.

Morones, J. R., Elechiguerra, J. L., Camacho, A., Holt, K., Kouri, J. B., Ramirez, J. T., and Yacaman, M. J. (2005). The bactericidal effect of silver nanoparticles. *Nanotechnology* **16**, 2346–2353.

Mulvaney, P. (1996). Surface Plasmon Spectroscopy of Nanosized Metal Particles. *Langimuir* **12**, 788–800.

Murray, C. B., Sun, S., Doyle, H., and Betley, T. (2001).Monodisperse 3d Transition Metal (Co, Ni, Fe) Nanoparticles and Their Assembly into Nanoparticle Superlattices. *MRS Bull.* **26** 985–991.

Pal, S., Tak, Y. K., and Song, J. M. (2007). Does the antibacterial activity of silver nanoparticles depend on the shape of the nanoparticle? A study of the Gram-negative bacterium *Escherichia coli. Appl. Environ. Microbial.* **73**, 1712–1720.

Philip, D., and Unni, C. (2011)..Extracellular biosynthesisofgoldandsilvernanoparticlesusing Krishna tulsi (*Ocimum sanctum*) leaf. *Physica E* **43**, 1318–1322.

Rajesh, W. R., Jaya, R. L., Niranjan, S. K., Vijay, D. M., and Sahebrao B. K. (2009). Phytosynthesis of Silver Nanoparticle Using *Gliricidiasepium* (Jacq.) *Curr. Nanosc.i* **5**, 117–122.

Shankar, S. S., Ahmad, A., and Sastry, M. (2003). *Geranium* leaf assisted biosynthesis of silver-nanoparticles. *Biotechnol. Prog.* **19**, 1627–1631.

Shankar, S. S., , A., Ankamwar, B., Singh, A., Ahmad, A., and Sastry, M. (2004a). Biological Synthesis of Triangular Gold Nanoprisms. *Nature Mater* **3**, 482–488.

Shankar, S. S., Rai, A., Ahmad, A., and Sastry, M. (2004b). Rapid synthesis of Au, Ag, and bimetallicAu core–Ag shell nanoparticles using Neem (*Azadirachtaindica*) leaf broth. *J. Colloid Interface Sci.* **275**, 496–502.

Sinha, S., Pan, I., Chanda, P., and Sen, S. K. (2009). Nanoparticles fabrication using ambient biological.Resources. *J. Appl. Bioscien.* **19**, 1113–1130.

Sondi, I., and Salopek-sondi, B. (2004). Silver nanoparticles as antimicrobial agent: a case study on *E. coli* as a model for Gram-negative bacteria. *J. Colloid Inter. Sci.* **275**, 177–182.

Song, J. Y., Jang, H. K., and Kim, B. S. (2009). Biological synthesis of gold nanoparticles using *Magnolia kobus*and *Diopyros kaki* leaf extract, *Process Biochemistry Process Biochem* **44**, 1133–1138.

Velmurugan, N., Gnana Kumar, G., Han, S. S., Nahm, K. S., and Lee, Y. S. (2009). Synthesis and characterization of potential fungicidal silvenano-sized particles and chitosan membrane containing silver particles. *Iran. Polym. J.* **18**, 383–92.

8

Auffray, C., Sieweke, M. H., and Geissmann, F. (2009). Blood monocytes: Development, heterogeneity, and relationship with dendritic cells. *Annu. Rev. Immunol.* **27**, 669-692.

Bastus, N. G., Sanchez-Tillo, E., Pujals, S., Farrera, C., Kogan, M. J., Giralt, E., Celada, A., Lloberas, J., and Puntes, V. (2009a). Peptides conjugated to gold nanoparticles induce macrophage activation. *Mol. Immunol.* **46**(4), 743-748.

Bastus, N. G., Sanchez-Tillo, E., Pujals, S., Farrera, C., Lopez, C., Giralt, E., Celada, A., Lloberas, J., and Puntes, V. (2009b). Homogeneous conjugation of peptides onto gold nanoparticles enhances macrophage response. *ACS Nano* **3**(6), 1335-1344.

Brinkmann, V., Reichard, U., Goosmann, C., Fauler, B., Uhlemann, Y., Weiss, D. S., Weinrauch, Y., and Zychlinsky, A. (2004). Neutro-phil extracellular traps kill bacteria. *Science* **303**(5663), 1532-1535.

Cohen, M. S. (1994). Molecular events in the activation of human neutrophils for microbial killing. *Clin. Infect. Dis.* **18** Suppl 2, S170-179.

Fernandez-Carneado, J., Kogan, M. J., Castel, S., and Giralt, E. (2004). Potential peptide carriers: Amphipathic proline-rich peptides derived from the N-terminal domain of gamma-zein. *Angew Chem. Int. Ed. Engl.* **43**(14), 1811-1814.

Gref, R., Minamitake, Y., Peracchia, M. T., Trubetskoy, V., Torchilin, V., and Langer, R. (1994). Biodegradable long-circulating polymeric nanospheres. *Science* **263**(5153), 1600-1603.

Kanwar, J. R., Kanwar, R. K., Burrow, H., and Baratchi, S. (2009). Recent advances on the roles of NO in cancer and chronic inflammatory disorders. *Curr. Med. Chem.* **16**(19), 2373-2394.

Kimling, J., Maier, M., Okenve, B., Kotaidis, V., Ballot, H., and Plech, A. (2006). Turkevich method for gold nanoparticle synthesis revisited. *J. Phys. Chem. B* **110**(32),15700-15707.

Lee, S., Cha, E. J., Park, K., Lee, S. Y., Hong, J. K., Sun, I. C., Kim, S. Y., Choi, K., Kwon, I. C., Kim, K., and Ahn, C. H. (2008). A near-infrared-fluorescence-quenched gold-nanoparticle imaging probe for *in vivo* drug screening and protease activity determination. *Angew Chem. Int. Ed. Engl.* **47**(15), 2804-2807.

Mosser, D. M. (2003). The many faces of macrophage activation. *J. Leukoc. Biol.* **73**(2), 209-212.

Nishanth. R. P., Jyotsna, R. G., Schlager, J. J., Hussain, S. M., and Reddanna, P. (2011). Inflammatory responses of RAW 264.7 macrophages upon exposure to nanoparticles: Role of ROS-NFkappaB signaling pathway. *Nanotoxicology* **5**(4), 502-516.

Roslavtseva, S. and Ivanova, G. (1975). Specific features of resistance development of houseflies to organophosphate insecticides. *Environ. Qual. Saf. Suppl.* **3**, 447-449.

Schwarzer, E., De Matteis, F., Giribaldi, G., Ulliers, D., Valente, E., and Arese, P. (1999). Hemozoin stability and dormant induction of heme oxygenase in hemozoin-fed human monocytes. *Mol. Biochem. Parasitol.* **100**(1), 61-72.

Vadiveloo, P. K. (1999). Macrophages--proliferation, activation, and cell cycle proteins. *J. Leukoc. Biol.* **66**(4), 579-582.

von Kockritz-Blickwede, M., Goldmann, O., Thulin, P., Heinemann, K., Norrby-Teglund, A., Rohde, M., and Medina, E. (2008). Phagocytosis-independent antimicrobial activity of mast cells by means of extracellular trap formation. *Blood* **111**(6), 3070-3080.

Xaus, J., Comalada, M., Valledor, A. F., Cardo, M., Herrero, C., Soler, C., Lloberas, J., and Celada, A. (2001). Molecular mechanisms involved in macrophage survival, proliferation, activation or apoptosis. *Immunobiology* **204**(5), 543-550.

Zhang, Q., Hitchins, V. M., Schrand, A. M., Hussain, S. M., and Goering, P. L. (2010). Uptake of gold nanoparticles in murine macrophage cells without cytotoxicity or production of proinflammatory mediators. *Nanotoxicology* **5**(3), 284-295.

9

Abu-Dahab, R., Schäfer, U. F., and Lehr, C. M. (2001). Lectin-functionalized liposomes for pulmonary drug delivery: Effect of nebulization on stability and bioadhesion. *European Journal of Pharmaceutical Sciences* **14**(1), 3746.

Ahlin, P., Kristl, J., Kristl, A., and Vrecer, F. (2002). Investigation of polymeric nanoparticles as carriers of enalaprilat for oral administration. *International Journal of Pharmaceutics* **239**(12), 113120.

Ahmad, Z. and Khuller, G. K. (2008). Alginate-based sustained release drug delivery systems for tuberculosis. *Expert Opinion in Drug Delivery* **5**(12), 13231334.

Ahmad, Z., Pandey, R., Sharma, S., and Khuller, G. K. (2005a). Evaluation of antitubercular drug loaded alginate nanoparticles against experimental tuberculosis. *Nanoscience* **1**(2), 8185.

Ahmad, Z., Pandey, R., Sharma, S., and Khuller, G. K. (2006a). Pharmacokinetic and pharmacodynamic behavior of antitubercular drugs encapsulated in alginate nanoparticles at two doses. *International Journal of Antimicrobial Agents* **27**(5), 409416.

Ahmad, Z., Pandey, R., Sharma, S., and Khuller, G. K. (2006b). Alginate nanoparticles as antituberculosis drug carriers: Formulation development, pharmacokinetics and therapeutic potential. *Indian Journal of Chest Disease and Allied Sciences* **48**(3), 171176.

Ahmad, Z., Pandey, R., Sharma, S., and Khuller, G. K. (2008). Novel chemotherapy for tuberculosis: Chemotherapeutic potential of econazole- and moxifloxacin-loaded PLG nanoparticles. *International Journal of Antimicrobial Agents* **31**(2), 142146.

Ahmad, Z., Sharma, S., and Khuller, G. K. (2005b). Inhalable alginate nanoparticles as antitubercular drug carriers against experimental tuberculosis. *International Journal of Antimicrobial Agents* **26**(4), 298303.

Ahmad, Z., Sharma, S., and Khuller, G. K. (2005c). *In vitro* and *ex vivo* antimycobacterial potential of azole drugs against *M. tuberculosis* H37Rv. *FEMS Microbiology Letters* **251**(1), 1922.

Ahmad, Z., Sharma, S., and Khuller, G. K. (2006c). Azole antifungals as novel chemotherapeutic agents against murine tuberculosis. *FEMS Microbiology Letters* **261**(2), 181186.

Ahmad, Z., Sharma, S., and Khuller, G. K. (2006e). The potential of azole antifungals against latent/persistent tuberculosis. *FEMS Microbiology Letters* **258**(2), 200203.

Ahmad, Z., Sharma, S., and Khuller, G. K. (2007). Chemotherapeutic evaluation of alginate nanoparticle-encapsulated azole antifungal and antitubercular drugs against murine tuberculosis. *Nanomedicine* **3**(3), 239243.

Ahmad, Z., Sharma, S., Khuller, G. K., Singh, P., Faujdar, J., and Katoch, V. M. (2006d). Antimycobacterial activity of econazole against multidrug-resistant strains of *Mycobacterium tuberculosis*. *International Journal of Antimicrobial Agents* **28**(6), 543544.

Alvarez-Román, R., Naik, A., Kalia, Y. N., Guy, R. H., and Fessi, H. (2004). Enhancement of topical delivery from biodegradable nanoparticles. *Pharmaceutical Research* **21**(10), 18181825.

AshaRani, P. V., Low Kah Mun, G., Hande, M. P., and Valiyaveettil, S. (2009). Cytotoxicity and genotoxicity of silver nanoparticles in human cells. *American Chemical Society Nano* **3**(2), 279–290.

Bala, I., Hariharan, S., and Kumar, M. N. (2004). PLGA nanoparticles in drug delivery: The state of the art. *Critical Reviews in Therapeutic Drug Carrier Systems* **21**(5), 387422.

Baram-Pinto, D., Shukla, S., Perkas, N., Gedanken, A., and Sarid, R. (2009). Inhibition of *Herpes simplex* virus type 1 infection by silver nanoparticles capped with mercaptoethane sulfonate. *Bioconjugate Chemistry* **20**(8), 1497–1502.

Barnard, D. L., Sidwell, R. W., Gage, T. L., Okleberry, K. M., Matthews, B., and Holan, G. (1997). Anti-respiratory syncytial virus activity of dendrimer polyanions. *Antiviral Research* **34**(2), 88–88.

Barrow, E. L. W., Winchester, G. A., Staas, J. K., Quenelle, D. C., and Barrow, W. W. (1998). Use of microsphere technology for sustained and targeted delivery of rifampin to *Mycobacterium tuberculosis*-infected mice. *Antimicrobial Agents and Chemotherapy* 42(10), 26822689.

Barry, C. E. and Duncan, K. (2004). Tuberculosisstrategies towards antiinfectives for a chronic disease. *Drug Discovery Today* 1(4), 491496.

Bastian, I., Rigouts, L., Van Deun, A., and Portaels, F. (2000). Directly observed treatment, short course strategy and multidrug-resistant tuberculosis: Are any modifications required? *Bulletin World Health Organization* 78(2), 238251.

Bernkop-Schnurch, A. (2005). Mucoadhesive polymers: Strategies, achievements and future challenges. *Advanced Drug Delivery Reviews* **57**(11), 1553–1555.

Bilati, U., Pasquarello, C., Corthals, G. L., Hochstrasser, D. F., Allémann, E., and Doelker, E. (2005). Matrix-assisted laser desorption/ ionization time-of-flight mass spectrometry for quantitation and molecular stability assessment of insulin entrapped within PLGA nanoparticles. *Journal of Pharmaceutical Sciences* **94**(3), 688694.

Blanzat, M., Turrin, C. O., Aubertin, A. M., Couturier-Vidal, C., Caminade, A. M., Majoral, J. P., Rico-Lattes, I., and Lattes, A. (2005). Dendritic catanionic assemblies: *In vitro* anti-HIV activity of phosphorus-containing dendrimers bearing galbeta1cer analogues. *Chembiochem* 6(12), 2207–2213.

Blanzat, M., Turrin, C. O., Perez, E., Rico-Lattes, I., Caminade, A. M., and Majoral, J. P. (2002). Phosphorus-containing dendrimers bearing galactosylceramide analogs: Self-assembly properties. *Chemical Communications (Cambridge)* **17**, 1864–1865.

Boisselier, E. and Astruc, D. (2009). Gold nanoparticles in nanomedicine: Preparations, imaging, diagnostics, therapies and toxicity. *Chemical Society Reviews* 38(6), 17591782.

Bosman, A. W., Janssen, H. M., and Meijer, E. W. (1999). About dendrimers: Structure, physical properties, and applications. *Chemical Reviews* 99(7), 1665–1688.

Bowman, M-C., Ballard, T. E., Ackerson, C. J., Feldheim, D. L., Margolis, D. M., and Melander, C. (2008). Inhibition of HIV fusion with multivalent gold nanoparticles. *Journal of American Chemical Society* **130**(22), 6896–6897.

Braydich-Stolle, L., Hussain, S., Schlager, J. J., and Hofmann, M. C. (2005). *In vitro* cytotoxicity of nanoparticles in mammalian germline stem cells. *Toxicological Sciences* **88**(2), 412–419.

Buchanan, C. M., Buchanan, N. L., Edgar, K. J., Little, J. L., Ramsey, M. G., Ruble, K. M., Wacher, V. J., and Wempe, M. F. (2007). Pharmacokinetics of saquinavir after intravenous and oral dosing of saquinavir:hydroxybutenyl-Î²-cyclodextrin formulations. *Biomacromolecules* 9(1), 305–313.

Bulut-Oner, F., Capan, Y., Kas, S., Oner, L., and Hincal, A. A. (1989). Sustained release isoniazid tablets. I- Formulation and *in vitro* evaluation. *Farmaco* 44(7–8), 739–752.

Caminero, J. A., Sotgiu, G., Zumla, A., and Migliori, G. B. (2010). Best drug treatment for multidrug-resistant and extensively drug-resistant tuberculosis. *Lancet Infectious Diseases* 10(9), 621–629.

Canizal, G., Ascencio, J. A., Gardea-Torresday, J., and Yacamán, M. J. (2001). Multiple twinned gold nanorods grown by bio-reduction techniques. *Journal of NanoparticleResearch* **3**(5), 475–481.

Chattopadhyay, N., Zastre, J., Wong, H. L., Wu, X. Y., and Bendayan, R. (2008). Solid lipid nanoparticles enhance the delivery of the HIV protease inhibitor, atazanavir, by a human brain endothelial cell line. *Pharmeceutical Research* **25**(10), 2262–2271.

Chickering, III D. E., Jacob, J. S., Desai, T.A., Harrison, M., Harris, W. P., Morrel, C. N., Chaturvedi, P., and Mathiowitz, E. (1997). Bioadhesive microspheres:III. An *in vivo* transit and bioavailability study of drug loaded alginate and poly (fumaric-co-sebacic anhydride) microspheres. *Journal of Controlled Release* 48(1), 35–46.

Choi, Y., Yoshida, T., Mimura, T., Kaneko, Y., Nakashima, H., Yamamoto, N., and Uryu, T. (1996). Synthesis of sulfated octadecyl ribo-oligosaccharides with potent anti-AIDS virus activity by ring opening polymerization of a 1,4-anhydroribose derivative. *Carbohydrate Research* 282(1), 113–123.

Clark, M. A., Hirst, B. H., and Jepson, M. A. (2000). Lectin-mediated mucosal delivery of drugs and microparticles. *Advanced Drug Delivery Reviews* 43(2–3), 207–223.

Cone, R. A. (2009). Barrier properties of mucus. *Advanced Drug Delivery Reviews* 61(2), 75–85.

Cui, J. H., Goh, J. S., Park, S. Y., Kim, P. H., and Le, B. J. (2001). Preparation and physical characterization of alginate microparticles using air atomization method. *Drug Development and Industrial Pharmacy* 27(4), 309–319.

Das, D. and Lin, S. (2005). Double-coated poly (butylcyanoacrylate) nanoparticulate delivery systems for brain targeting of dalargin via oral administration. *Journal of Pharmaceutical Sciences* 94(6), 1343–1353.

Dembri, A., Montisci, M. J., Gantier, J. C., Chacun, H., and Ponchel, G. (2001). Targeting of 3'-azido 3'-deoxythymidine (AZT)-loaded poly(isohexylcyanoacrylate) nanospheres to the gastrointestinal mucosa and associated lymphoid tissues. *Pharmaceutical Research* 18(4), 467–473.

Demicheli, C., Ochoa, R., Da Silva, J. B. B., Falcao, C. A. B., Rossi-Bergmann, B., de Melo, A. L., Sinisterra, R. D., and Frezard, F. (2004). Oral delivery of meglumineantimoniate–cyclodextrin complex for treatment of leishmaniasis. *Antimicrobial Agents and Chemotherapy* 48(1), 100–103.

Destache, C. J., Belgum, T., Christensen, K., Shibata, A., Sharma, A., and Dash, A. (2009). Combination antiretroviral drugs in PLGA nanoparticle for HIV-1. *BioMed Central Infectious Diseases* 9, 198.

Dobson, J. (2007). Toxicological aspects and applications of nanoparticles in paediatric respiratory disease. *Paediatric Respiratory Reviews* 8(1), 62–66.

Doroud, D., Zahedifard, F., Vatanara, A., Najafabadi, A. R., and Rafati, S. (2011a). Cysteine proteinases type I, encapsulated in solid lipid nanoparticles induces substantial protection against *L. major* infection in C57BL/6 mice. *Parasite Immunology*, March 16 [Epub ahead of print, PMID: 21410716].

Doroud, D., Zahedifard, F., Vatanara, A., Najafabadi, A. R., Taslimi, Y., Vahabpour, R., Torkashvand, F., Vaziri, B., and Rafati, S. (2011b). Delivery of a cocktail DNA vaccine encoding cysteine proteinases type I, II and III with solid lipid nanoparticles potentiate protective immunity against *Leishmania major* infection. *Journal of Controlled Release*, April 19 [Epub ahead of print, PMID: 21530597].

du Toit, L. C., Pillay, V., and Choonara, Y. E. (2010). Nano-microbicides: Challenges in drug delivery, patient ethics and intellectual property in the war against HIV/AIDS. *Advanced Drug Delivery Reviews* 62(4–5), 532–546.

Durand, R., Paul, M., Rivollet, D., Fessi, H., Houin, R., Astier, A., and Deniau, M. (1997a). Activity of pentamidine-loaded poly(D,L-lactide) nanoparticles against *Leishmania infantum* in a murine model. *Parasite* 4(4), 331–336.

Durand, R., Paul, M., Rivollet, D., Houin, R., Astier, A., and Deniau, M. (1997b). Activity of pentamidine-loaded methacrylate nanoparticles against *Leishmania infantum* in a mouse model.

Dutt, M. and Khuller, G. K. (2001). Therapeutic efficacy of poly (DL-lactide-co-glycolide) encapsulated antitubercular drugs against *Mycobacterium tuberculosis* infection induced in mice. *Antimicrobial Agents and Chemotherapy* 45(1), 363–366.

Dutta, T. and Jain, N. K. (2007). Targeting potential and anti-HIV activity of lamivudineloaded mannosylated poly (propyleneimine) dendrimer. *Biochimica et Biophysica Acta* 1770(4), 681–686.

Dutta, T., Garg, M., and Jain, N. K. (2008). Targeting of efavirenz loaded tuftsin conjugated poly(propyleneimine) dendrimers to HIV infected macrophages *in vitro. European Journal of Pharmaceutical Sciences* 34(2–3), 181–189.

Elechiguerra, J. L., Burt, J. L., Morones, J. R., Camacho-Bragado, A., Gao, X., Lara, H. H., and Yacaman, M. J. (2005). Interaction of silver nanoparticles with HIV-1. *Journal of Nanobiotechnology* **3**, 6.

Espuelas, M., Legrand, P., Loiseau, P. M., Bories, C., Barratt, G., and Irache, J. M. (2002). *In vitro* antileishmanial activity of amphotericin B loaded in poly(e-caprolactone) nanospheres. *Journal of Drug Targeting* **10**(8), 593–599.

Ferreira, L. S., Ramaldes, G. A., Nunan, E. A., and Ferreira, L. A. (2004). *In vitro* skin permeation and retention of paromomycin from liposomes for topical treatment of the cutaneous leishmaniasis. *Drug Development and Industrial Pharmacy* **30**(3), 289–296.

Fiegel, J., Garcia-Contreras, L., Thomas, M., Verberkmoes, J., Elbert, K., Hickey, A., and Edwards, D. (2008). Preparation and *in vivo* evaluation of a dry powder for inhalation of capreomycin. *Pharmaceutical Research* **25**(4), 805–811.

Frankenburg, S., Glick, D., Klaus, S., and Barenholz, Y. (1998). Efficacious topical treatment for murine cutaneous leishmaniasis with ethanolic formulations of amphotericin B. *Antimicrobial Agents and Chemotherapy* **42**(12), 3092–3096.

Frézard, F., Martins, P. S., Bahia, A. P., Le Moyec, L., de Melo, A. L., Pimenta, A. M., Salerno, M., da Silva, J. B., and Demicheli, C. (2008). Enhanced oral delivery of antimony from meglumine antimoniate/beta-cyclodextrin nanoassemblies. *International Journal of Pharmaceutics* **347**(1–2), 102–108.

Fundarò, A., Cavalli, R., Bargoni, A., Vighetto, D., Zara, G. P., and Gasco, M. R. (2000). Nonstealth and stealth solid lipid nanoparticles (SLN) carrying doxorubicin: Pharmacokinetics and tissue distribution after i.v. administration to rats. *Pharmacological Research* **42**(4), 337–343.

Gajbhiye, V., Palanirajan, V. K., Tekade, R. K., and Jain, N. K. (2009). Dendrimers astherapeutic agents: A systematic review. *Journal of Pharmacy and Pharmacology* **61**(8), 989–1003.

Gangadharam, P. R, Kailasam, S., Srinivasan, S., and Wise, D. L. (1994). Experimental chemotherapy of tuberculosis using single dose treatment with isoniazid in biodegradable polymers. *Journal of Antimicrobial Chemotherapy* **33**(2), 265–271.

Gangadharam, P. R., Ashtekar, D. R., Farhi, D. C., Wise, D. L. (1991). Sustained release of isoniazid *in vivo* from a single implant of a biodegradable polymer.*Tubercle* **72**(2), 115–122.

Garcia-Contreras, L., Sung, J. C., Muttil, P., Padilla, D., Telko, M., Verberkmoes, J. L., Elbert, K. J., Hickey, A. J., and Edwards, D. A. (2010). Dry powder PA-824 aerosols for treatment of tuberculosis in guinea pigs. *Antimicrobial Agents and Chemotherapy* **54**(4), 1436–1442.

Gaspar, M. M., Cruz, A., Fraga, A. G., Castro, A. G., Cruz, M. E., and Pedrosa, J. (2008). Developments on drug delivery systems for the treatment of mycobacterial infections. *Current Topics in Medicinal Chemistry* **8**(7), 579–591.

Gaspar, R., Oppredoes, F., Preat, V., and Roland, M. (1992a). Drug targeting with polyalkylcyanoacrylate nanoparticles: *In vitro* activity of primaquine-loaded nanoparticles against intracellular *Leishmania donovani*. *Annals of Tropical Medicine and Parasitology* **86**(1), 41–49.

Gaspar, R., Préat, V., and Roland, M. (1991). Nanoparticles of polyisohexylcyanoacrylate (PIHCA) as carriers of primaquine: Formulation, physico-chemical characterization and acute toxicity. *International Journal of Pharmaceutics* **68**(1–3), 111–119.

Gaspar, R., Preat, V., Oppredoes, F., and Roland, M. (1992b). Macrophage activation by polymeric nanoparticles of polyalkylcyanoacrylates: Activity against intracellular *Leishmania donovani* associated with hydrogen peroxide production. *Pharmaceutical Research* **9**(6), 782–787.

Ginsburg, A. S., Grosset, J. H., and Bishai, W. R. (2003). Fluoroquinolones, tuberculosis, and resistance. *Lancet Infectious Diseases* **3**(7), 432–442.

González-Rodríguez, M. L., Holgado, M. A., Sánchez-Lafuente, C., Rabasco, A. M., and Fini A. (2002). Alginate/chitosan particulate systems for sodium diclofenac release. *International Journal of Pharmaceutics* **232**(1–2), 225–234.

Goodman, C. M., McCusker, C. D., Yilmaz, T., and Rotello, V. M. (2004). Toxicity of gold nanoparticles functionalized with cationic and anionic side chains. *Bioconjugate Chemistry* **15**(4), 897–900.

Gruda, I. and Dussault, N. (1988). Effect of the aggregation state of amphotericin Bon its interaction with ergosterol. *Biochemistry and Cell Biology* **66**(3), 177–183.

Gunaseelan, S., Gunaseelan, K., Deshmukh, M., Zhang, X., and Sinko, P. J. (2010). Surface modifications of nanocarriers for effective intracellular delivery of anti-HIV drugs. *Advanced Drug Delivery Reviews* 62(4–5), 518–531.

Guzmán, M., Aberturas, M. R., Rodríguez-Puyol, M., and Molpeceres, J. (2000). Effect of nanoparticles on digitoxin uptake and pharmacologic activity in rat glomerular mesangial cell cultures. *Drug Delivery* 7(4), 215–222.

Ham, A. S., Cost, M. R., Sassi, A. B., Dezzutti, C. S., and Rohan, L. C. (2009). Targeted delivery of PSC-RANTES for HIV-1 prevention using biodegradable nanoparticles. *Pharmaceutical Research* 26(3), 502–511.

Han, S., Yoshida, D., Kanamoto, T., Nakashima, H., Uryu, T., and Yoshida, T. (2010). Sulfated oligosaccharide cluster with polylysine core scaffold as a new anti-HIV dendrimer. *Carbohydrate Polymers* 80(4), 1111–1115.

Harouse, J. M., Bhat, S., Spitalnik, S. L., Laughlin, M., Stefano, K., Silberberg, D. H., and Gonzalez-Scarano, F. (1991). Inhibition of entry of HIV-1in neural cell lines by antibodies against galactosyl ceramide. *Science* 253(5017), 320–323.

Harouse, J. M., Kunsch, C., Hartle, H. T., Laughlin, M. A., Hoxie, J. A., Wigdahl, B., and Gonzalez-Scarano, F. (1989). CD4-independent infection of human neural cells by human immunodeficiency virus type 1. *Journal of Virology* 63(6), 2527–2533.

Heiati, H., Tawashi, R., and Phillips, N. C. (1998). Solid lipid nanoparticles as drug carriers: II. Plasma stability and biodistribution of solid lipid nanoparticles containing the lipophilic prodrug 3'-azido-3'-deoxythymidine palmitate in mice. *International Journal of Pharmeceutics* 174(1–2), 71–80.

Heiati, H., Tawashi, R., Shivers, R. R., and Phillips, N. C. (1997). Solid lipid nanoparticles as drug carriers. I. Incorporation and retention of the lipophilic prodrug 3'-azido-3'-deoxythymidine palmitate. *International Journal of Pharmeceutics* 146(1), 123–131.

Hejazi, R. and Amiji, M. (2003). Chitosan-based gastrointestinal delivery systems. *Journal of Controlled Release* 89(2), 151–165.

Herwaldt, B. L. (1999). Leishmaniasis. *Lancet* 354(9185), 1191–1199.

Horisawa, E., Hirota Kawazoe, T. S., Yamada, J., Yamamoto, H., Takeuchi, H., and Kawashima, Y. (2002). Prolonged anti-inflammatory action of DL-lactide/glycolide copolymer nanospheres containing betamethazone sodium phosphate for an intra-articular delivery system in antigen-induced arthritic rabbit. *Pharmaceutical Research* 19(4), 403–410.

Hussain, S. M., Hess, K. L., Gearhart, J. M., Geiss, K. T., and Schlager, J. J. (2005). In vitro toxicity of nanoparticles in BRL 3A rat liver cells. *Toxicology In Vitro* 19(7), 975–983.

International Journal of Parasitology 27(11), 1361–1367.

Imbuluzqueta, E., Elizondo, E., Gamazo, C., Moreno-Calvo, E., Veciana, J., Ventosa, N., and Blanco-Prieto, M. J. (2011). Novel bioactive hydrophobic gentamicin carriers for the treatment of intracellular bacterial infections. *Acta Biomaterialia* 7(4), 1599–1608.

Jain, K. K. (2003). Nanodiagnostics: Application of nanotechnology in moleculardiagnostics. *Expert Review of Molecular Diagnostics* 3(2), 153–161.

Jain, R., Shah, N. H., Malick, A. W., and Rhodes, C. T. (1998). Controlled drug delivery by biodegradable poly(ester) devices: Different preparative approaches. *Drug Development and Industrial Pharmacy* 24(8), 703–727.

Jaiswal, J., Gupta, S. K., and Kreuter, J. (2004). Preparation of biodegradable cyclosporine nanoparticles by high-pressure emulsification-solvent evaporation process. *Journal of Controlled Release* 96(1), 169–178.

Jenning, V., Lippacher, A., and Gohla, S. H. (2002). Medium scale production of solid lipid nanoparticles (SLN) by high pressure homogenization. *Journal of Microencapsulation* 19(1), 1–10.

Jiang, Y-H., Emau, P., Cairns, J. S., Flanary, L., Morton, W. R., McCarthy, T. D., and Tsai, C-C. (2005). SPL7013 gel as a topical microbicide for prevention of vaginal transmission of SHIV89.6P in macaques. *AIDS Research and Human Retroviruses* 21(3), 207–213.

Jiao, Y., Ubrich, N., Marchand-Arvier, M., Vigneron, C., Hoffman, M., Lecompte, T., and

Maincent, P. (2002). *In vitro* and *in vivo* evaluation of oral heparin-loaded polymeric nanoparticles in rabbits. *Circulation* 105(2), 230–235.

Johnson, C. M., Pandey, R., Sharma, S., Khuller, G. K., Basaraba, R. J., Orme, I. M., and Lenaerts, A. J. (2005). Oral therapy using nanoparticle-encapsulated antituberculosis drugs in guinea pigs infected with *Mycobacterium tuberculosis*. *Antimicrobial Agents and Chemotherapy* 49(10), 4335–4338.

Joseph, I. and Venkataram, S. (1995). Indomethacin sustained release from alginate-gelatin or pectin-gelatin coacervates. *International Journal of Pharmaceutics* 126(1–2), 161–168.

Joshi, S. A., Chavhan, S. S., and Sawant, K. K. (2010). Rivastigmine-loaded PLGA and PBCA nanoparticles: Preparation, optimization, characterization, *in vitro* and pharmacodynamic studies. *European Journal of Pharmacology and Biopharmaceutics* 76(2), 189–199.

Kabanov, A. V. and Batrakova, E. V. (2004). New technologies for drug delivery across the blood brain barrier. *Current Pharmaceutical Design* 10(12), 1355–1363.

Katti, M. K. (2004). Pathogenesis, diagnosis, treatment, and outcome aspects of cerebral tuberculosis. *Medical Science Monitoring* 10(9), RA215–229.

Kawata, K., Osawa, M., and Okabe, S. (2009). *In vitro* toxicity of silver nanoparticlesat noncytotoxic doses to HepG2 human hepatoma cells. *Environmental Science and Technology* 43(15), 6046–6051.

Kayser, O., Olbrich, C., Yardley, V., Kiderlen, A. F., and Croft, S. L. (2003). Formulation of amphotericin B as nanosuspension for oral administration. *International Journal of Pharmaceutics* 254(1), 73–75.

Khalil, N. M., Carraro, E., Cótica, L. F., and Mainardes, R. M. (2011). Potential of polymeric nanoparticles in AIDS treatment and prevention. *Expert Opinion in Drug Delivery* 8(1), 95–112.

Kim, B. D., Na, K., and Choi, H. K. (2005). Preparation and characterization of solid lipid nanoparticles (SLN) made of cacao butter and curdlan. *European Journal of Pharmaceutical Sciences* 24(2–3), 199–205.

Kim, Y. S., Kim, J. S., Cho, H. S., Rha, D. S., Kim, J. M., Park, J. D., Choi, B. S., Lim, R.,

Chang, H. K., Chung, Y. H., Kwon, I. H., Jeong, J., Han, B. S., and Yu, I. J. (2008). Twenty-eight-day oral toxicity, genotoxicity, and gender-related tissue distribution of silver nanoparticles in Sprague-Dawley rats. *Inhalation Toxicology* 20(6), 575–583.

Kisich, K. O., Gelperina, S., Higgins, M. P., Wilson, S., Shipulo, E., Oganesyan, E., and Heifets, L. (2007). Encapsulation of moxifloxacin within poly (butylcyanoacrylate) nanoparticles enhances efficacy against intracellular *Mycobacterium tuberculosis*. *International Journal of Pharmaceutics* 345(1–2), 154–162.

Kovochich, M., Marsden, M. D., and Zack, J. A. (2011). Activation of latent HIV using drug-loaded nanoparticles. *PLoS One* 6(4), e18270.

Kumar, A., Patel, G., and Menon, S. K. (2009). Fullerene isoniazid conjugate- a tuberculostat with increased lipophilicity: Synthesis and evaluation of antimycobacterial activity. *Chemical Biology and Drug Design* 73(5), 553–557.

Kumar, G., Sharma, S., Shafiq, N., Pandhi, P., Khuller, G. K., and Malhotra, S. (2011). Pharmacokinetics and tissue distribution studies of orally administered nanoparticles encapsulated ethionamide used as potential drug delivery system in management of multi-drug resistant tuberculosis. *Drug Delivery* 18(1), 65–73.

Kuo, Y-C. (2005). Loading efficiency of stavudine on polybutylcyanoacrylate and methylmethacrylate-sulfopropylmethacrylate copolymer nanoparticles. *International Journal of Pharmeceutics* 290(1–2), 161–172.

Kuo, Y.-C. and Chen, H.-H. (2006). Effect of nanoparticulate polybutylcyanoacrylate and methylmethacrylate–sulfopropylmethacrylate on the permeability of zidovudine and lamivudine across the *in vitro* blood–brain barrier. *International Journal of Pharmaceutics* 327(1–2), 160–169.

Kuo, Y-C. and Chen, H-H. (2009). Entrapment and release of saquinavir using novel cationic solid lipid nanoparticles. *International Journal of Pharmaceutics* 365(1–2), 206–213.

Kuo, Y-C. and Kuo, C-Y. (2008). Electromagnetic interference in the permeabilityof saquinavir across the blood-brain barrier using nanoparticulatecarriers. *International Journal of Pharmeceutics* 351(1–2), 271–281.

Kuo, Y-C. and Su, F-L. (2007). Transport of stavudine, delavirdine, and saquinaviracross the blood-brain barrier by polybutylcyanoacrylate, methylmethacrylate-sulfopropylmethacrylate, and solid lipid nanoparticles. *International Journal of Pharmeceutics* **340**(1–2), 143–152.

Kurmi, B. D., Kayat, J., Gajbhiye, V., Tekade, R. K., and Jain, N. K. (2010). Micro- and nanocarrier-mediated lung targeting. *Expert Opinion in Drug Delivery* **7**(7), 781–794.

Lai, S. K., O'Hanlon, D. E., Harrold, S., Man, S. T., Wang, Y. Y., Cone, R., and Hanes, J. (2007). Rapid transport of large polymeric nanoparticles in fresh undiluted human mucus. *Proceedings of the National Academy of Sciences U S A* **104**(5), 1482–1487.

Lai, S. K., Wang, Y. Y., and Hanes, J. (2009a). Mucus-penetrating nanoparticles for drug and gene delivery to mucosal tissues. *Advanced Drug Delivery Reviews* **61**(2), 158–171.

Lai, S. K., Wang, Y. Y., Wirtz, D., and Hanes, J. (2009b). Micro- and macrorheology of mucus. *Advanced Drug Delivery Reviews* **61**(2), 86–100.

Lala, S., Gupta, S., Sahu, N. P., Mandal, D., Mondal, N. B., Moulik, S. P., and Basu, M. K. (2006). Critical evaluation of the therapeutic potential of bassic acid incorporated in oil-in-water microemulsions and poly-D,L-lactide nanoparticles against experimental leishmaniasis. *Journal of Drug Targeting* **14**(4), 171–179.

Lalloo, U. G. and Ambaram, A. (2010). New antituberculous drugs in development. *Current HIV/AIDS Report* **7**(3), 143–151.

Lambert, H. P. (1999). Historical notes on infectious disease. In: *Clinical Infectious DiseaseA Practical Approach*, R. K. Root, F. Waldvogel, L. Corey, and W. E. Stamm (Eds.), Oxford University Press, Inc., New York, USA, Chapter 1, pp. 1–6.

Lamprecht, A., Ubrich, N., Yamamoto, H., Schäfer, U., Takeuchi, H., Maincent, P., Kawashima, Y., and Lehr, C. M. (2001). Biodegradable nanoparticles for targeted drug delivery in treatment of inflammatory bowel disease. *Journal of Pharmacology and Experimental Therapeutics* **299**(2), 775–781.

Lannuccelli, V., Coppi, G., and Cameroni, R. (1996). Biodegradable intraoperative system for bone infection treatment. I. The drug/polymer interaction. *International Journal of Pharmaceutics* **143**(2), 195–201.

Lara, H. H., Ayala-Nunez, N. V., Ixtepan-Turrent, L., and Rodriguez-Padilla, C. (2010). Mode of antiviral action of silver nanoparticles against HIV-1. *Journal of Nanobiotechnology* **8**, 1.

Laxminarayan, R. and Jamison, D. (2010). Global burden of disease: causes, levels, and intervention strategies. In: *Oxford Textbook of Medicine*, D. A. Warrell, T. M. Cox, and J. D. Firth (Eds.), 5th ed., Oxford University Press, Inc., New York, USA, Volume 1, Section 3.1, pp. 73–79.

Lehr, C. M. (2000). Lectin-mediated drug delivery: The second generation of bioadhesives. *Journal of Controlled Release* **65**(1–2), 19–29.

Lis, H. and Sharon, N. (1986). Lectins as molecules and as tools. *Annual Review of Biochemistry* **55**, 35–67.

Lobenberg, R., Maas, J., and Kreuter, J. (1998). Improved body distribution of ^{14}C-labelled AST bound to nanoparticles in rats determined by radioluminography. *Journal of Drug Targeting* **5**(3), 171–179.

Lockman, P. R., Koziara, J. M., Mumper, R. J., and Allen, D. D. (2004). Nanoparticle surface charges alter blood-brain barrier integrity and permeability. *Journal of Drug Targeting* **12**(9–10), 635–641.

Loftsson, T., Brewster, M. E., and Masson, M. (2004). Role of cyclodextrins in improving oral-drug delivery. *American Journal of Drug Delivery* **2**(4), 261–275.

Lopes, E., Pohlman, A. R., Bassani, V., and Guterres, S. S. (2000). Polymeric colloidal systems containing ethionamide: Preparation and physicochemical characterization. *Pharmazie* **55**(7), 527–530.

Lu, L., Sun, R. W., Chen, R., Hui, C. K., Ho, C. M., Luk, J. M., Lau, G. K. and Che, C. M. (2008). Silver nanoparticles inhibit hepatitis B virus replication. *Antiviral Therapy* **13**(2), 253–262.

Lucinda-Silva, R. M. and Evangelista, R. C. (2003). Microspheres of alginate-chitosan containing isoniazid. *Journal of Microencapsulation* **20**(2), 145–152.

Macri, R. V., Karlovská, J., Doncel, G. F., Du, X., Maisuria, B. B., Williams, A. A., Sugandhi, E. W., Falkinham, J. O. 3rd, Esker, A. R., and

Gandour, R. D. (2009). Comparing anti-HIV, antibacterial, antifungal, micellar, and cytotoxic properties of tricarboxylato dendritic amphiphiles. *Bioorganic and Medicinal Chemistry* **17**(8), 3162–3168.

Mainardes, R. M. and Evangelista, R. C. (2005). PLGA nanoparticles containing praziquantel: effect of formulation variables on size distribution. *International Journal of Pharmaceutics* **290**(1–2), 137–144.

Mainardes, R. M., Gremiao, M. P., Brunetti, I. L., da Fonseca, L. M., and Khalil, N. M. (2009). Zidovudine-loaded PLA and PLA-PEG blend nanoparticles: Influence of polymer type on phagocytic uptake by polymorphonuclear cells. *Journal of Pharmaceutical Sciences* **98**(1), 257–267.

Mallipeddi, R. and Rohan, L. C. (2010). Nanoparticle-based vaginal drug delivery systems for HIV prevention. *Expert Opinion in Drug Delivery* **7**(1), 37–48.

Manosroi, A., Konkaneramit, L., and Manosroi, J. (2004). Stability and transdermal absorption of topical amphotericin B liposome formulations. *International Journal of Pharmaceutics* **270**(1–2), 279–286.

McCarthy, T. D., Karellas, P., Henderson, S. A., Giannis, M., O'Keefe, D. F., Heery, G., Paull, J. R., Matthews, B. R., and Holan, G. (2005). Dendrimers as drugs: Discovery and preclinical and clinical development of dendrimer-based microbicides for HIV and STI prevention. *Molecular Pharmacology* **2**(4), 312–318.

McNamara, L. A. and Collins, K. L. (2011). Hematopoietic stem/precursor cells as HIV reservoirs. *Current Opinion in HIV and AIDS* **6**(1), 43–48.

Medda, S., Jaisankar, P., Manna, R. K., Pal, B., Giri, V. S., and Basu, M. K. (2003). Phospholipid microspheres: A novel delivery mode for targeting antileishmanial agent in experimental leishmaniasis. *Journal of Drug Targeting* **11**(2), 123–128.

Ménez, C., Legrand, P., Rosilio, V., Lesieur, S., and Barratt, G. (2007). Physicochemical characterization of molecular assemblies of miltefosine and amphotericin B. *Molecular Pharmacology* **4**(2), 281–288.

Meyerhoff, A. (1999). US Food and Drug Administration approval AmBisome (liposomal amphotericin B) for treatment of viseral leishamiasis. *Clinical Infectious Diseases* **28**(1), 42–48.

Morello, M., Krone, C. I., Dickerson, S., Howerth, E., Germishuizen, W. A., Wong, Y. L., Edwards, D., Bloom, B. R., and Hondalus, M. K. (2009). Dry powder pulmonary insufflation in the mouse for application to vaccine or drug studies. *Tuberculosis (Edinburgh)* **89**(5), 371–377.

Moretton, M. A., Glisoni, R. J., Chiappetta, D. A., and Sosnik, A. (2010). Molecular implications in the nanoencapsulation of the antituberculosis drug rifampicin within flower-like polymeric micelles. *Colloids and Surfaces B: Biointerfaces* **79**(2), 467–479.

Moulard, M., Lortat-Jacob, H., Mondor, I., Roca, G., Wyatt, R., Sodroski, J., Zhao, L., Olson, W., Kwong, P. D., and Sattentau, Q. J. (2000). Selective interactions of polyanions with basic surfaces on human immunodeficiency virus type 1 gp120. *Journal of Virology* **74**(4), 1948–1960.

Mrsny, R. J. (2009). Lessons from nature: "Pathogen-Mimetic" systems for mucosal nanomedicines. *Advanced Drug Delivery Reviews* **61**(2), 172–192.

Muhuri, G. and Pal, T. K. (1991). Computation of release kinetics of isoniazid microcapsules. *Bollettino Chimico Farmaceutico* **130**(5), 169–171.

Muller, R. H. and Keck, C. M. (2004). Challenges and solutions for the delivery of biotech drugs- a review of drug nanocrystal technology and lipid nanoparticles. *Journal of Biotechnology* **113**(1–3), 151–170.

Muller, R. H., Jacobs, C., and Kayser, O. (2001). Nanosuspensions as particulate drug formulations in therapy. Rational for development and what we can expect for the future. *Advanced Drug Delivery Reviews* **47**(1), 3–19.

Nanjwade, B. K., Singh, J., Parikh, K. A. and Manvi, F. V. (2010). Preparation and evaluation of carboplatin biodegradable polymeric nanoparticles. *International Journal of Pharmaceutics* **385**(1–2), 176–180.

Nuermberger, E. L., Yoshimatsu, T., Tyagi, S., Williams, K., Rosenthal, I., O'Brien, R. J., Vernon,

A. A., Chaisson, R. E., Bishai, W. R., and Grosset, J. H. (2004). Moxifloxacin-containing regimens of reduced duration produce a stable cure in murine tuberculosis. *American Journal of Respiratory and Critical Care Medicine* **170**(10), 1131–1134.

Oganesian, E. A., Bud'ko, A. P., Stukalov, IuV., Liubimov, II., Biketov, S. F., Sveshnikov, P. G., Kheifets, L. B., and Gelperina, S. E. (2005). Development and estimation of nanosomal rifampicin. *Antibiotiki i Khimioterapii=a* 50(8–9), 15–19.

Ohashi, K., Kabasawa, T., Ozeki, T., and Okada, H. (2009). One-step preparation of rifampicin/poly (lactic-co-glycolic acid) nanoparticle-containing mannitol microspheres using a four-fluid nozzle spray drier for inhalation therapy of tuberculosis. *Journal of Controlled Release* 135(1), 19–24.

Oka, H., Onaga, T., Koyama, T., Guo, C. T., Suzuki, Y., Esumi, Y., Hatano, K., Terunuma, D., and Matsuoka, K. (2009). Syntheses and biological evaluations of carbosilane dendrimers uniformly functionalized with sialyl [alpha](2–3) lactose moieties as inhibitors for human influenzaviruses. *Bioorganic and Medicinal Chemistry* 17(15), 5465–5475.

Pandey, R. and Khuller, G. K. (2004a). Polymer based drug delivery systems for mycobacterial infections. *Current Drug Delivery* 1(3), 195–201.

Pandey, R. and Khuller, G. K. (2004b). Subcutaneous nanoparticle based antitubercular chemotherapy in an experimental model. *Journal of Antimicrobial Chemotherapy* 54(1), 266268.

Pandey, R. and Khuller, G. K. (2004c). Chemotherapeutic potential of alginate chitosan microspheres as antitubercular drugs. *Journal of Antimicrobial Chemotherapy* 53(4), 635–640.

Pandey, R. and Khuller, G. K. (2005a). Antitubercular inhaled therapy: Opportunities, progress and challenges. *Journal of Antimicrobial Chemotherapy* 55(4), 430–435.

Pandey, R. and Khuller, G. K. (2005b). Solid lipid particle based inhalable sustained drug delivery system against experimental tuberculosis. *Tuberculosis (Edinburgh)* 85(4), 227–234.

Pandey, R. and Khuller, G. K. (2006). Oral nanoparticle-based antituberculosis drug delivery to the brain in an experimental model. *Journal of Antimicrobial Chemotherapy* 57(6), 1146–1152.

Pandey, R. and Khuller, G. K. (2007). Nanoparticle-based oral drug delivery system for an injectable antibiotic-streptomycin. Evaluation in a murine tuberculosis model. *Chemotherapy* 53(6), 437–441.

Pandey, R., Ahmad, Z., Sharma, S., and Khuller, G. K. (2005a). Nano-encapsulation of azole antifungals: Potential applications to improve oral drug delivery. *International Journal of Pharmaceutics* 301(1–2), 268–276.

Pandey, R., Ahmed, Z., Sharma, S., and Khuller, G. K. (2003a). Nanoparticle encapsulated antitubercular drugs as a potential oral drug delivery system against murine tuberculosis. *Tuberculosis (Edinburgh)* 83(6), 373–378.

Pandey, R., Sharma, A., Zahoor, A., Sharma, S., Khuller, G. K., and Prasad, B. (2003b). Poly (DL-lactide-co-glycolide) nanoparticle based inhalable sustained drug delivery system for experimental tuberculosis. *Journal of Antimicrobial Chemotherapy* 52(6), 981–986.

Pandey, R., Sharma, S., and Khuller, G. K. (2005b). Oral solid lipid nanoparticle-based antitubercular chemotherapy. *Tuberculosis (Edinburgh)* 85(5), 415–420.

Pandey, R., Sharma, S., and Khuller, G. K. (2006a). Chemotherapeutic efficacy of nanoparticle encapsulated antitubercular drugs. *Drug Delivery* 13(4), 287–294.

Pandey, R., Sharma, S., and Khuller, G. K. (2006b). Oral poly(lactide-co-glycolide) nanoparticle based antituberculosis drug delivery: Toxicological and chemotherapeutic implications. *Indian Journal of Experimental Biology* 44(6), 459–467.

Patton, D. L., Cosgrove Sweeney, Y. T., McCarthy, T. D., and Hillier, S. L. (2006). Preclinical safety and efficacy assessments of dendrimer-based (SPL7013) microbicide gel formulations in an onhuman primate model. *Antimicrobial Agents and Chemotherapy* **50**(5), 1696–1700.

Pérez-Anes, A., Stefaniu, C., Moog, C., Majoral, J. P., Blanzat, M., Turrin, C-O., Caminade, A-M., and Rico-Lattes, I. (2010). Multivalent catanionic GalCer analogs derived from first generation dendrimeric phosphonic acids. *Bioorganic and Medicinal Chemistry* **18**(1), 242–248.

Porcel, E., Liehn, S., Remita, H., Usami, N., Kobayashi, K., Furusawa, Y., Sech, C. L., and Lacombe, S. (2010). Platinum nanoparticles: A promising material for future cancer therapy? *Nanotechnology* 21(8), 85103.

Prego, C., García, M., Torres, D., and Alonso, M. J. (2005). Transmucosal macromolecular drug delivery. *Journal of Controlled Release* 101(1–3), 151–162.

Pulliam, B., Sung, J. C., and Edwards, D. A. (2007). Design of nanoparticle-based dry powder pulmonary vaccines. *Expert Opinion in Drug Delivery* 4(6), 651–663.

Rajaonarivony, M., Vauthier, C., Couarraze, G., Puisieux, F., and Couvreur, P. (1993). Development of a new drug carrier made from alginate. *Journal of Pharmaceutical Sciences* 82(9), 912–917.

Rao, K. S., Ghorpade, A., and Labhasetwar, V. (2009). Targeting anti-HIV drugs to the CNS. *Expert Opinion in Drug Delivery* 6(8), 771–784.

Ravi Kumar, M. N. (2000). Nano and microparticles as controlled drug delivery devices. *Journal of Pharmacy and Pharmaceutical Sciences* 3(2), 234–258.

Rekha, M. R. and Sharma, C. P. (2009). Synthesis and evaluation of lauryl succinyl chitosan particles towards oral insulin delivery and absorption. *Journal of Controlled Release* 135(2), 144–151.

Rodrigues, J. M., Croft, S. L., Fessi, H., Bories, C., and Devissaguet, J. P. (1994). The activity and ultrastructural localization of primaquine-loaded poly(D,L-lactide) nanoparticles in *Leishmania donovani* infected mice. *Tropical Medicine and Parasitology* 45(3), 223–228.

Rodrigues, J. M. Jr., Fessi, H., Bories, C., Puisieux, F., and Devissaguet, J. P. (1995). Primaquine-loaded poly(lactide) nanoparticles: Physicochemical study and acute tolerance in mice. *International Journal of Pharmaceutics* 126(1–2), 253–260.

Rogers, J., Parkinson, C., Choi, Y., Speshock, J., and Hussain, S. (2008). A preliminary assessment of silver nanoparticle inhibition of monkeypox virus plaque formation. *Nanoscale Research Letters* 3(4), 129–133.

Roy, P., Das, S., Bera, T., Mondol, S., and Mukherjee, A. (2010). Andrographolide nanoparticles in leishmaniasis: Characterization and *in vitro* evaluations. *International Journal of Nanomedicine* 5, 1113–1121.

Roy, R., Zanini, D., Meunier, S. J., and Romanowska, A. (1993). Solid-phase synthesis of dendritic sialoside inhibitors of influenza A virus haemagglutinin. *Journal of the Chemical Society: Chemical Communications* 24, 1869–1872.

Rupp, R., Rosenthal, S. L., and Stanberry, L. R. (2007). VivaGel (SPL7013 Gel): A candidate dendrimer – microbicide for the prevention of HIV and HSV infection. *International Journal of Nanomedicine* 2(4), 561–566.

Santiangelo, R., Paderu, P., Delmas, G., Chen, Z-W., Mannino, R., Zarif, L., and Perlin, D. S. (2000). Efficacy of oral cochleate-amphotericin B in mouse model of systemic candidiasis. *Antimicrobial Agents and Chemotherapy* 44(9), 2356–2360.

Saraogi, G. K., Gupta, P., Gupta, U. D., Jain, N. K., and Agrawal, G. P. (2010). Gelatin nanocarriers as potential vectors for effective management of tuberculosis. *International Journal of Pharmaceutics* 385(1–2), 143–149.

Saraogi, G. K., Sharma, B., Joshi, B., Gupta, P., Gupta, U. D., Jain, N. K., and Agrawal, G. P. (2011). Mannosylated gelatin nanoparticles bearing isoniazid for effective management of tuberculosis. *Journal of Drug Targeting* 19(3), 219–227.

Semete, B., Booysen, L., Lemmer, Y., Kalombo, L., Katata, L., Verschoor, J., and Swai, H. S. (2010). *In vivo* evaluation of the biodistribution and safety of PLGA nanoparticles as drug delivery systems. *Nanomedicine* 6(5), 662–671.

Shah, L. and Amiji, M. (2006). Intracellular delivery of saquinavir in biodegradable polymeric nanoparticles for HIV/AIDS. *Pharmeceutical Research* 23(11), 2638–2645.

Shahiwala, A. and Amiji, M. M. (2007). Nanotechnology-based delivery systems in HIV/AIDS therapy. *Future HIV Therapy* 1(1), 49–59.

Sharma, A., Pandey, R., Sharma, S., and Khuller, G. K. (2004a). Chemotherapeutic efficacy of poly (DL-lactide-co-glycolide) nanoparticle encapsulated antitubercular drugs at sub-therapeutic dose against experimental tuberculosis. *International Journal of Antimicrobial Agents* 24(6), 599–604.

Sharma, A., Sharma, S., and Khuller, G. K. (2004b). Lectin functionalized poly (lactide-co-glycolide) nanoparticles as oral/aerosolized antitubercular drug carriers for treatment of tuberculosis. *Journal of Antimicrobial Chemotherapy* 54(4), 761–766.

Sondi, I. and Salopek-Sondi, B. (2004). Silver nanoparticles as antimicrobial agent: A case study on *E. coli* as a model for Gram-negative bacteria. *Journal of Colloid and Interface Science* 275(1), 177–182.

Sosnik, A., Carcaboso, A. M., Glisoni, R. J., Moretton, M. A., and Chiappetta, D. A. (2010). New old challenges in tuberculosis: Potentially effective nanotechnologies in drug delivery. *Advanced Drug Delivery Reviews* 62(4–5), 547–559.

Sun, L., Singh, A. K., Vig, K., Pillai, S. R., and Singh, S. R. (2008). Silver nanoparticles inhibit replication of respiratory syncytial virus. *Journal of Biomedical Nanotechnology* 4, 149–158.

Sun, R. W., Chen, R., Chung, N. P., Ho, C. M., Lin, C. L., and Che, C. M. (2005). Silver nanoparticles fabricated in Hepes buffer exhibit cytoprotective activities toward HIV-1 infected cells. *Chemical Communications (Cambridge)* 28(40), 5059–5061.

Sun, Z., Zhang, J., Song, H., Zhang, X., Li, Y., Tian, M., Liu, Y., Zhao, Y., and Li, C. (2010). Concomitant increases in spectrum and level of drug resistance in *Mycobacterium tuberculosis* isolates. *International Journal of Tuberculosis and Lung Disease* 14(11), 1436–1441.

Sung, J. C., Garcia-Contreras, L., Verberkmoes, J. L., Peloquin, C. A., Elbert, K. J., Hickey, A. J., and Edwards, D. A. (2009b). Dry powder nitroimidazopyran antibiotic PA-824 aerosol for inhalation. *Antimicrobial Agents and Chemotherapy* 53(4), 1338–1343.

Sung, J. C., Padilla, D. J., Garcia-Contreras, L., Verberkmoes, J. L., Durbin, D., Peloquin, C. A., Elbert, K. J., Hickey, A. J., and Edwards, D. A. (2009a). Formulation and pharmacokinetics of self-assembled rifampicin nanoparticle systems for pulmonary delivery. *Pharmaceutical Research* 26(8), 1847–1855.

Svenson, S. and Tomalia, D. A. (2005). Dendrimers in biomedical applications–reflectionson the field. *Advanced Drug Delivery Reviews* 57(15), 2106–2129.

Takka, S. and Acartürk, F. (1999). Calcium alginate microparticles for oral administration: I: Effect of sodium alginate type on drug release and drug entrapment efficiency. *Journal of Microencapsulation* 16(3), 275–290.

Takka, S., Ocak, O. H., and Acartürk, F. (1998). Formulation and investigation of nicardipine HCl-alginate gel beads with factorial design-based studies. *European Journal of Pharmaceutical Sciences* 6(3), 241–246.

Telwatte, S., Moore, K., Johnson, A., Tyssen, D., Sterjovski, J., Aldunate, M., Gorry, P. R., Ramsland, P. A., Lewis, G. R., Paull, J. R., Sonza, S., and Tachedjian, G. (2011). Virucidal activity of the dendrimer microbicide SPL7013 against HIV-1. *Antiviral Research*, April 1 [Epub ahead of print, PMID: 21459115].

Thakur, C. P. and Narayan, S. A. (2004). A comparative evaluation of amphotericin B and sodium antimony gluconate, as first-line drugs in the treatment of Indian visceral leishmaniasis. *Annals of Tropical Medicine and Parasitology* 98(2), 129–138.

Thirawong, N., Thongborisute, J., Takeuchi, H., and Sriamornsak, P. (2008). Improved intestinal absorption of calcitonin by mucoadhesive delivery of novel pectin-liposome nanocomplexes. *Journal of Controlled Release* 125(3), 236–245.

Tønnesen, H. H. and Karlsen, J. (2002). Alginate in drug delivery systems. *Drug Development and Industrial Pharmacy* 28(6), 621–630.

Torres-Santos, E. C., Rodrigues, J. M. J., Moreira, D. L., Kaplan, M. A. C., and Rossi-Bergman, B. (1999). Improvement of *in vitro* and *in vivo* antileishmanial activities of 2′,6′-dihydroxy-4′-methoxychalcone by entrapment in poly (D,L-lactide) nanoparticles. *Antimicrobial Agents and Chemotherapy* 43(7), 1776–1778.

Tosi, G., Rivasi, F., Gandolfi, F., Costantino, L., Vandelli, M. A., and Forni, F. (2005). Conjugated poly (D,L-lactide-co-glycolide) for the preparation of *in vivo* detectable nanoparticles. *Biomaterials* 26(19), 4189–4195.

Ul-Ain, Q., Sharma, S., and Khuller, G. K. (2003a). Chemotherapeutic potential of orally administered poly (lactide-co-glycolide) microparticles containing isoniazid, rifampicin and pyrazinamide against experimental tuberculosis. *Antimicrobial Agents and Chemotherapy* 47(9), 3005–3007.

Ul-Ain, Q., Sharma, S., Khuller, G. K., and Garg, S. K. (2003b). Alginate based oral drug delivery system for tuberculosis: Pharmacokinetics and therapeutic effects. *Journal of Antimicrobial Chemotherapy* 51(4), 931–938.

Verma, A. K., Pandey, R. P., Chanchal, A., and Sharma, P. (2011). Immuno-potentiating role of encapsulated proteins of infectious diseases in biopolymeric nanoparticles as a potential delivery system. *Journal of Biomedical Nanotechnology* 7(1), 63–64.

Vyas, S. P., Kannan, M. E., Jain, S., Mishra, V., and Singh, P. (2004). Design of liposomal aerosol for improved delivery of rifampicin to alveolar macrophages. *International Journal of Pharmaceutics* 269(1), 37–49.

Vyas, T. K., Shah, L., and Amiji, M. M. (2006). Nanoparticulate drug carriers fordelivery of HIV/AIDS therapy to viral reservoir sites. *Expert Opinion in Drug Delivery* 3(5), 613–628.

Wang, C. and Hickey, A. J. (2010). Isoxyl aerosols for tuberculosis treatment: preparation and characterization of particles. *AAPS Pharmaceutical Sciences and Technology* 11(2), 538–549.

Wang, J., Wang, L., Sun, Y., Zhu, X., Cao, Y., Wang, X., Zhang, H., and Song, D. (2010). Surface plasmon resonance biosensor based on Au nanoparticle in titania sol-gel membrane. *Colloids and Surfaces B: Biointerfaces* 75(2), 520–525.

Weber, N., Ortega, P., Clemente, M. I., Shcharbin, D., Bryszewska, M., de la Mata, F. J., Gómez, R. and Muñoz-Fernández, M. A. (2008). Characterization of carbosilanedendrimers as effective carriers of siRNA to HIV-infected lymphocytes. *Journal of Controlled Release* 132(1), 55–64.

Weers, J. G., Bell, J., Chan, H. K., Cipolla, D., Dunbar, C., Hickey, A. J., and Smith, I. J. (2010). Pulmonary formulations: What remains to be done? *Journal of Aerosol Medicine: Pulmonary Drug Delivery* 23(S2), S5–S23.

Wei, D., Sun, W., Qian, W., Ye, Y., and Ma, X. (2009). The synthesis of chitosan-basedsilver nanoparticles and their antibacterial activity. *Carbohydrate Research* 344(17), 2375–2382.

Whitehead, L., Collett, J. H., and Fell, J. T. (2000). Amoxycillin release from a floating dosage form based on alginates. *International Journal of Pharmaceutics* 210(1–2), 45–49.

Woitiski, C. B., Neufeld, R. J., Veiga, F., Carvalho, R. A., and Figueiredo, I. V. (2010). Pharmacological effect of orally delivered insulin facilitated by multilayered stable nanoparticles. *European Journal of Pharmaceutical Sciences* 41(3–4), 556–563.

World Health Organization, (2003). Treatment of tuberculosis: Guidelines for national programmes, 3 ed. Geneva, WHO, WHO/CDS/TB/2003.313.

Yang, H., Parniak, M. A., Isaacs, C. E., Hillier, S. L., and Rohan, L. C. (2008). Characterization of cyclodextrin inclusion complexes of the anti-HIV non-nucleoside reverse transcriptase inhibitor UC781. *AAPS Journal* 10(4), 606–613.

Yang, S., Zhu, J., Lu, Y., Liang, B., and Yang, C. (1999). Body distribution of camptothecin solid lipid nanoparticles after oral administration. *Pharmeceutical Research* 16(5), 751–757.

Yu, B. T., Sun, X., and Zhang, Z. R. (2003). Enhanced liver targeting by synthesis of N1-stearyl-5-Fu and incorporation into solid lipid nanoparticles. *Archives of Pharmaceutical Research* 26(12), 1096–1101.

Yu Chang, S-S., Lee, C-L., and Wang, C. R. C. (1997). Gold nanorods: Electrochemicalsynthesis and optical properties. *Journal of Physical Chemistry B* 101(34), 6661–6664.

Zara, G. P., Bargoni, A., Cavalli, R., Fundarò, A., Vighetto, D., and Gasco, M. R. (2002a). Pharmacokinetics and tissue distribution of idarubicin-loaded solid lipid nanoparticles after duodenal administration to rats. *Journal of Pharmaceutical Sciences* 91(5), 1324–1333.

Zara, G. P., Cavalli, R., Bargoni, A., Fundaro, A., Vighetto, D., and Gasco, M. R. (2002b). Intravenous administration to rabbits of non-stealth and stealth doxorubicin-loaded solid lipid nanoparticles at increasing concentrations of stealth agent: Pharmacokinetics and distribution of doxorubicin in brain and other tissues. *Journal of Drug Targeting* 10(4), 327–335.

Zara, G. P., Cavalli, R., Fundarò, A., Bargoni, A., Caputo, O., and Gasco, M. R. (1999). Pharmacokinetics of doxorubicin incorporated in solid lipid nanospheres (SLN). *Pharmacological Research* 40(3), 281–286.

Zhao, J., Bowman, L., Zhang, X., Vallyathan, V., Young, S. H., Castranova, V., and Ding, M. (2009). Titanium dioxide (TiO2) nanoparticles induce JB6 cell apoptosis through activation of the Caspase-8/bid and mitochondrial pathways. *Journal of Toxicology and Environmental Health, Part A:Current Issues* **72**(19), 1141–1149.

Zhou, Y., Yu, S. H., Cui, X. P., Wang, C. Y., and Chen, Z. Y. (1999). Formation of silver nanowires by a novel solid-liquid phase arc discharge method. *Chemistry of Materials* **11**(3), 545–546.

Zhou, J., Shu, Y., Guo, P., Smith, D. D., and Rossi, J. J. (2011). Dual functional RNA nanoparticles containing phi29 motor pRNA and anti-gp120 aptamer for cell-type specific delivery and HIV-1 inhibition. Methods, January 20 [Epub ahead of print, PMID: 21256218].

10

Agarwal, A., Saraf, S., Asthana, A., Gupta U., Gajbhiye V., and Jain, N. K. (2008). Ligand based dendritic systems for tumor targeting. *International Journal of Pharmaceutics*, **350**, 3–13.

Ah Kim, H., Lee, S., Park, J. H., Lee, S., Lee, B.W., Ihm, S.H., Kim, T.I., Kim, S.W., Ko, K. S., and Lee M. (2009). Enhanced protection of Ins-1 beta cells from apoptosis under hypoxia by delivery of DNA encoding secretion signal peptide-linked exendin-4. *Journal of Drug Targeting*, **17**, 242–248.

Albrecht, V., Wiehe, A., Roeder, B., and Neuberger, W. (2005). CeramOptec Industries, Inc., assignee; US Patent Application 2005/0281777.

Balicki, D., Reisfeld, R. A., Pertl, U., Beutler, E., and Lode, H. N. (2000). Inventors, Histone H2A-mediated transient cytokine gene delivery induces efficient antitumor esponses in murine neuroblastoma. *Proceedings of National Academy of Sciences of USA*, **97**, 1500–11504.

Balogh, L., Hagnauer, G., Tomalia, D., and Mcmanus, A., (2001). Inventors, The government of USA, assignee; US6224898.

Battah, S. H., Chee, C. E., Nakanishi, H., Gerscher, S., MacRobert, A. J., and Edwards, C. (2001). Synthesis and biological studies of 5-aminolevulinic acid-containing dendrimers for

photodynamic therapy. *Bioconjugate Chemistry*, **12**, 980–988.

Bernstein, D. I., Stanberry, L. R., Sacks, S., Ayisi, N. K., Gong, Y. H., Ireland, J., Mumper, R. J., Holan, G., Matthews, B., McCarthy, T., and Bourne, N. (2003). Evaluations of unformulated and formulated dendrimer-based microbicide candidates in mouse and guinea pig models of genital herpes. *Antimicrobial Agents Chemotherapy*, **47**, 3784–3788.

Bharali, D. J., Khalil, M., Gurbuz, M., Simone, T. M., and Mousa, S. A. (2009). Nanoparticles and cancer therapy: a concise review with emphasis on dendrimers. *Int. J. Nanomedicine*, **4**, 1–7.

Bosman, A. W., Janssen, H. M., and Meijer, E. W. (1999). About Dendrimers: structure, physical properties, and applications. *Chemical Reviews*, **99**, 1665–1688.

Boswell, C. A., Eck, P. K., Regino, C. A., Bernardo, M., Wong, K. J., Milenic, D. E., Choyke, P. L., and Brechbiel, M. W. (2008). Synthesis, characterization, and biological evaluation of integrin alphavbeta3-targeted PAMAM dendrimers. *Molecular Pharmaceutics*, **5**, 527–539.

Bourne, M. W., Margerun, L., Hylton, N., Campion, B., Lai, J. J., Derugin, N., and Higgins, C. B. (1996). Evaluation of the effects of intravascular MR contrast media (gadolinium dendrimer) on 3D time of flight magnetic resonance angiography of the body. *Journal of Magnetic Resonance Imaging*, **6**, 305–310.

Branderhorst, H. M., Liskamp, R. M., Visser, G. M., and Pieters, R. J. Strong inhibition of cholera toxin binding by galactose dendrimers. *Chemical Communications* (Camb), **47**, 5043–5045.

Chafekar, S. M., Malda, H., Merkx, M., Meijer, E. W., Viertl, D., Lashuel, H. A., Baas, F., and Scheper, W. (2007). Branched KLVFF tetramers strongly potentiate inhibition of beta-amyloid aggregation. *Chembiochem*, **8**, 1857–1864.

Chen, C. Z., Beck-Tan, N. C., Dhurjati, P., van Dyk, T. K., LaRossa, R. A., and Cooper, S. L. (2000). Quaternary ammonium functionalized poly(propylene imine) dendrimers as effective antimicrobials: structure-activity studies. *Biomacromolecules*, **1**, 473–480.

Chen, C. Z., Beck-Tan, N. C., Dhurjati, P., van Dyk, T. K., LaRossa, R. A., and Cooper, S. L.

(2000). Quaternary ammonium functionalized poly(propylene imine) dendrimers as effective antimicrobials: structure-activity studies. *Biomacromolecules*, **1**, 473–480.

Chisholm, E. J., Vassaux, G., Martin-Duque, P., Chevre, R., Lambert, O., Pitard, B., Merron, A., Weeks, M., Burnet, J., Peerlinck, I., Dai, M.-S., Alusi, G., Mather, S. J., Bolton, K., Uchegbu, I. F., Schatzlein, A. G., and Baril, P. (2009). Cancer-specific Transgene Expression Mediated by Systemic Injection of Nanoparticles. *Cancer Research*, **69**, 2655–2662.

Chonco, L., Bermejo-Martin, J. F., Ortega, P., Shcharbin, D., Pedziwiatr, E., Klajnert, B., de la Mata, F. J., Eritja, R., Gómez, R., Bryszewska, M., and Muñoz-Fernandez Ma-A. (2007). Water-soluble carbosilane dendrimers protect phosphorothioate oligonucleotides from binding to serum proteins. *Organic & Biomolecular Chemistry*, **5**, 1886–1893.

Cooper, S. and Chen, C. (2002). Inventors University of Delaware (Newark, DE), assignee; US6440405.

Cooper, S. and Chen, C. (2003). Inventors University of Delaware (Newark, DE), assignee; US6579906.

Cramer, S., Moore, J., Kundu, A., Li, Y., and Jayaraman, G., (1995). Inventors Heslin & Rothenberg Attorney, US5478924.

Cromer, J. R., Wood, S. J., Miller, K. A., Nguyen, T., and David, S. A. (2005). Functionalized dendrimers as endotoxin sponges. Bioorg. *Med. Chem. Lett.*, **15**, 1295–1298.

D'Emanuele, A., Jevprasesphant, R., Penny, J., and Attwood, D. (2004). The use of a dendrimer-propranolol prodrug to bypass efflux transporters and enhance oral bioavailability. *Journal of Controlled Release*, **95**, 447–453.

Devarakonda, B., Hill, R. A., Liebenberg, W., Brits, M., and de Villiers, M. M. (2005). Comparison of the aqueous solubilization of practically insoluble niclosamide by polyamidoamine (PAMAM) dendrimers and cyclodextrins. *International Journal of Pharmaceutics*, **304**, 193–209.

Devarakonda, B., Otto, D. P., Judefeind, A., Hill, R. A., and de Villiers, M. M. (2007). Effect of pH on the solubility and release of furosemide from polyamidoamine (PAMAM) dendrimer complex-

es. *International Journal of Pharmaceutics*, **345**, 142–153.

Diallo, M. (2009). Inventor *No assignee*, US Patent Application 2009/0223896.

Donalisio, M., Rusnati, M., Civra, A., Bugatti, A., Allemand, D., Pirri, G., Giuliani, A., Landolfo, S., and Lembo, D. (2010). Identification of a dendrimeric heparan sulfate-binding peptide that inhibits infectivity of genital types of human papillomaviruses. *Antimicrobial Agents Chemotherapy*, **54**, 4290–4299.

Duan, X., McLaughlin, C., Griffith, M., and Sheardown, H. (2007). Biofunctionalization of collagen for improved biological response: scaffolds for corneal tissue engineering. *Biomaterials*, **28**, 78–88.

Dufes, C., Nicol, Keith W., Bilsland, A., Proutski, I., Uchegbu, I. F., and Schatzlein, A. G. (2005). Synthetic Anticancer Gene Medicine Exploits Intrinsic Antitumor Activity of Cationic Vector to Cure Established Tumors. *Cancer Research*, **65**, 8079–8084.

Dufes, C., Uchegbu, I., and Schatzlein, A. (2005). Dendrimers in gene delivery. *Advanced Drug Delivery Reviews*, **57**, 2177–2202.

Dunphy, I., Vinogradov, S. A., and Wilson, D. F. (2002). Oxyphor R2 and G2: phosphors for measuring oxygen by oxygen-dependent quenching of phosphorescence. *Analitical Biochemistry*, **310**, 191–198.

Eliyahu, H., Barenholz, Y., and Domb, A. J. (2005). Polymers for DNA Delivery. *Molecules*, **10**, 34–64.

Eliyahu, H., Servel, N., Domb, A. J., and Barenholz, Y. (2002). Lipoplex-induced hemagglutination: potential involvement in intravenous gene delivery. *Gene Therapy*, **9**, 850–858.

Esumi, K., Houdatsu, H., and Yoshimura, T. (2004). Antioxidant action by gold-PAMAM dendrimer nanocomposites. *Langmuir*, **20**, 2536–2538.

Feigin, V. L. (2005). Stroke epidemiology in the developing world. *Lancet*, **365**, 2160–2161.

Fischer, M. and Vogtle, F. (1999). *Dendrimers: From Design to Application - A. Progress Report* Angewande Chemistry International Edition English, **38**, 884–905.

Florence, A., Sakthivel, T., Wilderspin, A., and Toth, I., (2001). Inventors The school of Pharmacy University (GB), assignee; US6194543.

Florence, A. T., Wilderspin, A. F., Toth, I., Bayele, H. K., and Sakthivel, T., Inventors (1999).

Frechet, J. M. (1994). Functional polymers and dendrimers: reactivity, molecular architecture, and interfacial energy. *Science*, 263, 1710–1715.

Gazumyan, A., Mitsner, B., and Ellestad, G. A. (2000). Novel anti-RSV dianionic dendrimer-like compounds: design, synthesis and biological evaluation. *Curr. Pharm. Des.*, 6, 525–546.

German, M. S. and Szoka, F.C., Jr., (1998). Inventors *The Regents of the University of California*, USA, assignee; US5830730.

Getts, R., inventor (2002). Inventors No assignee, US Patent application 2002/0051981.

Gillies, E. R., and Fréchet, J. M. (2005). Dendrimers and dendritic polymers in drug delivery. *Drug Discovery Today*, 10, 35–43.

Gong, E., Matthews, B., McCarthy, T., Chu, J., Holan, G., Raff, J., and Sacks, S. (2005). Evaluation of dendrimer SPL7013, a lead microbicide candidate against herpes simplex viruses. *Antiviral Research*, 68, 139–146.

Gong, Y., Matthews, B., Cheung, D., Tam, T., Gadawski, I., Leung, D., Holan, G., Raff, J., and Sacks, S. (2002). Evidence of dual sites of action of dendrimers: SPL-2999 inhibits both virus entry and late stages of herpes simplex virus replication. *Antiviral Research*, 55, 319–329.

Han, L., Zhang, A., Wang, H., Pu, P., Kang, C., and Chang, J. (2010). Tat-BMPs-PAMAM conjugates enhance therapeutic effect of small interference RNA on U251 glioma cells in vitro and *in vivo*. *Human Gene Therapy*, 21, 417–426.

Harada, Y., Iwai, M., Tanaka, S., Okanoue, T., Kashima, K., Maruyama-Tabata, H., Hirai, H., Satoh, E., Imanishi, J., and Mazda, O. (2000). Highly efficient suicide gene expression in hepatocellular carcinoma cells by Epstein-Barr virus-based plasmid vectors combined with polyamidoamine dendrimers. *Cancer Gene Therapy*, 7, 27–36.

Hawker, C. J. and Frechet, J. M. J. (1990). Preparation of Polymers with Controlled Molecular architecture. A New Convergent Approach to Dendritic Macromolecules. *Journal of American Chemical Society*, 112, 7638-7647.

Haxton, K. J., and Burt, H. M. (2009). Polymeric drug delivery of platinum-based anticancer agents. *Journal of Pharmaceutical Sciences*, 98, 2299–2316.

Heegaard, P. and Boas, U. (2006). Inventors Danmarks Fodevareforskning (DK), assignee; US Patent Application 2006/0127350.

Heegaard, P. M. H., Pedersen, H. G., Flink, J., and Boas, U. (2004). Amyloid aggregates of the prion peptide PrP106–126 are destabilised by oxidation and by the action of dendrimers. *FEBS Letters*, 577, 127–133.

Heegaard, P. M. and Boas, U. (2006). Dendrimer based anti-infective and anti-inflammatory drugs. *Recent Patents in Antiinfection Drug Discovery*, 1, 331–351.

Heegaard, P. M., Boas, U., and Sorensen, N. S. (2010). Dendrimers for vaccine and immunostimulatory uses. *Bioconjugate Chemistry*, 21, 405–418.

Huang, R., Ke, W., Han, L., Liu, Y., Shao, K., Ye L., Lou, J., Jiang, C., and Pei, Y. (2009). Brain-targeting mechanisms of lactoferrin-modified DNA-loaded nanoparticles. *Journal of Cerebral Blood Flow Metabolism*, 29, 1914–1923.

Huang, R. Q., Qu, Y. H., Ke, W. L., Zhu, J. H., Pei, Y. Y., and Jiang, C. (2007). Efficient gene delivery targeted to the brain using a transferrin-conjugated polyethyleneglycol-modified polyamidoamine dendrimer. *FASEB Journal*, 21, 1117–1125.

Hubbell, J., Elbert, D., and Herbert, C. (2008). Inventors California Institute of Technology (Pasadena, CA, US), assignee; US7316845.

Hudde, T., Rayner, S. A., Comer, R. M., Weber, M., Isaacs, J. D., Waldmann, H., Larkin, D. F. P., and George, A. J. T. (1999). Activated polyamidoamine dendrimers, a non-viral vector for gene transfer to the corneal endothelium. *Gene Therapy*, 6, 939–943.

Inoue, Y., Kurihara, R., Tsuchida, A., Hasegawa, M., Nagashima, T., Mori, T., Niidome, T., Katayama, Y., and Okitsu, O. (2008). Efficient delivery of siRNA using dendritic poly(L-lysine) for loss-of-function analysis, *Journal of Controlled Release*, 126, 59–66.

Jacobson, K., Kim, Y., Klutz, A., Hechler, B., and Gachet, C. (2009). Inventors The Government of USA, assignee; US patent application 2009/0012035.

Jiménez, J. L., Clemente, M. I., Weber, N. D., Sanchez, J., Ortega, P., de la Mata, F. J., Gómez, R., García, D., López-Fernández, L. A., and Muñoz-Fernández, M. A. (2010). Carbosilane dendrimers to transfect human astrocytes with small interfering RNA targeting human immunodeficiency virus. *BioDrugs*, 24, 331–343.

Jimenez, O. and Moll, F. (2005). Inventors US Patent Application 2005/0175669.

Johnson, T. A., Stasko, N. A., Matthews, J. L., Cascio, W. E., Holmuhamedov, E. L., Johnson, C. B., and Schoenfisch, M. H. (2010). Reduced ischemia/reperfusion injury via glutathione-initiated nitric oxide-releasing dendrimers. *Nitric Oxide*, 22, 30–36.

Kaminskas, L. M., Kelly, B. D., McLeod, V. M., Boyd, B. J., Krippner, G. Y., Williams, E. D., and Porter, C. J. (2009). Pharmacokinetics and tumor disposition of PEGylated, methotrexate conjugated poly-l-lysine dendrimers. *Molecular Pharmaceutics*, 6, 1190–1204.

Ke, W., Shao, K., Huang, R., Han, L., Liu, Y., Li, J., Kuang, Y., Ye, L., Lou, J., and Jiang, C. (2009). Gene delivery targeted to the brain using an Angiopep-conjugated polyethyleneglycol-modified polyamidoamine dendrimer. *Biomaterials*, 30, 6976–6985.

Kellar, K. E., Henrichs, P. M., Hollister, R., Koenig, S. H., Eck, J., and Wie, D. (1997). High relaxivity linear Gd(DTPA)-polymer conjugates: the role of hydrophobic interactions. *Magnetic Resonance Medicine*, 38, 712–716.

Kensinger, R. D., Catalone, B. J., Krebs, F. C., Wigdahl, B., and Schengrund, C. L. (2004). Novel polysulfated galactose-derivatized dendrimers as binding antagonists of human immunodeficiency virus type 1 infection. *Antimicrobial Agents Chemotherapy*, 48, 1614–1623.

Kim, H. A., Lee, B. W., Kang, D., Kim, J. H., Ihm, S. H., and Lee, M. (2009). Delivery of hypoxia-inducible VEGF gene to rat islets using polyethylenimine. *Journal of Drug Targeting*, 17, 1–9.

Kim, I. D., Lim, C. M., Kim, J. B., Nam, H. Y., Nam, K., Kim, S. W., Park, J. S., Lee, J. K. (2010). Neuroprotection by biodegradable PAMAM ester (e-PAM-R)-mediated HMGB1 siRNA delivery in primary cortical cultures and in the postischemic brain. *Journal of Controlled Release*, 142, 422–430.

Kim, Y. and Zimmerman S. C. (1998). Applications of dendrimers in bio-organic chemistry. *Current Opinion in Chemical Biology*, 2, 733–742.

King, J. and Hill J. (2006). Inventors King Technology Inc. (Hopkins, MN, US), assignee; US7048864.

King, J. and Hill J. (2007). Inventors King Technology Inc. (Hopkins, MN, US), assignee; US7264739.

King, J. and Hill, J. (2009). Inventors KWG Technology (Hopkins, MN, US), assignee; US7507335.

King, M., Duan, X., and Sheardown, H. (2004). Partitioning of model toxins to hydrophobically terminated DAB dendrimers. *Biotechnology & Bioengineering*, 86, 512–519.

Klajnert, B., Cladera, J., and Bryszewska, M. (2006c). Molecular interactions of dendrimers with amyloid peptides: pH dependence. *Biomacromolecules*, 7, 2186–2191.

Klajnert, B., Cortijo-Arellano, M., Bryszewska, M., and Cladera, J. (2006a). Influence of heparin and dendrimers on the aggregation of twoamyloid peptides related to Alzheimer's and prion diseases. *Biochemical et Biophysical Research Communications*, 339, 577–582.

Klajnert, B., Cortijo-Arellano, M., Cladera, J., and Bryszewska, M. (2006b). Influence of dendrimer's structure on its activity against amyloid fibril formation. *Biochemical et Biophysical Research Communications*, 345, 21–28.

Klajnert, B., Cortijo-Arellano, M., Cladera, J., Majoral, J. P., Caminade, A. M., and Bryszewska, M. (2007). Influence of phosphorus dendrimers on the aggregation of theprion peptide PrP 185-208, Biochemical et Biophysical Research Communications, 364, 20–25.

Klajnert, B., Janiszewska, J., Urbanczyk-Lipkowska, Z., Bryszewska, M., Shcharbin, D., and Labieniec, M. (2006). Biological properties of low molecular mass peptide dendrimers. *International Journal of Pharmaceutics*, 309, 208–217.

Kobayashi, H. and Brechbiel, M. W. (2003). Dendrimer-based macromolecular MRI contrast agents: characteristics and application. *Molecular Imaging*, 2, 1–10.

Kobayashi, H. and Brechbiel, M. W. (2005). Nano-sized MRI contrast agents with dendrimer cores. *Advanced Drug Delivery Reviews*, **57**, 2271–2286.

Kobayashi, H., Kawamoto, S., Jo, S. K., Bryant, H. L. Jr., Brechbiel, M. W., and Star, R. A. (2003). Macromolecular MRI contrast agents with small dendrimers: pharmacokinetic differences between sizes and cores. *Bioconjugate Chemistry*, **14**, 388–394.

Kobayashi, H., Kawamoto, S., Saga, T., Sato, N., Hiraga, A., Ishimori, T., Akita, Y., Mamede, M. H., Konishi, J., Togashi, K., and Brechbiel, M. W. (2001). Novel liver macromolecular MR contrast agent with a polypropylenimine diaminobutyl dendrimer core: comparison to the vascular MR contrast agent with the polyamidoamine dendrimer core. *Magnetic Resonance Medicine*, **46**, 795–802.

Konda, S. D., Aref, M., Brechbiel, M., and Wiener, E.C. (2000). Development of a tumor-targeting MR contrast agent using the high-affinity folate receptor: work in progress. *Investigative Radiology*, **35**, 50–57.

Kono, K., Kojima, C., Hayashi, N., Nishisaka, E., Kiura, K., Watarai, S., and Harada, A. (2008). Preparation and cytotoxic activity of poly(ethylene glycol)-modified poly(amidoamine) dendrimers bearing adriamycin. *Biomaterials*, **29**, 1664–1675.

Kono, K., Liu, M., and Fréchet, J.M. (1999). Design of dendritic macromolecules containing folate or methotrexate residues. *Bioconjugate Chemistry*, **10**, 1115–1121.

Kubota, S. (2002). Inventor DendriMolecular, Inc. (US), assignee; US6410680.

Kurtoglu, Y. E., Navath, R. S., Wang, B., Kannan, S., Romero, R., and Kannan, R. M. (2009). Poly(amidoamine) dendrimer-drug conjugates with disulfide linkages for intracellular drug delivery. *Biomaterials*, **30**, 2112–2121.

Lebedev, A. Y., Cheprakov, A. V., Sakadžić, S., Boas, D. A., Wilson, D. F., and Vinogradov, S. A. (2009). Dendritic phosphorescent probes for oxygen imaging in biological systems. *ACS Applications in Material Interfaces*, **1**, 1292–1304.

Lee, C. Y., Sharma, A., Cheong, J. E., and Nelson, J. L. (2009). Synthesis and antioxidant

properties of dendritic polyphenols. *Bioorganic Medical Chemistry Letters*, **19**, 6326–6330.

Lee, C. Y., Sharma, A., Uzarski, R. L., Cheong, J. E., Xu, H., Held, R. A., Upadhaya, S. K., and Nelson, J. L. (2011). Potent antioxidant dendrimers lacking pro-oxidant activity. *Free Radical in Biology and Medicine*, **50**, 918–925.

Li, Z., Huang, P., Zhang, X., Lin, J., Yang, S., Liu, B., Gao, F., Xi, P., Ren, Q., and Cui, D. (2010). RGD-conjugated dendrimer-modified gold nanorods for *in vivo* tumor targeting and photothermal therapy. *Molecular Pharmaceutics*, **7**, 94–104.

Lin, S., Yu, K. S., Singh, P., and Diamond, S. (1999). Inventor Dade Behring Inc. (US), assignee; US5861319.

Majoral, J. P., Caminade, A. M., Laurent, R., and Sutra, P. (2002). Phosphorus-containing dendrimers. From material science to biology. *Heteroatom Chemistry*, **13**, 474–485.

Majoral, J. P., Meunier, B., Caminade, A. M., Loup, Ch., and Zanta-Boussif, M. A. (2005). Inventors Centre National de La Recherche Scientifique-CNRS, assignee; US6969528.

Malik, N. and Duncan, R. (2004). Inventors The Dow Chemical Company (Midland, MI), assignee; US6790437.

Malik, N., Duncan, R., Tomalia, D., and Esfand, R., inventors (2006). Dendritic Nanotechnologies, Inc. (Mt. Pleasant, MI, US), assignee; US7005124.

Malik, N., Evagorou, E. G., and Duncan, R. (1999). Dendrimer-platinate: A novel approach to cancer chemotherapy. *Anticancer Drugs*, **10**, 767–776.

Mansfield, M. L. and Klushin, L. I. (1993). Monte Carlo studies of dendrimer macromolecules. *Macromolecules*, **26**, 4262–4268.

Maruyama-Tabata, H., Harada, Y., Matsumura, T., Satoh, E., Cui, F., Iwai, M., Kita, M., Hibi, S., Imanishi, J., Sawada, T., and Mazda, O. (2000). Effective suicide gene therapy in vivo by EBV-based plasmid vector coupled with polyamidoamine dendrimers. *Gene Therapy*, **7**, 53–60.

Matsunaga, T., Takeyama, H., Yoza, B., Fukushima, K., and Satou, S. (2008). Inventors Yokogawa Electric Corporation (Musashino-shi, Tokyo, JP), assignee; US7405042.

Matthews, B. and Holan, G. (2002). Inventors Starpharma Limited (Parkville, AU), assignee; US6464971.

Matthews, O. A., Shipway, A. N., and Stoddart, J. F. (1998). Dendrimers—Branching out from Curiosities into New Technologies. *Progress in Polymer Science*, **23**, 1–56.

McCarthy, T. D., Karellas, P., Henderson, S. A., Giannis, M., O'Keefe, D. F., Heery, G., Paull, J. R., Matthews, B. R., and Holan, G. (2005). Dendrimers as drugs: discovery and preclinical and clinical development of dendrimer-based microbicides for HIV and STI prevention. *Molecular Pharmaceutics*, **2**, 312–318.

Medina, S. H. and El-Sayed, M. E. (2009). Dendrimers as carriers for delivery of chemotherapeutic agents. Chemical Reviews, **109**, 3141–3157.

Migdal, C. (1990). Inventor Texaco Inc. (US), assignee; US4938885.

Milowska, K., Malachowska, M., and Gabryelak, T. (2011). PAMAM G4 dendrimers affect the aggregation of α-synuclein. *International Journal of Biological Macromolecules*, **48**, 742–746.

Moll, III F., Ferzli, C., Lin, S., and Singh, P. (2000). Inventor Dade Behring Inc. (US), assignee; US6121056.

Murat, M. and Grest, G. S. (1996). Molecular Dynamics Study of Dendrimer Molecules in Solvents of Varying Quality. *Macromolecules*, **29**, 1278–285.

Myc, A., Douce, T. B., Ahuja, N., Kotlyar, A., Kukowska-Latallo, J., Thomas, T. P., Baker, J. R. Jr. (2008). Preclinical antitumor efficacy evaluation of dendrimer-based methotrexate conjugates. *Anticancer Drugs*, **19**, 143–149.

Na, M., Yiyun, C., Tongwen, X., Yang, D., Xiaomin, W., Zhenwei, L., Zhichao, C., Guanyi, H., Yunyu, S., and Longping, W. (2006). Dendrimers as potential drug carriers. Part II. Prolonged delivery of ketoprofen by in vitro and in vivo studies. *European Journal of Medical Chemistry*, **41**, 670–674.

Nagahori, N., Lee, R. T., Nishimura, S., Page, D., Roy, R., and Lee, Y. C. (2002). Inhibition of adhesion of type 1 fimbriated Escherichia coli to highly mannosylated ligands. *ChemBioChem*, **3**, 836–844.

Najlah, M., Freeman, S., Attwood, D., and D'Emanuele, A. (2007). *In vitro* evaluation of dendrimer prodrugs for oral drug delivery. *International Journal of Pharmaceutics*, **336**, 183–190.

Nakanishi, H., Mazda, O., Satoh, E., Asada, H., Morioka, H., Kishida, T., Nakao, M., Mizutani, Y., Kawauchi, A., Kita, M., Imanishi, J., and Miki, T. (2003). Nonviral genetic transfer of Fas ligand induced significant growth suppression and apoptotic tumor cell death in prostate cancer in vivo. *Gene Therapy*, **10**, 434–442.

Nazmi, A., Dutta, K., and Basu, A. (2010). Antiviral and neuroprotective role of octaguanidinium dendrimer-conjugated morpholino oligomers in Japanese encephalitis. *Plos Neglected Tropical Diseases*, **4**, e892.

Newkome, G. R., Childs, B. J., Rourk, M. J., Baker, G. R., and Moorefield, C. N. (1998-1999). Dendrimer construction and macromolecular property modification via combinatorial methods. *Biotechnology & Bioengineering*, **61**, 243–253.

Newkome, G. R., Yao, Z., Baker, G. R., and Gupta, V. K. (1985). Cascade Molecules: A New Approach to Micelles. A [27]-Arborol. *Journal of Organic Chemistry*, **50**, 2004–2006.

Newkome, G. R., Yao, Z. Q., Baker, G. R., Gupta, V. K., Russo, P. S., and Saunders, M. J. (1986). Chemistry of micelles series. Part 2. Cascade molecules. Synthesis and characterization of a benzene[9]3-arborol. *Journal of American Chemical Society*, **108**, 849–850.

Nishikawa, K., Matsuoka, K., Kita, E., Okabe, N., Mizuguchi, M., Hino, K., Miyazawa, S., Yamasaki, C., Aoki, J., Takashima, S., Yamakawa, Y., Nishijima, M., Terunuma, D., Kuzuhara, H., and Natori, Y. (2002). A therapeutic agent with oriented carbohydrates for treatment of infections by Shiga toxin-producing Escherichia coli O157:H7. *Proceedings of National Academy of Sciences of USA*, **99**, 7669–7674.

Nishiyama, N., Stapert, H. R., Zhang, G. D., Takasu, D., Jiang, D. L., Nagano, T., Aida, T., and Kataoka, K. (2003). Light-harvesting ionic dendrimer porphyrins as new photosensitizers for photodynamic therapy. *Bioconjugate Chemistry*, **14**, 58–66.

Niven, R., Pearlman, R., Wedeking, T., Mackeigan, J., Noker, P., Simpson-Herren, L., and

Smith, J. G. (1998). Biodistribution of Radiolabeled Lipid-DNA Complexes and DNA in Mice. *Journal of Pharmaceutical Sciences*, **87**(1998) 1292–1299.

Nwe, K., Bryant, L. H. Jr., and Brechbiel, M. W. (2010). Poly(amidoamine) dendrimer based MRI contrast agents exhibiting enhanced relaxivities derived via metal preligation techniques. *Bioconjugate Chemistry*, **21**, 1014–1017.

Nwe, K., Milenic, D., Bryant, L. H., Regino, C. A., and Brechbiel, M. W. (2011). Preparation, characterization and in vivo assessment of Gd-albumin and Gd-dendrimer conjugates as intravascular contrast-enhancing agents for MRI. *Journal of Inorganic Biochemistry*, **105**, 722–727.

Oka, H., Onaga, T., Koyama, T., Guo, C. T., Suzuki, Y., Esumi, Y., Hatano, K., Terunuma, D., and Matsuoka, K. (2008). Sialyl alpha(2->3) lactose clusters using carbosilane dendrimer core scaffolds as influenza hemagglutinin blockers. *Bioorganic & Medical Chemistry Letters*, **18**, 4405–4408.

Oka, H., Onaga, T., Koyama, T., Guo, C. T., Suzuki, Y., Esumi, Y., Hatano, K., Terunuma, D., and Matsuoka, K. (2009). Syntheses and biological evaluations of carbosilane dendrimers uniformly functionalized with sialyl alpha(2->3) lactose moieties as inhibitors for human influenza viruses. *Bioorganic & Medical Chemistry*, **17**, 5465–5475.

Ortega, P., Bermejo, J. F., Chonco, L., de Jesus, E., de la Mata, F. J., Fernandez, G., Flores, J., Gomez, R., Serramia, M. J., and Munoz-Fernandez, M. A. (2006). Novel water soluble carbosilane dendrimers: synthesis and biocompatibility. *European Journal of Inorganic Chemistry*, **7**, 1388–1396.

Paddle, B. M. (2003). Therapy and prophylaxis of inhaled biological toxins. *Journal of Applied Toxicology*, **23**, 139–170.

Pan, B., Cui, D., Sheng, Y., Ozkan, C., Gao, F., He, R., Li, Q., Xu, P., and Huang, T. (2007). Dendrimer-Modified Magnetic Nanoparticles Enhance Efficiency of Gene Delivery System. *Cancer Research*, **67**, 8156–8163.

Pan, B., Cui, D., Xu, P., Ozkan, C., Feng, G., Ozkan, M., Huang, T., Chu, B., Li, Q., He, R., and Hu, G. (2009). Synthesis and characterization of polyamidoamine dendrimer-coated multi-walled carbon nanotubes and their application in gene delivery systems. *Nanotechnology*, **20**, 125101.

Patil, M. L., Zhang, M., Taratula, O., Garbuzenko, O. B., He, H., and Minko, T. (2009). Internally Cationic Polyamidoamine PAMAM-OH Dendrimers for siRNA Delivery: Effect of the Degree of Quaternization and Cancer Targeting. *Biomacromolecules*, **10**, 258–266.

Pedziwiatr-Werbicka, E., Ferenc, M., Zaborski, M., Gabara, B., Klajnert, B., and Bryszewska, M. (2011). Characterization of complexes formed by polypropylene imine dendrimers and anti-HIV oligonucleotides. *Colloids and Surfaces B*, **83**, 360–366.

Pérez-Anes, A., Stefaniu, C., Moog, C., Majoral, J. P., Blanzat, M., Turrin, C. O., Caminade, A. M., and Rico-Lattes, I. Multivalent catanionic GalCer analogs derived from first generation dendrimeric phosphonic acids. *Bioorganic & Medical Chemistry*, **18**, 242–248.

Razinkov, V., Gazumyan, A., Nikitenko, A., Ellestad, G., and Krishnamurthy, G. (2001). RFI-641 inhibits entry of respiratory syncytial virus via interactions with fusion protein. *Chemical Biology*, **8**, 645–659.

Rekas, A., Lo, V., Gadd, G. E., Cappai, R., and Yun, S. I. (2009). PAMAM dendrimers as potential agents against fibrillation of alpha-synuclein, a Parkinson's disease-related protein. *Macromolecular Biosciences*, **9**, 230–238.

Rojo, J. and Delgado, R. (2004). Glycodendritic structures: promising new antiviral drugs. *Journal of Antimicrobial Chemotherapy*, **54**, 579–581.

Santhakumaran, L. M., Thomas, T., and Thomas, T. J. (2004). Enhanced cellular uptake of a triplex-forming oligonucleotide by nanoparticle formation in the presence of polypropylenimine dendrimers. *Nucleic Acids Research*, **32**, 2102–2112.

Santos, J. L., Oramas, E., Pêgo, A. P., Granja, P. L., and Tomás, H. (2009). Osteogenic differentiation of mesenchymal stem cells using PAMAM dendrimers as gene delivery vectors. *Journal of Controlled Release*, **134**, 141–148.

Sarin, H. (2009). Recent progress towards development of effective systemic chemotherapy for the treatment of malignant brain tumors. *Journal of Translational Medicine*, **7**, 77.

Sato, N., Kobayashi, H., Hiraga, A., Saga, T., Togashi, K., Konishi, J., and Brechbiel, M.W. (2001). Pharmacokinetics and enhancement patterns of macromolecular MR contrast agents with various sizes of polyamidoamine dendrimer cores. *Magnetic Resonance Medicine*, **46**, 1169–1173.

School of Pharmacy, University of London (London, GB), assignee; US7081495.

Semchikov ,Yu. D. (1998). Dendrimers – new class of polymers. *Soros Obrazovatelnyj Zhurnal*, **12**, 45–51.

Shakhbazau, A., Isayenka, I., Kartel, N., Goncharova, N., Sevyaryn, I., Kosmacheva, S., Potapnev, M., Shcharbin, D., and Bryszewska, M. (2010a). Transfection efficiencies of PAMAM dendrimers correlate inversely with their hydrophobicity. *International Journal of Pharmaceutics*, **383**, 228–235.

Shakhbazau, A., Shcharbin, D., Isayenka, I., Goncharova, N., Sevyaryn, I., Kosmacheva, S., Potapnev, M., Ionov, M., Gabara, B., and Bryszewska, M. (2010b). Use of polyamidoamine dendrimers to engineer BDNF-producing human mesenchymal stem cells. *Molecular Biology Reports*, **37**, 2003–2008.

Shcharbin, D. and Bryszewska, M. (2006). Complex formation between endogenous toxin bilirubin and polyamidoamine dendrimers. A spectroscopic study. *Biochimica et Biophysica Acta*, **1760**, 1021–1026.

Shcharbin, D., Klajnert, B., Mazhul, V., and Bryszewska, M. (2003). Estimation of PAMAM dendrimers binding capacity by fluorescent probe ANS. *Journal of Fluorescence*, **13**, 519–524.

Shcharbin, D., Pedziwiatr, E., and Bryszewska, M. (2009). How to Study Dendriplexes I: characterization (review). *Journal of Controlled Release*, **135**, 186–197.

Shcharbin, D., Pedziwiatr, E., Blasiak, J., and Bryszewska, M. (2010). How to study dendriplexes II: Transfection and cytotoxicity. *Journal of Controlled Release*, **141**, 110–127.

Shcharbin, D., Pedziwiatr, E., Chonco, L., Bermejo-Martín, J. F., Ortega, P., de la Mata, F. J., Eritja, R., Gómez, R., Klajnert, B., Bryszewska, M., and Muñoz-Fernandez, M. A. (2007). Analysis of interaction between dendriplexes and bovine serum albumin. *Biomacromolecules*, **8**, 2059–2062.

Shcharbin, D., Pedziwiatr, E., Nowacka, O., Kumar, M., Zaborski, M., Ortega, P., de la Mata, F. J., Gómez, R., Muñoz-Fernandez, M. A., and Bryszewska, M. (2011). Carbosilane dendrimers NN8 and NN16 form a stable complex with siGAG1. *Colloids and Surfaces B*, **83**, 388–391.

Singh, P., Moll III F., Cronin, P., Lin, S., Ferzli, C., Koski, K., and Saul, R., (1999). Inventors Dade Behring Inc. (US), assignee; US5898005.

Solassol, J., Crozet, C., Perrier, V., Leclaire, J., Béranger, F., Caminade, A. M., Meunier, B., Dormont, D., Majoral, J. P., and Lehmann, S. (2004). Cationic phosphorus-containing dendrimers reduce prion replication both in cell culture and in mice infected with scrapie. *Journal of General Virology*, **85**, 1791–1799.

Spangler, B. and Spangler, C. (2006). Inventors No assignee, US7138121.

Supattapone, S., Nguyen, H. O. B., Cohen, F. E., Prusiner, S. B., and Scott, M. R. (1999). Elimination of prions by branched polyamines and implications for therapeutics. *Proceedings of National Academy of Sciences of USA*, **96**, 14529–14534.

Supattapone, S., Piro, J. R., and Rees, J. R. (2009). Complex polyamines: unique prion disaggregating compounds. *CNS & Neurological Disorders – Drug Targets*, **8**, 323–328.

Supattapone, S., Wille, H., Uyechi, L., Safar, J., Tremblay, P., Szoka, F. C., Cohen, F. E., Prusiner, S., and Scott, M. R. (2001). Branched Polyamines Cure Prion-Infected Neuroblastoma Cells. *Journal of Virology*, **75**, 3453–3461.

Szoka, F. C.Jr. and Haensler, J. (1997). Inventors No assignee; US5661025.

Tack, F., Bakker, A., Maes, S., Dekeyser, N., Bruining, M., Elissen-Roman, C., Janicot, M., Janssen, H. M., De Waal, B. F. M., Fransen, P. M., Lou, X., Meijer, E. W., Arien, A., Brewster, M. E. (2006a). Dendrimeric poly(propyleneimines) as effective delivery agents for DNAzymes: Toxicity, in vitro transfection and in vivo delivery, *Journal of Controlled Release*, **116**, e26–e28.

Tack, F., Bakker, A., Maes, S., Dekeyser, N., Bruining, M., Elissen-Roman, C., Janicot, M., Janssen, H. M., De Waal, B. F. M., Fransen, P. M., Lou, X., Meijer, E. W., Arien, A., and Brewster,

M. E. (2006b). Dendrimeric poly(propylene-imines) as effective delivery agents for DNAzymes: Dendrimer synthesis, stability and oligonucleotide complexation. *Journal of Controlled Release*, **116**, e24–e26.

Tam, J. P., Lu, Y. A., and Yang, J. L. (2002). Antimicrobial dendrimeric peptides. *European Journal of Biochemistry*, **269**, 923–932.

Tan, M. L., Choong, P. F., and Dass, C. R. (2009). Review: doxorubicin delivery systems based on chitosan for cancer therapy. *Journal of Pharmacy and Pharmacology*, **61**, 131–142.

Tanaka, S., Iwai, M., Harada, Y., Morikawa, T., Muramatsu, A., Mori, T., Okanoue, T., Kashima, K., Maruyama-Tabata, H., Hirai, H., Satoh, E., Imanishi, J., and Mazda, O. (2000). Targeted killing of carcinoembryonic antigen (CEA)-producing cholangiocarcinoma cells by polyamidoamine dendrimer-mediated transfer of an Epstein-Barr virus (EBV)-based plasmid vector carrying the CEA promoter. *Gene Therapy*, **7**, 1241–1249.

Taratula, O., Garbuzenko, O. B., Kirkpatrick, P., Pandya, I., Savla, R., Pozharov, V. P., He, H., and Minko, T. (2009). Surface-engineered targeted PPI dendrimer for efficient intracellular and intratumoral siRNA delivery. *Journal of Controlled Release*, **140**, 284–293.

Thompson, J. P. and Schengrund, C. L. (1998). Inhibition of the adherence of cholera toxin and the heat-labile enterotoxin of Escherichia coli to cell-surface GM1 by oligosaccharide-derivatized dendrimers. *Biochemical Pharmacology*, **56**, 591–597.

Tomalia, D. A. (1995). Dendrimer molecules. *Scientific American*, **272**, 62–66.

Tomalia, D. A. (1996). Starburst(R) dendrimers - nanoscopic supermolecules according dendritic rules and principles. *Macromolecular Symposia*, **101**, 243–255.

Tomalia, D. A. and Majoros, I. J. (2006). Inventors The Regents of the University of Michigan (Ann Arbor, MI, US), assignee; US7078461.

Tomalia, D. A., Baker, H., Dewald, J., Hall, M., Kallos, G., Martin, S., Roeck, J., Ryder, J., and Smith, P. (1986). Dendritic macromolecules: synthesis of starburst dendrimers. *Macromolecules*, **19**, 2466–2468.

Toyokuni, T., Hakomori, S., and Singhal, A.K. (1994). Synthetic carbohydrate vaccines: synthesis and immunogenicity of Tn antigen conjugates. *Bioorganic & Medical Chemistry*, **2**, 1119–1132.

Tripathi, P. K., Khopade, A. J., Nagaich, S., Shrivastava, S., Jain, S., and Jain, N. K. (2002). Dendrimer grafts for delivery of 5-fluorouracil. *Pharmazie*, **57**, 261–264.

Uchegbu, I., Munro, A., Schatzlein, A. G., Gray, A. I., and Zinselmeyer, B. (2005). Inventors No assignee; US Patent Application 20050019923.

Vallittu, P., Lassila, L., Skrifvars, M., Viljanen, E., Yli-urpo, A. (2008). Inventors Stick Tech OY (Turko, FI), assignee; US7354969.

Vandamme, T. F. and Brobeck, L. (2005). Poly(amidoamine) dendrimers as ophthalmic vehicles for ocular delivery of pilocarpine nitrate and tropicamide. *J. Control. Release*, **102**(2005), 23–38.

Vincent L., Varet J., Pille, J. Y., Bompais, H., Opolon, P., Maksimenko, A., Malvy, C., Mirshahi, M., Lu, H., Vannier, J. P., Soria, C., and Li, H. (2003). Efficacy of dendrimer-mediated angiostatin and TIMP-2 gene delivery on inhibition of tumor growth and angiogenesis: in vitro and in vivo studies. *International Journal of Cancer*, **105**, 419–429.

Vinogradov, S. and Wilson, D. (1998). Inventors Trustees of the University of Pennsylvania (US), assignee; US5837865.

Vlasov, G. P. (2003). Biodegradable starburst carbon chain polymer-protein and lysine dendrite conjugates: Adjustment of immune properties, DNA bonding and delivery. *Macromolecular Symposia*, **197**, 331–343.

Vlasov, G. P. (2006). Starlike branched and hyperbranched biodegradable polymer systems as DNA carriers. *Russian Journal of Bioorganic Chemistry*, **32**, 205–218.

Weber, N., Ortega, P., Clemente, M. I., Shcharbin, D., Bryszewska, M., de la Mata, F. J., Gómez, R., and Muñoz-Fernández, M. A. (2008). Characterization of carbosilane dendrimers as effective carriers of siRNA to HIV-infected lymphocytes. *Journal of Controlled Release*, **132**, 55–64.

Weissleder, R., Bogdanov, A. Jr., Tung, C. H., and Weinmann, H. J. (2001). Size optimization of synthetic graft copolymers for in vivo angiogenesis imaging. *Bioconjugate Chemistry*, **12**, 213–219.

Wiener, E. C., Brechbiel, M. W., Brothers, H., Magin, R. L., Gansow, O. A., Tomalia, D. A., and Lauterbur, P. C. (1994). Dendrimer-based metal chelates: a new class of magnetic resonance imaging contrast agents. *Magnetic Resonance Medicine*, **31**, 1–8.

Wiener, E. C., Konda, S., Shadron, A., Brechbiel, M., and Gansow, O. (1997). Targeting dendrimer–chelates to tumors and tumor cells expressing the high-affinity folate receptor. *Investigative Radiology*, **32**, 748–754.

Witvrouw, M., Fikkert, V., Pluymers, W., Matthews, B., Mardel, K., Schols, D., Raff, J., Debyser, Z., De Clercq, E., Holan, G., and Pannecouque, C. (2000). Polyanionic (i.e., polysulfonate) dendrimers can inhibit the replication of human immunodeficiency virus by interfering with both virus adsorption and later steps (reverse transcriptase/integrase) in the virus replicative cycle. *Molecular Pharmacology*, **58**, 1100–1108.

Wright, C. (1998). Inventor Novavax, Inc. (US), assignee; US5795582.

Xu, H., Regino, C. A., Koyama, Y., Hama, Y., Gunn, A. J., Bernardo, M., Kobayashi, H., Choyke, P. L., and Brechbiel, M. W. (2007). Preparation and preliminary evaluation of a biotin-targeted, lectin-targeted dendrimer-based probe for dual-modality magnetic resonance and fluorescence imaging. *Bioconjugate Chemistry*, **18**, 1474–1482.

Zhu, S., Hong, M., Tang, G., Qian, L., Lin, J., Jiang, Y., and Pei, Y. (2010). Partly PEGylated polyamidoamine dendrimer for tumor-selective targeting of doxorubicin: the effects of PEGylation degree and drug conjugation style. *Biomaterials*, **31**, 1360–1371.

Zhuo, R. X., Du, B., and Lu, Z. R. (1999). In vitro release of 5-fluorouracil with cyclic core dendritic polymer. *Journal of Controlled Release*, **57**, 249–257.

11

Alberts, B., Johnson, A., Lewis, J., Raff, M., Roberts, K., and Walter, P. (2002). *Molecular biology of the cell*. 4th revised edition. Garland Science, New York.

Angelova, M., Soléau, S., Meléard, P., Faucon, J., and Bothorel, P. (1992). Preparation of giant vesicles by external AC fields. Kinetics and application, Prog. *Colloid Polym. Sci.* **89**, 127–131.

Antunes, F. E., Marques, E. F., Miguel, M. G., and Lindman, B. (2009). Polymer–vesicle association. *Adv. Colloid Interface Sci.* **147**, 18–35.

Barenholz, Y. (2001). Liposome application: problems and prospects. *Curr. Opinion Coll. Interface Sci.* **6**(1), 66–77.

Bickel, T., Marques, C. M., and Jeppesen, C. (2000). Pressure patches for membranes: The induced pinch of a grafted polymer. *Phys. Rev. E* 62, 1124–1127.

Bordi, F., Sennato, S., and Truzzolillo, D. (2009). Polyelectrolyte-induced aggregation of liposomes: A new cluster phase with interesting applications. *J. Phys.: Condens. Matter* 21, 203102–203128.

Brooks, J., Marques, C., and Cates, M. (1991). Role of adsorbed polymer in bilayer elasticity. *Europhys. Lett.* **14**(7), 713–718.

Brugnerotto, J., Desbrières, J., Roberts, G., and Rinaudo, M. (2001). Characterization of chitosan by steric exclusion chromatography. *Polymer* **42**, 9921–9927.

Cametti, C. (2008). Polyion-induced aggregation of oppositely charged liposomes and charged colloidal particles: The many facets of complex formation in low-density colloidal systems. *Chem. Phys. Lipids* **155**, 63–73.

Campillo, C., Pépin-Donat, B., and Viallat, A. (2007). Responsive viscoelastic giant lipid vesicles filled with a poly(N-isopropylacrylamide) artificial cytoskeleton. *Soft Matter* **3**(11), 1421–1427.

Campillo, C. C., Schröder, A. P., Marques, C. M., and Pépin-Donat, B. (2008). Volume transition in composite poly(NIPAM)-giant unilamellar vesicles. *Soft Matter* **4**(12), 2486–2491.

Campillo, C. C., Schröder, A. P., Marques, C. M., and Pépin-Donat, B. (2009). Composite gel-filled giant vesicles: Membrane homogeneity and mechanical properties. *Mat. Sci. Eng. C-Bio. S.* **29**(2), 393–397.

Charitat, T., Lecuyer, S., and Fragneto, G. (2008). Fluctuations and destabilization of single phospholipid bilayers. *Biointerphases* **3**(2), FB3–15.

Clément, F. and Joanny, J. F. (1997). Curvature elasticity of an adsobed polymer layer. *J. Phys. II (France)* **7**(7), 973–980.

Delorme, N. and Fery, A. (2006). Direct method to study membrane rigidity of small vesicles based on atomic force microscope force spectroscopy. *Phys. Rev. E* **74**, 030901.

Dimova R., Pouligny B., and Dietrich C. (2000). Pretransitional effects in dimyristoylphosphatidylcholine vesicle membranes: Optical dynamometry study. *Biophys. J.* **79**, 340–356.

Ding, W. X., Qi, X. R., Fu, Q., and Piao, H. S. (2007). Pharmacokinetics and pharmacodynamics of sterylglucoside-modified liposomes for levonorgestrel delivery via nasal route. *Drug Delivery* **14**, 101–104.

Döbereiner, H. G. (2000), Properties of giant vesicles. *Curr. Opinion Coll. Interface Sci.* **5**, 256–263, and references herein.

Döbereiner, H. G., Evans, E., Kraus, M., Seifert, U., and Wortis, M. (1997). Mapping vesicle shapes into the phase diagram: A comparison of experiment and theory. *Phys. Rev. E* **55**(4), 4458–4474.

Dobrynin, A. V., Deshkovski, A., and Rubinstein, M. (2000). Adsorption of polyelectrolytes at an oppositely charged surface. *Phys. Rev. Lett.* **84**, 3101–3104.

Drummond, D. C., Meyer, O., Hong, K., Kirpon, D. B., and Papahadjopoulos, D. (1999). Optimizing liposomes for delivery of chemotherapeutic agents to solid tumors. *Pharmacol. Rev.* **51**(4), 691–743.

Dubreuil, F., Quemeneur, F., Fery, A., Rinaudo, M., and Pépin-Donat, B. (in preparation). Elastic properties of chitosan-coated lipid vesicles studied by AFM.

Edwards, K. A. and Baeumner, A. J. (2006). Analysis of liposomes, *Talanta* **68**, 1432–1441.

Elsabee, M., Morsi, R., and Al-Sabagh, A. (2009). Surface active properties of chitosan and its derivatives. *Colloids Surf. B* **74**, 1–16.

Faivre, M., Campillo, C., Pépin-Donat, B., and Viallat, A (2006). Responsive giant vesicles filled with poly (N-isopropylacrylamide) sols or gels. *Prog. Coll. Pol. Sci.* **133**, 42–44.

Fery, A. and Weinkamer, R. (2007). Mechanical properties of micro and nanocapsules: Single capsule measurements. *Polymer* **48**, 7221–7235.

Filipovica-Grcï, J., Skalko-Basnet, N., and Jalsenjak, I. (2001). Mucoadhesive chitosan-coated liposomes: characteristics and stability. *J. Microencapsulation* **18**(1), 3–12.

Frette, V., Tsafrir, I., Guedeau-Boudeville, M. A., Jullien, L., Kandel, D., and Stavans, J. (1999). Coiling of cylindrical membrane stacks with anchored polymers. *Phys. Rev.Lett.* **83**, 2465–2468.

Gibbs, B. F., Kermasha, S., Alli, I., and Mulligan, C. N. (1999). Encapsulation in the food industry: A review. *Int. J. Food. Sci. Nutr.* **50**(3), 213–224.

Gregory, J. (1972). Rates of flocculation of latex particles by cationic polymers. *J. Colloid Interface Sci.* **42**(2), 448–456.

Guo, J., Ping, Q., Jiang, G., Huanga, L., and Tonga, Y. (2003). Chitosan coated liposomes: Characterization and interaction with leuprolide. *Int. J. Pharm.* **260**, 167–173.

Helfer, E., Harlepp, S., Bourdieu, L., Robert, J., MacKintosh, F. C., and Chatenay, D. (2001). Buckling of actin-coated membranes under application of a local force. *Phys. Rev.Lett.* **87**(8), 088103.

Helfrich, W. (1973). Elastic properties of lipid bilayers: Theory and possible experiments. *Z. Naturforsch. C* **28**, 693–703.

Henriksen, I., Smistad, G., and Karlsen, J. (1994). Interactions between liposomes and chitosan. *Int. J. Pharm.* **101**(3), 227–236.

Henriksen, I., Vhgen, S., Sande, S., Smistad, G., and Karlsen, J. (1997). Interactions between liposomes and chitosan II: Effect of selected parameters on aggregation and leakage. *Int. J. Pharm.* **146**, 193–204.

Hoffmann,, U., Rotsch, C., Parak, W., and Radmacher, M. (1997). Investigating the cytoskeleton of chicken cardiocytes with the atomic force microscope. *J. Struct. Biol.* **119**(2), 84–91.

Jesorka, A., Markström, M., and Orwar, O. (2005). Controlling the internal structure of giant unilamellar vesicles by means of reversible temperature dependent Sol-Gel transition of internalized Poly(N-isopropyl acrylamide). *Langmuir* **21**, 1230–1237.

Kaasgaard, T. and Andresen, T. L. (2010). Liposomal Cancer Therapy: Exploiting Tumor Characteristics. *Expert opinion on drug delivery* 7(2), 225–243.

Kaasgaard, T., Leidy, C., Crowe, J. H., Mouritsen, O. G., and Jorgensen, K. (2003). Temperature-Controlled Structure and Kinetics of Ripple Phases in One- and Two-Component Supported Lipid Bilayers. *Biophys. J.* **85**, 350–360.

Katifori, E., Alben, S., Cerda, E., Nelson, D. R., and Dumais, J. (2010). Foldable structures and the natural design of pollen grains. *Proc. Natl. Acad. Sci. USA* **109**, 7635–7639.

Kawakami, K., Nishihara, Y., and Hirano, K. J. (2001). Effect of hydrophilic polymers on physical stability of liposome dispersions. *Phys. Chem. B* **105**, 2374–2385.

Kennedy, J. F., Phillips, G. O., Williams, P. A., and Hascall, V. C. (Eds.) (2002). *Hyaluronan, vol. 1: Chemical, biochemical and biological aspects; Hyaluronan, vol 2: Biomedical, medical and clinical aspects*. Woodhead Pub., Abington (UK).

Khor, E. and Lim, L. (2003). Implantable applications of chitin and chitosan. *Biomaterials* **24**, 2339–2349.

Kim, Y. and Sung, W. (2001). Membrane curvature induced by polymer adsorption. *Phys. Rev. E* **63**, 041910.

Kiser, P., Wilson, G., and Needham, D. (1998). A synthetic mimic of the secretory granule for drug delivery. *Nature*, **394**(6692), 459–462.

Knorr, R. L., Staykova, M., Gracia, R. S., and Dimova, R. (2010). Wrinkling and electroporation of giant vesicles in the gel phase. *Soft Matter* 6, 1990–1996.

Kocsis, J. F., Llanos, G., and Holmer, E. (2000). Heparin-coated stents. *J. Long-Term Eff. Med. Implants* 10, 19–45.

Kogan, G., Soltés, L., Stern, R., and Gemeiner, P. (2007). Hyaluronic acid: A natural biopolymer with a broad range of biomedical and industrial applications. *Biotechnol. Lett* 29, 17–25.

Koynova, R. and Caffrey, M. (1998). Phases and phase transitions of the phosphatidylcholines. *Biochim. Biophys. Acta* **1376**, 91–145.

Kremer, S., Campillo, C., Pépin-Donat, B., Viallat, A., and Brochard-Wyart, F. (2008). Nanotubes from gelly vesicles. *EurPhys. Lett.* **82**(4), 48002–48005.

Kremer, S., Campillo, C., Quemeneur, F., Rinaudo, M., Pépin-Donat, B., and Brochard-Wyart, F. (2011). Nanotubes from asymmetrically decorated vesicles. *Soft Matter* 7(3), 946–951.

Lee, J., Petrov, P., and Döbereiner, H. G. (1999). Curvature of zwitterionic membranes in transverse ph gradients. *Langmuir* **15**, 8543–8546.

Lidmar, J., Mirny, L., and Nelson, D. (2003). Virus shape and buckling transition in sperical shells. *Phys. Rev. E* **68**(5), 051910.

Lim, C., Zhoua, E., and Quek, S. (2006). Mechanical models for living cells—A review, *J. Biomechanics* **39**, 195–216.

Lim, G. L., Wortis, M., and Mukhopadhyay, R. (2008). *Soft Matter vol. 4: Lipid bilayers and red blood cells*. G. Gompper and M. Schick (Eds.). Wiley-VCH GmbH & Co., Weinheim (Germany).

Lipowsky, R. (1997). Flexible membranes with anchored polymers. *Colloids and Surfaces* 128, 255–264.

Lipowsky, R. and Sackmann, E. (1995). *Structure and dynamics of membranes*. Handbook of biological physics (Vol 1A and 1B). Elsevier Science, Amsterdam.

Liu, A. and Fletcher, D. (2009). Biology under construction: *In vitro* reconstitution of cellular function. *Nat. Rev. Mol. Cell Biol.* 10, 644–650.

Liu, K. K. (2006). Deformation behavior of soft particles: A review. *J. Phys. D: Appl. Phys.* **39**, R189–199.

Luzzati, V. and Husson, F. (1962). The structure of the liquid crystalline phases of lipid-water systems. *J. Cell Biol.* 12(2), 207–219.

MacEwan, S. R., Callahan, D. J., and Chilkoti, A. (2010). Stimulus-responsive macromolecules and nanoparticles for cancer drug delivery. *Nanomedicine* 5(5), 793–806.

Mady, M., Darwish, M., Khalil, S., and Khalil, W. (2009). Biophysical studies on chitosan-coated liposomes. *Eur. Biophys. J.* 38, 1127–1133.

Malmsten, M. (2003). Protein adsorption in intravenous drug delivery. In *Biopolymers at Interfaces*. Dekker, New York.

Markström, M., Gunnarsson, A., Orwar, O., and Jesorka, A. (2007). Dynamic microcompartmentalization of giant unilamellar vesicles by sol–gel transition and temperature induced shrinking/swelling of poly(N-isopropyl acrylamide). *Soft Matter* **3**, 587–595.

Mazeau, K. and Vergelati, C. (2002). Atomistic modeling of the adsorption of benzophenone onto cellulosic surfaces. *Langmuir* **18**, 1919–1927.

Mertins, O. and Dimova, R. (2011). Binding of chitosan to phospholipid vesicles studied with isothermal titration calorimetry. *Langmuir* 27, 5506–5515.

Mertins, O., Lionzo, M., Micheletto, Y., Pohlmann, A., and da Silveira, N. (2008). Chitosan effect on the mesophase behaviour of phosphatidylcholine supramolecular systems. *Mater. Sci. Eng. C* 29, 463–469.

Mertins, O., Schneider, P., Pohlmann, A., and da Silveira, N. (2010). Interaction between phospholipids bilayer and chitosan in liposomes investigated by ^{31}P NMR spectroscopy. *Colloids Surf. B* **75**(1), 294–299.

Mukhopadhyay, R., Lim, G., and Wortis, M. (2002). Echinocyte shapes: Bending, stretching, and shear determine spicule shape and spacing. *Biophys. J.* 82, 1756–1772.

Needham, D. and Evans, E. (1988). Structure and mechanical properties of giant lipid (DMPC) vesicle bilayers from 20°C below to 10°C above the liquid crystal-crystalline phase transition at 24 °C. *Biochemistry* 27, 8261–8269.

Nikolov, V., Lipowsky, R., and Dimova, R. (2007). Behaviour of giant vesicles with anchored DNA molecules. *Biophys. J.* **92**, 4356–4368.

Noireaux, V. and Libchaber, A. (2004). A vesicle bioreactor as a step toward an artificial cell assembly. *Proc. Natl. Acad. Sci. U. S. A.* **101**, 17669–17674.

Olbrich, K., Rawicz, W., Needham, D., and Evans, E. (2000). Water permeability and mechanical strength of polyunsturated lipid bilayers. *Biophys. J.* **79**, 321–327.

Osinkina, L., Markström, M., Orwar, O., and Jesorka, A. (2010). A method for heat-stimulated compression of Poly(N-isopropyl acrylamide)

hydrogels inside single giant unilamellar vesicles. *Langmuir* **26**, 1–4.

Pavinatto, A., Pavinatto, F., Barros-Timmons, A., and Oliveira, N. O. Jr. (2010). Electrostatic interactions are not sufficient to account for chitosan bioactivity. *ACS Appl. Mater. Interfaces* **2**, 246–251.

Peer, D. and Margalit, R. (2004). Tumor-targeted hyaluronan nano-liposomes increase the antitumor activity of liposomal doxorubicin in syngeneic and human xenograft mouse tumor models. *Neoplasia* 6, 343–353.

Perugini, P., Genta, I., Pavanetto, F., Conti, B., Scalia, S., and Baruffini, A. (2000). Study on glycolic acid delivery by liposomes and microspheres. *Int. J. Pharm.* **196**(1), 51–61.

Pospieszny, H., Struszczyk, H., Chirkov, S. N., and Atabekov, J. G. (1994). *New applications of chitosan in agriculture.* Bremerhaven, Wirtschaftsverlag NW, Germany.

Quemeneur, F., Rammal, A., Rinaudo, M., and Pépin-Donat, B. (2007). Large and giant vesicles "decorated" with chitosan: Effects of pH, salt, and glucose stress, and surface adhesion. *Biomacromolecules* **8**, 2512–2519.

Quemeneur, F., Rinaudo, M., and Pépin-Donat, B. (2008a). Influence of molecular weight and pH on adsorption of chitosan at the surface of large and giant vesicles. *Biomacromolecules* **9**, 396–402.

Quemeneur, F., Rinaudo, M., and Pépin-Donat, B. (2008b). Influence of polyelectrolyte chemical structure on their interaction with lipid membrane of zwitterionic liposomes. *Biomacromolecules* **9**, 2237–2243.

Quemeneur, F. (2010). *Relationship between mechanical parameters and behaviour under external stresses in lipid vesicles with modified membranes.* Ph D. Thesis. University of Grenoble, France, and University of Konstanz, Germany.

Quemeneur, F., Mertins, O., Rinaudo, M., Schröder, A. P., Marques, C. M., and Pépin-Donat, B. (in preparation). Stability of the polyelectrolyte coating on zwitterionic liposomes.

Quemeneur, F., Rinaudo, M., Maret, G., and Pépin-Donat, B. (2010). Decoration of lipid vesicles by polyelectrolytes: mechanism and structure. *Soft Matter* **6**, 4471–4481.

Quemeneur, F., Quilliet, C., Faivre, M., Viallat, A., and Pépin-Donat, B. (2011). Gel-phase vesicles buckle into specic shapes. *Phys. Rev.Lett.* under revision.

Rinaudo, M. (2006). Chitin and chitosan: Properties and applications. *Prog. Polym. Sci.* **31**, 603–632.

Rinaudo, M. (2008). Main properties and current applications of some polysaccharides as biomaterials. *Polym. Int.* **57**(3), 397–430.

Rinaudo, M. (2009). Polyelectrolyte properties of a plant and animal polysaccharide. *Struct. Chem.*, 20(2), 277–289.

Ringsdorf, H., Sackmann, E., Simon, J., and Winnik, F. M. (1993). Interactions of liposomes and hydrophobically-modified poly(N-isopropylacrylamides) an attempt to model the cytoskeleton. *Biochim. Biophys. Acta* 1153, 335–344.

Schild, H. G. (1992). Poly(N-Isopropylacrylamide): Experiment, theory and application. *Prog. Colloid Polym. Sci.* 17, 163–249.

Shafir, A. and Andelman, D. (2007). Bending moduli of charged membranes immersed in polyelectrolyte solutions. *Soft Matter* **3**, 644–650.

Simon, J., Khuner, M., Ringsdorf, H., and Sackmann, E. (1995). Polymer-induced shape changes and capping in giant liposomes. *Chem. Phys. Lipids* 76(2), 241–258.

Stauch, O., Schubert, R., Savin, G., and Burchard, W. (2002a). Structure of artificial cytoskeleton containing liposomes in aqueous solution studied by static and dynamic light scattering. *Biomacromolecules* **3**, 565–578.

Stauch, O., Uhlmann, T., Fröhlich, M., Thomann, R., El-badry, M., Kim, Y., and Schubert, R. (2002b). Mimicking a cytoskeleton by Coupling Poly(N-isopropylacrylamide) to the inner leaflet of liposomal membranes: Effects of photopolymerization on vesicle shape and polymer architecture. *Biomacromolecules* **3**, 324–332.

Surace, C., Arpicco, S., Dufay-Wojcicki, A., Marsaud, V., Bouclier, C., Clay, D., Cattel, L., Renoir, J. M., and Fattal, E. (2009). Lipoplexes targeting the CD44 hyaluronic acid receptor for efficient transfection of breast cancer cells. *Molecular Pharmaceutics* 6(4), 1062–1073.

Taglienti, A., Cellesi, F., Crescenzi, V., Sequi, P., Valentini, M., and Tire, N. (2006). Investigating the interactions of hyaluronan derivatives with biomolecules. the use of diffusional NMR techniques. *Macomol. Biosci.* **6**, 611–622.

Takeuchi, H., Matsui, Y., Sugihara, H., Yamamoto, H., and Kawashima, Y. (2005). Effectiveness of submicron-sized, chitosan-coated liposomes in oral administration of peptide drugs. *Int. J. Pharm.* **303**(1–2), 160–170.

Thongborisute, J., Takeuchi, H., Yamamoto, H., and Kawashima, Y. (2006). Visualization of the penetrative and mucoadhesive properties of chitosan and chitosan-coated liposomes through the rat intestine. *J. Liposome Res.* **16**, 127–141.

Tribet, C. and Vial, F. (2008). Flexible macromolecules attached to lipid bilayers: impact on fluidity, curvature, permeability and stability on the membranes. *Soft Matter* **4**, 68–81.

Tsafrir, I., Caspi, Y., Guedeau-Boudeville, M.-A., Arzi, T., and Stavans, J. (2003). Budding and tubulation in highly oblate vesicles by anchored amphiphilic molecules. *Phys. Rev. Lett.* **91**(13), 138102.

Tsafrir, I., Sagi, D., Arzi, T., Guedeau-Boudeville, M. A., Frette, V., Kandel, D., and Stavans, J. (2001). Pearling Instabilities of Membrane Tubes with Anchored Polymers. *Phys. Rev. Lett.* **86**(6), 1138–1141.

Uhrich, K. E., Cannizzaro, S. M., Langer, R. S., and Shakesheff, K. M. (1999). Polymeric systems for controlled drug release. *Chemical Reviews* **99**(11), 3181–3198.

Vasir, J. K., Reddy, M. K., and Labhasetwar, V. D. (2005). Nanosystems in drug targeting: Opportunities and challenges. *Current Nanoscience* 1(1), 47–64.

Velegol, D. and Thwar, P. (1984). Analytical model for the effect of surface charge nonuniformity on colloidal interactions. *Langmuir* 17, 7687–7693.

Volodkin, D., Ball, V., Schaaf, P., Voegel, J. C., and Mohwald, H. (2007). Complexation of phosphocholine liposomes with polylysine. Stabilization by surface coverage versus aggregation. *Biochim. Biophys. Acta* 1768, 280–290.

Xu, T., Zhang, N., Nichols, H. L., Shi, D., and Wen X. (2007). Modification of nanostructured materials for biomedical applications. *Mater. Sci. Eng. C* 27, 579–594.

Yokoyama, M. (2005). Drug targeting with nano-sized carrier systems. *J. Artif. Organs* **8**, 77–84.

Zhang, J. and Wang, S. (2009). Topical use of co-enzyme Q(10)-loaded liposomes coated with tri-methylchitosan: Tolerance, precorneal retention and anti-cataract effect. *Int. J. Pharm.* **372**(1–2), 66–75.

12

Ahn, J. H., Choi, S. J., Han, J. W., Park, T. J., Lee, S. Y., and Choi, Y. K. (2010). Double gate nanowire field effect Transistor for a biosensor. *Nano Letters* **10**(8), 2934–2938.

Baronas, R., Ivanauskas, F., and Kulys, J. (2010). *Mathematical modeling of biosensors: an introduction for Chemists and Mathematicians*. Springer Dordrecht, Heidelberg, London, New York.

Chiu, T. C., and Huang, C. C. (2009). Aptamer-Functionalized Nano-Biosensors. *Sensors* **9**(12), 10356–10388.

Christine, P. (2008). An artificial ion channel biosensor to identify potential anti-HIV drugs. *Analytical Chemistry* **80**(15) 5677.

Cornell, B. A., Braach-Maksvytis, V. L. B., King, L. G., Osman, P. D. J., Raguse, B., Wieczorek, L., and Pace, R. J. (1997). A biosensor that uses ion channel switches. *Nature* **387**(6633), 580–583.

Doyle, D. A., Cabral, J. M., Pfuetzner, R. A., Kuo, A., Gulbis, J. M., Cohen, S. L., Chait, B. T., and MacKinnon, R. (1998). The structure of the potassium channel: Molecular basis of K+ conduction and selectivity. *Science* **280**(5360), 69–77.

Drummond, A. J., Ashton, B., Buxton, S., Cheung, M., Cooper, A., Heled, J., Kearse, M., Moir, R., Stones-Havas, S., Sturrock, S., Thierer, T., and Wilson, A. (2010). Geneious v5.3, Available from http://www.geneious.com.

Hille, B. (2001). *Ion Channels of Excitable Membranes*. Sinauer Associates, Inc., Sunderland, Massachusetts, USA, 3rd edition.

Hodgkin, A. H. and Huxley, A. F. (1952a). The components of membrane conductance in the giant axon of Loligo. *Journal of Physiology* **116**(4), 473–496.

Hodgkin, A. H. and Huxley, A. F. (1952b). Currents carried by sodium and potassium ions through the membrane of the giant axon of Lo-ligo. *Journal of Physiology* **116**(4), 449–472.

Hodgkin, A. H. and Huxley, A. F. (1952c).The dual effect of membrane potential on sodium conductance in the giant axon of Loligo. *Journal of Physiology* **116**(4), 497–506.

Hodgkin, A. H. and Huxley, A. F. (1952d). A quantitative description of membrane current and its application to conduction and excitation in nerve. *Journal of Physiology* **117**(4), 500–544.

Hwang, H., Schatz, G. C., and Ratner, M. (2006). Ion current calculations based on three dimensional Poisson-Nernst-Planck theory for a cyclic peptide nanotube. *Jourmnal of Physical Chemistry B* **110**(13), 6999–7008.

Hwang, H., Schatz, G. C., and Ratner, M. A. (2007). Kinetic lattice grand canonical Monte Carlo simulation for ion current calculations in a model ion channel system. *The Journal of Chemical Physics* **127**(2), 024706.

Joseph, S., Mashl, R. J., Jacobsson, E., and Aluru, N. R. (2003). *Ion Channel Based Biosensors: Ionic Transport in Carbon Nanotubes*. **1**, 158–161.

Kim, D. S., Park, H. J., Park, J. E., Shin, J. K., Kang, S. W., Seo, H. I., and Lim, G. (2005). MOSFET-Type Biosensor for Detection of Streptavidin–Biotin Protein Complexes. *Sensors and Materials* **17**(5), 259–268.

Krishnamurthy, V.; Monfared, S. M., and Cornell, B. (2010). Ion channel Biosensors—Part I: Construction, Operation, and Clinical Studies. *IEEE Transactions on Nanotechnology* **9**(3) 303–312.

Maxwell, D. J., Taylor, J. R., and Nie, S. (2002). Self-Assembled Nanoparticle Probes for Recognition and Detection of Biomolecules. *JACS* **124**(32), 9606–9612.

Millar, C., Asenov, A, and Roy, S. (2005). Self-Consistent Particle Simulation of Ion Channels. *Journal of Computational and Theoretical Nanoscience* **2**(1), 56–67.

Nair, P., and Alam, M. (2007). Design Considerations of Silicon Nanowire Biosensors. *IEEE T-ED* **54**(12), 3400–3408.

Nair, P., and Alam, M. (2008). Screening-limited response of nanobiosensors. *Nano Letters* **8**(5), 1281–1285.

Neher, E. and Sakmann, B. (1976). Single-channel currents recorded from membrane of denervated frog muscle fibres. *Nature* **260**(5554), 799–802.

Ooe, K., Hamamoto, Y., Kadokawa, T. and Hirano, Y. (2008). Development of the MOSFET type Enzyme biosensor using GOx and ChOx. *Journal of Robotics and Mechatronics* **20**(1), 38–46.

Papke, D., Toghraee, R., Ravailoi, U., and Raj, A. (2009). "BioMOCA Suite", doi: 10254/nano-hub-r3981.8

Radak, B., Hwang, H., Schatz, G. C. and Ratner, M. A. (2011), 'PNP cyclic Peptide Ion Channel Model, doi: 10254/nanohub-r2469.4.

Tan, S. J., Lao, I. K., and Ji, H. M. (2006). Microfluidic design for bio-sample delivery to silicon nanowire biosensor—a simulation study. *Journal of Physics Conference Series* **34**, 626.

Urisu, T., Asano, T., Zhang, Z., Uno, H., Tero, R., Junkyu, H., Hiroko, I., Arima, Y., Iwata, H., Shibasaki, K., and Tominaqa, M. (2008). Incubation type Si-based ion channel biosensor. *Analytical and Bioanalytical Chemistry* **391**(8), 2703–2709

Wanekaya, A. K., Chen, W., Myung, N. V., and Mulchandani, A. (2006). Nanowire- based electrochemical biosensors. *Electroanalysis* **18**(6), 533–550.

Zhong, Q., Jiang, Q., Moore, P. B., Newns, D. M., and Klein, M. L. (1998). Molecular dynamics simulation of a synthetic ion channel. *Biophysical Journal* **74**(1), 3–10

Zhou, Y., Morais-Cabral, J. H., Kaufman, A., and MacKinnon, R. (2001). Chemistry of ion coordination and hydration revealed by a K+ channel-Fab complex at 2.0 A resolution. *Nature* **414**(6859), 43–48.

13

Ali, J., Ali, M., Baboota, S., Sahani, J. K., Ramassamy, C., Dao, L., and Bhavna (2010). Potential of nanoparticulate drug delivery systems by intranasal administration. *Current Pharmaceutical Design* **16**(14), 1644–1653.

Bekisz, J., Schmeisser, H., Hernandez, J., Goldman, N. D., and Zoon, K. C. (2004). Human interferons alpha, beta and omega. *Growth Factors* **22**(4), 243–251.

Benedict, C., Frey, W. H. 2nd, Schioth, H. B., Schultes, B., Born, J., and Hallschmid, M. (2010). Intranasal insulin as a therapeutic option in the treatment of cognitive impairments. *Experimental Gerontology* 16 September, 2010 [Epub ahead of print]

Botelho, S., Estanislau, C., and Morato, S. (2007). Effect of under- and overcrowding on exploratory behavior in the elevated plus-maze. *Behavioral Processes* **74**(3), 357–362.

Cai, W., Khaoustov, V. I., Xie, Q., Pan, T., Le, W., and Yoffe, B. (2005). Interferon-alpha-induced modulation of glucocorticoid and serotonin receptors as a mechanism of depression. *Journal of Hepatology* **42**(6), 880–887.

Capuron, L., Neurauter, G., Musselman, D. L., Lawson, D. H., Nemeroff, C. B., Fuchs, D., and Miller, A. H. (2003). Interferon-alpha-induced changes in tryptophan metabolism. Relationship to depression and paroxetine treatment. *Biological Psychiatry* **54**(9), 906–914.

Chill, J. H., Quadt, S. R., Levy, R., Schreiber, G., and Anglister, J. (2003). The human type I interferon receptor: NMR structure reveals the molecular basis of ligand binding. *Structure* **11**(7), 791–802.

Dafny, N. and Jang, P. B. (2005). Interferon and the central nervous system. *European Journal of Pharmacology* **523**(1–3), 1–15. Review

Daniels, W. M. U., Pietersen, C. Y., Carstens, M. E., Daya, S., and Stein, D. (2000). Overcrowding induced anxiety and causes loss of serotonin 5HT-1a receptors in rats. *Metabolic Brain Disease* **15**(4), 287–295.

Hallschmid, M., Benedict, C., Born, J., and Kern, W. (2007). Targeting metabolic and cognitive pathways of the CNS by intranasal insulin administration. *Expert Opinion on Drug Delivery* **4**(4), 319–322.

Kaneko, N., Kudo, K., Mabuchi, T., Takemoto, K., Fujimaki, K., Wati, H., Iguchi, H., Tezuka, H., and Kanba, S. (2006). Suppression of cell proliferation by interferon-alpha through interleukin-1 production in adult rat dentate gyrus. *Neuropsychopharmacology* **31**(12), 2619–2626.

Kenis, G., Prickaerts, J., van, Os. J., Koek, G. H., Robaeys, G., Steinbusch, H. W., and Wichers, M. (2010). Depressive symptoms following interferon-alpha therapy: Mediated by immune-induced reductions in brain-derived neurotrophic factor? *The International Journal of Neuropsychopharmacology.* 29 July, 2010, 1–7. [Epub ahead of print].

Khaitov, R. M., Ignat'eva, G. A., and Sidorovich, G. A. (2000). *Immunology.* Moscow, Medicine, Russian, p. 432.

Kontsek, P. (1994). Human type I interferons: Structure and function. *Acta Virologica* **38**(6), 345–360, Review.

Loseva, E. V., Loginova, N. A., Birukova, L. M., Mats, V. N., and Pasikova, N. V. (2007a). Effect of small doses of interferon-alpha on food conditioning in young and ageing rats. *Rossiiskii Fiziologicheskii Zhurnal Imeni I.M. Sechenova* **93**(4), 386–393, Russian.

Loseva, E. V., Pasikova, N. V., Loginova, N. A., Birukova, L. M., and Mats, V. N. (2007b). Influence of small doses human interferon-alpha intranasal injection on behavior of rats of different age. *Zhurnal Vysshei Nervnoi Deiatelnosti Imeni I P Pavlova* **57**(3), 323–335, Russian.

Loseva, E. V., Loginova, N. A., and Akmaev, I. G. (2008). The role of interferon-alpha in regulation of nervous system functions. *Uspekhi Fiziologicheskikh Nauk* **39**(2), 32–46, Review, Russian.

Loseva, E. V., Loginova, N. A., and Akmaev, I. G. (2009a). Dose-dependent effects of neuroimmonomodulator interferon-alpha on behavior of humans and animals. *Rossiiskii Fiziologicheskii Zhurnal Imeni I.M. Sechenova* **95**(12), 1397–1406, Review, Russian.

Loseva, E. V., Loginova, N. A., Nekludov, V. V., Mats, V. N., Kurskaya, O. V., and Pasikovam N. V. (2009b). Effects of human and rat interferon-alpha on the behavior of rats of different ages. Comparative study of the homology of amino acid sequences. *Zhurnal Vysshei Nervnoi Deiatelnosti Imeni I P Pavlova* **59**(4), 461–472, Russian.

Lotrich, F. E. (2009). Major depression during interferon-alpha treatment: Vulnerability and prevention.. *Dialogues in Clinical Neuroscience* **11**(4), 417–425.

Makino, M., Kitano, Y., Komiyama, C., Hirohashi, M., and Takasuna, K. (2000a). Involvement of central opioid systems in human interferon-alpha induced immobility in the mouse forced swimming test. *British Journal of Pharmacology* **130**(6), 1269–1274.

Makino, M., Kitano, Y., Komiyama, C., Hirohashi, M., Kohno, M., Moriyama, M., and Takasuna, K. (2000b). Human interferon-alpha induces immobility in the mouse forced swimming test: involvement of the opioid system. *Brain Research* **852**(2), 482–484.

Mayr, N., Zeitlhofer, J., Deecke, L., Fritz, E., Ludwig, H., and Gisslinger, H. (1999). Neurological function during long-term therapy with recombinant interferon alpha. *The Journal of Neuropsychiatry and Clinical Neurosciences* **11**(3), 343–348.

Moriyama, M. and Arakawa, Y. (2006). Treatment of interferon-alpha for chronic hepatitis C. *Expert Opinion on Pharmacotherapy* **7**(9), 1163–1179.

Naitoh, H., Nomura, S., Kunimi, Y., and Yamaoka, K. (1992). "Swimming-induced head twithing" in rats in the forced swimming test induced by overcrowding stress: A new marker in the animal model of depression? *The Keio Journal of Medicine,* **41**(4), 221–224.

Owens, M. G. and Nemeroff, C. B. (1993). The role of corticotropin-releasing factor in the pathophysiology of affective and anxiety disorders: Laboratory and clinical studies. *Ciba Foundation Symposium* **172**, 296–308; discussion 308–316, Review

Ozsoy, Y., Gungor, S., and Cevher, E. (2009). Nasal delivery of high molecular weight drugs. *Molecules* **14**(9), 3754–3779.

Pires, A., Fortuna, A., Alves, G., and Falcao, A. (2009). Intranasal drug delivery: How, why and what for? *Journal of Pharmacy & Pharmaceutical Sciences* **12**(3), 288–311.

Raison, C. L., Dantzer, R., Kelley, K. W., Lawson, M. A., Woolwine, B. J., Vogt, G., Spivey, J. R., Saito, K., and Miller, A. H. (2010). CSF concentrations of brain tryptophan and kynurenines during immune stimulation with IFN-alpha: Relationship to CNS immune responses and depression. *Molecular Psychiatry* **15**(4), 393–403. Epub 17 Novmber, 2009.

Raison, C. L., Demetrashvili, M., Capuron, L., and Miller, A. H. (2005). Neuropsychiatric adverse effects of interferon-alpha: Recognition and management. *CNS Drugs* 19(2), 105–123.

Sammut, S., Goodall, G., and Muscat, R. (2001). Acute interferon-alpha administration modulates sucrose consumption in the rat. *Psychoneuroendocrinology* 26(3), 261–272.

Sarkisova, K. Yu. and Kulikov, M. A. (2006). Behavioral characteristics of WAG/Rij rats susceptible and non-susceptible to audiogenic seizures. *Behavioural Brain Research* 166(1), 9–18.

Sarkisova, K. Yu., Midzianovskaia, I. S., and Kulikov, M. A. (2003). Depressive-like behavioral alterations and c-fos expression in the dopaminergic brain regions in WAG/Rij rats with genetic absence epilepsy. *Behavioural Brain Research* 144(1-2), 211–226.

Sato, T., Suzuki, E., Yokoyama, M., Semba, J., Watanabe, S., and Miyaoka, H. (2006). Chronic intraperitoneal injection of interferon-alpha reduces serotonin levels in various regions of rat brain, but does not change levels of serotonin transporter mRNA, nitrite or nitrate. *Psychiatry and Clinical Neurosciences* 60(4), 499–506.

Thorne, R. G., Emory, C. R., Ala, T. A., and Frey, W. H. 2nd (1995). Quantitative analysis of the olfactory pathway for drug delivery to the brain. *Brain Research* 692(1–2), 278–282.

Thorne, R. G., Hanson, L. R., Ross, T. M., Tung, D., and Frey, W. H. 2nd. (2008). Delivery of interferon-beta to the monkey nervous system following intranasal administration. *Neuroscience* 152(3), 785–797.

Wang, J., Campbell, I. L., and Zhang, H. (2008). Systemic interferon-alpha regulates interferon-stimulated genes in the central nervous system. *Molecular Psychiatry* 13(3), 293–301.

Wang, J., Dunn, A. J., Roberts, A. J., and Zhang, H. (2009). Decreased immobility in swimming test by homologous interferon-alpha in mice accompanied with increased cerebral tryptophan level and serotonin turnover. *Neuroscience Letters* 452(2), 96–100. Epub 24 Janury, 2009.

Yamada, T. and Yamanaka, I. (1995). Microglial localization of alpha-interferon receptor in human brain tissues. *Neuroscience Letters* 189(2), 73–76.

Yamano, M., Yuki, H., Yasuda, S., and Miyata, K. (2000). Corticotropin-releasing hormone receptors mediate consensus interferon-alpha YM643-induced depression-like behavior in mice. *The Journal of Pharmacology and Experimental Therapeutics* 292(1), 181–187.

Yuki, Y. and Kiyono, H. (2009). Mucosal vaccines: novel advances in technology and delivery. *Expert Review of Vaccines* 8(8), 1083–1097.

Zhang, H., Tian, Z., and Wang, J. (2010). Behavioral evaluation of transgenic mice with CNS expression of IFN-alpha by elevated plus-maze and Porsolt swim test. *Neuroscience Letters* 479(3), 287–291. Epub 4 June, 2010.

14

Aleksandrova, M. A. (2001). Biological foundations for neurotransplantation. *Ontogenez* 32(2), 106–113, Review, Russian.

Aleksandrova, M. A., Podgornyi, O. V., Marei, M. V., Poltavtseva, R. A., Tsitrin, E. B., Gulyaev, D. V., Cherkasova, L. V., Revishchin, A. V., Korochkin, L. I., Khrushchov, N. G., and Sukhikh, G. N. (2005). Characteristics of human neural stem cells *in vitro* and after transplantation into rat brain. *Bulletin of Experimental Biology and Medicine*, 139(1), 114–120.

Aleksandrova, M. A., Saburina, I. N., Poltavtseva, R. A., Revishchin, A. V., Korochkin, L. I., and Sukhikh, G. T. (2002). Behavior of human neural progenitor cells transplanted to the rat brain. Brain Research. *Developmental Brain Research* 134 (1–2), 143–148.

Aleksandrova, M. A., Sukhikh, G. T., Chailakhyan, R. K., Podgornyi, O. V., Marei, M. V., Poltavtseva, R. A., and Gerasimov, Y. V. (2006). Comparative analysis of differentiation and behavior of human neural and mesenchymal stem cells *in vitro* and *in vivo*. *Bulletin of Experimental Biology and Medicine* 141(1), 152–160.

Armstrong, R. J. and Svendsen, C. N. (2000). Neural stem cells: From cell biology to cell replacement. *Cell Transplantation* 9(2), 139–152.

Azizi, S. A., Stokes, D., Augelli, B. J., DiGirolamo, C., and Prockop, D. J. (1998). Engraftment and migration of human bone marrow stromal cells implanted in the brains of albino rats--similarities to astrocyte grafts. *Proceedings of* the *National Academy of Sciences of the United States of America* **95**(7), 3908–3913.

Bath, K. G. and Lee, F. S. (2010). Neurotrophic factor control of adult SVZ neurogenesis. *Developmental Neurobiology* **70**(5), 339–349.

Boksa, P., Krishnamurthy, A., and Brooks, W. (1995). Effects of a period of asphyxia during birth on spatial learning in the rat. *Pediatric Research* **37**(4), 489–496.

Burns, T. C., Verfaillie, C. M., and Low, W. C. (2009). Stem cells for ischemic brain injury: A critical review. *The Journal of Comparative Neurology* **515**(1), 125–144.

Chu, K., Jung, K. H., Kim, S. J., Lee, S. T., Park, H. K., Song, E. C., Kim, S. U., Kim, M., Lee, S. K., and Roh, J. K. (2008).Transplantation of human neural stem cells protect against ischemia in a preventive mode via hypoxia-inducible factor-1alpha stabilization in the host brain. *Brain Research* **1207**, 182–192.

Cipriani, P., Guiducci, S., Miniati, I., Cinelli, M., Urbani, S., Marrelli, A., Dolo, V., Pavan, A., Saccardi, R., Tyndall, A., Giacomelli, R., and Cerinic, M. M. (2007). Impairment of endothelial cell differentiation from bone marrow-derived mesenchymal stem cells: New insight into the pathogenesis of systemic sclerosis. *Arthritis and Rheumatism* **56**(6), 1994–2004.

Cummings, B. J., Uchida, N., Tamaki, S. J., Salazar, D. L., Hooshmand, M., Summers, R., Gage, F. H., and Anderson, A. J. (2005). Human neural stem cells differentiate and promote locomotor recovery in spinal cord-injured mice. *Proceedings of the National Academy of Sciences of the United States of America* **102**(39), 14069–14074.

Dezawa, M., Kanno, H., Hoshino, M., Cho, H., Matsumoto, N., Itokazu, Y., Tajima, N., Yamada, H., Sawada, H., Ishikawa, H., Mimura, T., Kitada, M., Suzuki, Y., and Ide, C. (2004). Specific induction of neuronal cells from bone marrow stromal cells and application for autologous transplantation. *The Journal of Clinical Investigation* **113**(12), 1701–1710.

Girman, S. V. and Golovina, I. L. (1989). The long-term effect of acute hypoxic hypoxia on shuttlebox avoidance learning in rats. *Zhurnal Vysshei Nervnoi Deiatelnosti Imeni I P Pavlova* **39**(2), 349–355, Russian.

Hymel, K. P., Makoroff, K. L., Laskey, A. L., Conaway, M. R., and Blackman, J. A. (2007). Mechanisms, clinical presentations, injuries, and outcomes from inflicted versus noninflicted head trauma during infancy: Results of a prospective, multicentered, comparative study. *Pediatrics* **119**(5), 922–929.

Jellinger, K. A. (2008). The pathology of "vascular dementia": A critical update. *Journal of Alzheimer's Disease* **14**(1), 107–123.

Jenny, B., Kanemitsu, M., Tsupykov, O., Potter, G., Salmon, P., Zgraggen, E., Gascon, E., Skibo, G., Dayer, A. G., and Kiss, J. Z. (2009). Fibroblast growth factor-2 overexpression in transplanted neural progenitors promotes perivascular cluster formation with a neurogenic potential. *Stem Cells* **27**(6), 1309–1317.

Jin, H. K. and Schuchman, E. H. (2003). Ex vivo gene therapy using bone marrow-derived cells: Combined effects of intracerebral and intravenous transplantation in a mouse model of Niemann-Pick disease. *Molecular Therapy* **8**(6), 876–885.

Kim, S. U. (2007). Genetically engineered human neural stem cells for brain repair in neurological diseases. *Brain and Development* **29**(4), 193–201.

Kurozumi, K., Nakamura, K., Tamiya, T., Kawano, Y., Ishii, K., Kobune, M., Hirai, S., Uchida, H., Sasaki, K., Ito, Y., Kato, K., Honmou, O., Houkin, K., Date, I., and Hamada, H. (2005). Mesenchymal stem cells that produce neurotrophic factors reduce ischemic damage in the rat middle cerebral artery occlusion model. *Molecular Therapy* **11**(1), 96–104.

Loseva. E. V. (2001).Neurotransplantation of the fetal tissue and compensatory-restorative processes in the recipient nervous system. *Uspekhi Fiziologicheskikh Nauk* **32**(1), 19–37, Review, Russian.

Loseva, E. V. and Alekseeva, T. G. (2007). Influences of an acoustic signal with ultrasound components on the acquisition of a defensive conditioned reflex in Wistar rats. *Neuroscience and Behavioral Physiology* **37**(5), 459–465.

Magaki, T., Kurisu, K., and Okazaki, T. (2005). Generation of bone marrow-derived neural cells in serum-free monolayer culture. *Neuroscience Letters* **384**(3), 282–287.

Mayer, H., Bertram, H., Lindenmaier, W., Korff, T., Weber, H., and Weich, H. (2005). Vascular endothelial growth factor (VEGF-A) expression in human mesenchymal stem cells: Autocrine and paracrine role on osteoblastic and endothelial differentiation. *Journal of Cellular Biochemistry* 95(4), 827–839.

Minguell, J. J., Fierro, F. A., Epuñan, M. J., Erices, A. A., and Sierralta, W. D. (2005). Nonstimulated human uncommitted mesenchymal stem cells express cell markers of mesenchymal and neural lineages. *Stem Cells and Development* 14(4), 408–414.

Moore, K. E., Mills, J. F., and Thornton, M. M. (2006). Alternative sources of adult stem cells: A possible solution to the embryonic stem cell debate. *Gender Medicine* 3(3), 161–168.

Muñoz-Elias, G., Marcus, A. J., Coyne, T. M., Woodbury, D., and Black, I. B. (2004). Adult bone marrow stromal cells in the embryonic brain: Engraftment, migration, differentiation, and long-term survival. *The Journal of Neuroscience* 24(19), 4585–4595.

Neuhuber, B., Gallo, G., Howard, L., Kostura, L., Mackay, A., and Fischer, I. (2004). Reevaluation of *in vitro* differentiation protocols for bone marrow stromal cells: Disruption of actin cytoskeleton induces rapid morphological changes and mimics neuronal phenotype. *Journal of Neuroscience Research* 77(2), 192–204.

Neuhuber, B., Timothy Himes, B., Shumsky, J. S., Gallo, G., and Fischer, I. (2005). Axon growth and recovery of function supported by human bone marrow stromal cells in the injured spinal cord exhibit donor variations. *Brain Research* 1035(1), 73–85.

Pearlman, A. L. and Sheppard, A. M. (1996). Extracellular matrix in early cortical development. *Progress in Brain Research* 108, 117–134.

Pessina, A. and Gribaldo, L. (2006). The key role of adult stem cells: Therapeutic perspectives. *Current Medical Research and Opinion* 22(11), 2287–2300.

Podgornyi, O. V., Kheifets, I. V., Aleksandrova, M. A., Loseva, E. V., Revishchin, A. V., Poltavtseva, R. A., Marey, M. V., Korochkin, L. I., and Sukhikh, G. T. (2004). Human neural stem cells normalize rat behavior after hypoxia. *Bulletin of Experimental Biology and Medicine* 137(4), 348–351.

Polezhaev, L. V. and Aleksandrova, M. A. (1983). Allotransplantation of embryonic brain tissue into the brains of adult mammals during hypoxic hypoxia. *Zhurnal Nevropatologii i Psikhiatrii Imeni S.S. Korsakova*, 83(7), 990–997, Russian

Polezhaev, L. V., Aleksandrova, M. A., Vitvitskii, V. N., and Cherkasova, L. V. (1993). *Transplantation of Brain Tissue in Biology and Medicine*. Moskva, Nauka, Russian.

Sarnowska, A., Braun, H., Sauerzweig, S., and Reymann, K. G. (2009). The neuroprotective effect of bone marrow stem cells is not dependent on direct cell contact with hypoxic injured tissue. *Experimental Neurology* 215(2), 317–327.

Smith, S., Neaves, W., and Teitelbaum, S. (2007). Adult versus embryonic stem cells: Treatments. *Science* 316(5830), 1422–1423.

Voronina, T. A. (2000). Hypoxia and memory. Specific features of nootropic agents effects and their use. *Vestnik Rossiiskoi Akademii Meditsinskikh Nauk* 9, 27–34, Review, Russian.

Wang, J. and Milner, R. (2006). Fibronectin promotes brain capillary endothelial cell survival and proliferation through alpha5beta1 and alphavbeta3 integrins via MAP kinase signalling. *Journal of Neurochemistry* 96(1), 148–159.

Wen, S., Li, H., and Liu, J. (2009). Dynamic signaling for neural stem cell fate determination. *Cell Adhesion & Migration* 3(1), 107–117.

Woodbury, D., Schwarz, E. J., Prockop, D. J., and Black, I. B. (2000). Adult rat and human bone marrow stromal cells differentiate into neurons. *J. Neurosci Res.* 61(4), 364–370.

Zhang, J., Li, Y., Chen, J., Yang, M., Katakowski, M., Lu, M., and Chopp, M. (2004). Expression of insulin-like growth factor 1 and receptor in ischemic rats treated with human marrow stromal cells. *Brain Research* 1030(1), 19–27.

Zhao, L. R., Duan, W.,M., Reyes, M., Keene, C. D., Verfaillie, C. M., and Low, W. C. (2002). Human bone marrow stem cells exhibit neural phenotypes and ameliorate neurological deficits after grafting into the ischemic brain of rats. *Experimental Neurology* 174(1), 11–20.

15

Abdul-Fattah, A. M., Truong-Le, V., Yee, L., Pan, E., Ao, Y., Kalonia, D. S., and Pikal, M. J.

(2007). Drying-induced variations in physical-chemical properties of amorphous pharmaceuticals and their impact on stability II. Stability of a vaccine. *Pharmaceutical Research* **24**(4), 715–727.

Abdul-Rahman, Y. A. K. and Crosby, E. J. (1973). Direct formation of particles from drops by chemical reaction with gases. *Chem.Eng. Sci.* **28**, 1273–1284.

Bhaskar Chauhan, Shyam Shimpi, and Anant Paradkar (2005). Preparation and evaluation of glibenclamide-polyglycolized glycerides solid dispersions with silicon dioxide by spray drying technique. *European Journal of Pharmaceutical Sciences* **26**, 219–230.

Bodmeier, R. and Chen, H. (1998). Preparation of biodegradable polylactide microparticles using a spray-drying technique. *J.Pharm. Pharmacol.* **40**, 754–757.

Charlesworth, D. H. and Marshall, W. R. Jr. (1960). Evaporation from drops containing dissolved solids. *AIChE Journal* **6**, 9–23.

Chawla, A., Taylor, K. M. G., Newton, J. M., and Johnson, M. C. R. (1994). Production of spray-dried salbutamol sulphate for use in dry powder aerosol formulations. *Int. J. Pharm* **108**, 233–240.

Choong-Koook Kim, Yong-Sang Yoon, and Jae Yang Kong (1995). Preparation and evaluation of flurbiprofen dry elixir as a novel dosage form using a spray drying technique. *International Journal of Pharmaceutics* **120**, 21–31.

Costa., A. L., Galassi, C., and Roncari, E. (2002). Direct synthesis of PMN samples by spray-drying. *Journal of the European Ceramic Society* **22**, 2093–2100.

Czugler, M., Eckle, E., and Stezowski, J. J. (1981). Crystal and molecular structure of a 2,6-tetradeca-O-methyl-/%cyclodextrinadamantanol 1: 1 inclusion complex. *J. Chem. Sot. Chem. Comm.* **24**, 1291–1292.

Dan, E. Dobry, Dana M. Settell., John M. Baumann, Rod J. Ray, Lisa J. Graham, and Ron A. Beyerinck (2009). A Model-Based Methodology for Spray-Drying Process Development. *J. Pharm Innov.* doi 10.1007/s12247-009-9064-4.

Dellamary, L. A., Tarara, T. E., Smith, D. J., Woelk, C. H., Adractas, A., Costello, M. L., Gill, H., and Weers, J. G., (2000). Hollow porous

particles in metered dose inhalers. *Pharm. Res.* **17**, 168–174.

Desai, K. G. H. and Park, H. J. (2005). Recent developments in microencapsulation of food ingredients. *Drying Technology* **23**, 1361–1394.

Dong Xun Li, Yu-Kyuong Oh, Soo-Jeong Lime, Jong Oh Kima, Ho Joon Yang, Jung Hoon Sunga, Chul Soon Yong, and Han-Gon Cho. (2008). Novel gelatin microcapsule with bioavailability enhancement of ibuprofen using spray-drying technique. *International Journal of Pharmaceutics* **355**, 277–284.

Drusch, S. (2006). Sugar beet pectin: A novel emulsifying wall component for microencapsulation of lipophilic food ingredients by spray-drying. *Food Hydrocolloids*. doi:10.1016/j.foodhyd.2006.08.007.

Dziezak, J. D. (1988). Microencapsulation and encapsulated ingredients. *Food Technology* **42**, 136–151.

Edwards, D. A., Caponetti, G., Hrkach, J., Lotan, N., Hanes, J., Ben-Jebria, A. et al. (2002). Aerodynamically light particles for pulmonary drug delivery. *USA Patent* **6**, 102, 399.

El-Sayed, T. M., Wallack, D. A., and King, C. J. (1990). Changes in particle morphology during drying of drops of carbohydrate solutions and food liquids. 1. Effects of composition and drying conditions. *Industrial & Engineering Chemistry Research* **29**, 2346–2354.

Franceschinis, E., Voinovich, D., Grassi, M., Perissutti, B., Filipovic-Grcic, J., Martinac, A., and Meriani-Merlo, F. (2005). Self-emulsifying pellets prepared by wet granulation in high-shear mixer: Influence of formulation variables and preliminary study on the *in vitro* absorption. *Int. J. Pharm* **291**, 87–97.

Gibbs, B. F., Kermasha, S., Alli, I., and Mulligan, C. N. (1999). Encapsulation in the food industry: A review. *Internatioanl Journal of Food Sciences and Nutrition* **50**, 213–224.

Gohel, M. C. (2005). A review of co-processed directly compressible excipients. *J. Pharm. Pharmaceut Sci.* **8**(1) 76–93.

Gohel, M. C. and Jogani, P. D. (2003). Exploration of melt granulation technique for the development of coprocessed directly compressible adjuvant containing lactose and microcrystalline cellulose. *Pharm. Dev. Technol* **8**(2) 175–185.

Gouin, S. (2004). Micro-encapsulation: Industrial appraisal of existing technologies and trends. *Trends in Food Science and Technology* **15**, 330–347.

Gupta, S. M. and Kulakarni, A. R. (1994). Synthesis and dielectric properties of lead magnesium niobate a review. Mater. *Chem. Phys* **39**, 98–109.

Hartwig Steckel. and Heike G. Brandes (2004). A novel spray-drying technique to produce low density particles for pulmonary delivery. *International Journal of Pharmaceutics* **278** 187–195.

Hauschild, K. and Picke, K. M. (2004). Evaluation of a new coprocessed compound based on lactose and maize starch for tablet formulation. *AAPS PharmSci* **6**(2), article 16.

Helena Cabral-Marques and Rita Almeida (2009). Optimization of spray–drying process variables for dry powder inhalation (DPI) formulations of corticosteroid I cyclodextrin inclusion complexes. *European journal of Pharmaceutics and Biopharmaceutics* **73**(1), 121–129.

Hickey, A. J., Martonen, T. B., and Yang, Y. (1996). Theoretical relationship of lung deposition to the fine particle fraction of inhalation aerosols. *Pharm. Acta Helv* **71**, 185–190.

Holm., R. Porter, C. J. H., Edwards, G. A., Müllertz, A., Kristensen, H. G., Charman, W. N. (2003). Examination of oral absorption and lymphatic transport of halofantrine in a triple-cannulated canine model after administration in selfmicroemulsifying drug delivery systems (SMEDDS) containing structured triglycerides. *Eur. J. Pharm. Sci* **20**, 91–97.

Humberstone, A. J. and Charman, W. N. (1997). Lipid-based vehicles for the oral delivery of poorly water soluble drugs. *Adv. Drug Deliv. Rev* **25**, 103–128.

Izutsu, K., Yoshioka, S., and Terao, T. (1993). Decreased protein-stabilizing effects of cryoprotectants due to crystallization. *Pharmaceutical Research* **10**, 1232–1237.

Jeffery, O. H. Sham., Yu Zhang., Warren H. Finlay., Wilson H. Roa., and Raimar Lobenberg. (2004). Formulation and characterization of spray-dried powders containing nanoparticles for aerosol delivery to the lung. *International Journal of Pharmaceutics* **269** 457–467.

Johnson, D. W. Jr. (1987). Innovations in ceramic powder preparation. In *Ceramic Powder Science*, ed. G. L. Messing, K. S. Mazdiyasni, J. W. McCauley, and R. A. Haber (Eds.). American Ceramic Society, Westerville, OH, pp. 3–19.

Kang, B. K., Lee, J. S., Chon, S. K., Jeong, S. Y., Yuk, S. H., Khang, G. Lee, H. B., and Cho, S. H. (2004). Development of self-microemulsifying drug delivery systems (SMEDDS) for oral bioavailability enhancement of simvastatin in beagle dogs. *Int. J. Pharm* **274**, 65–73.

Kata, M. and Lukacs, M. (1986). Enhancement of solubility of vinpocetine base with & cyclodextrin. *Pharmazie* **41**, 151–152.

Kawashima, Y. Lin., S. Y. Ueda, M., and Tekenaka, H. (1984). Preparation of directly compressible powders of a physical mixture and a complex of theophylline-phenobarbital using spray drying. *Inf. I Pharm* **18**, 335–343.

Khavkin, Y. (2004). *Theory and practice of swirl atomizers*. Taylor & Francis, New York.

Kikuchi, M., Hirayama, F., and Uekama, K. (1987). Improvement of chemical instability of carmoful in P-cyclodextrin solid complex by utilizing some organic acids. *Chem. Pharm. Bull* **35**, 315–319.

Kim, C. K., Shin, H. J., Yang, S. G., Kim, J. H., and Oh, Y. K. (2001). Once-a-day oral dosing regimen of cyclosporin A: combined therapy of cyclosporin A premicroemulsion concentrates and enteric coated solid-state premicroemulsion concentrates. *Pharm. Res* **18** 454–459.

King, A. H. (1995). Encapsulation of food ingredients: A review of available technology, focusing on hydrocolloids. In *Encapsulation and controlled release of food ingredients*. S. J. Risch and G. A. Reineccius (Eds.). ACS symposium series, vol. 590, American Chemical Society, Washington, DC, pp. 26–39.

Kuo, M. C. and Lechuga-Ballesteros, D. (2003). Dry powder compositions having improved dispersity. *USA Patent* **6**, 518, 239.

Kurozumi, M. Nambu, N., and Nagai, T. (1975). Inclusion compounds of non-steroidal antiinflammatory and other slightly water soluble drugs with and/3-cyclodextrins in powder form. *Chem. Pharm. Bull.* **23** 3062–3068.

Larry, R. B. (2005). Commercial challenges of protein drug delivery. *Expert Opinion on Drug Delivery* 2, 29–42.

Laurence C. Chow and Limin Sun (2004). Properties of Nanostructured Hydroxyapatite Prepared by a Spray Drying Technique. *Journal of Research of the National Institute of Standards and Technology* 109, 543–551.

Lawrence, M. J. and Rees, G. D. (2000). Microemulsion-based media as novel drug delivery system. *Adv. Drug Deliv. Rev.* 45 89–121.

Lin, S. X. Q. and Chen, X. D. (2002). Improving the glass-filament method for accurate measurement of drying kinetics of liquid droplets. *ChemicalEngineering Research and Design* 80, 401–410.

Lin, S. Y. and Yang, J. C. (1986). Inclusion complexation of warfarin with cyclodextrins to improve some pharmaceutical characteristics. *Pharm. Weekb. Ser. Ed* 8 223–228.

Liu, X. D., Atarashi, T., Furuta, T., Yoshii, H., Aishima, S., and Ohkawara, M. (2001). Microencapsulation of emulsified hydrophobic flavours by spray drying. *Drying Technology* 19, 1361–1374.

Lukasiewicz, S. J. (1989). Spray-drying ceramic powders. *J. Am. Ceram.Soc* 72(4), 617–624.

Masters, K. (1991). *Spray-drying handbook.* John Wiley & Sons, NY, 5th edition.

Maury, M., Murphy, K., Kumar, S., Shi, L., and Lee, G. (2005). Effects of process variables on the powder yield of spray-dried trehalose on a laboratory spraydryer. *Eur. J. Pharmac. and Biopharma* 59, 565–573.

Michael, J. K. (1993). Spray drying and spray congealing of pharmaceuticals. In *Encyclopedia of pharmaceutical technology.* Marcel Dekker INC, New York, vol. 14, pp. 207–221.

Nazzal, S. and Khan, M. A. (2006). Controlled release of a self-emulsifying formulation from a tablet dosage form: Stability assessment and optimization of some processing parameters. *Int. J. Pharm* 315, 110–121.

Nazzal, S., Nutan, M., Palamakula, A., Shah, R., Zaghloul, A. A., and Khan, M. A. (2002). Optimization of a self-nanoemulsified tablet dosage form of Ubiquinone using response surface methodology: Effect of formulation ingredients. *Int. J. Pharm* 240, 103–114.

Ove, B. Christiansen (2002). *Successful Spray Drying.*

Patel, R. P., Patel, M. P., and Suthar, A. M. (2009). Spray drying technology: An overview. *Indian Journal of Science and Technology*, vol. 2 No.10 ISSN: 0974–6846.

Patrice, Tewa-Tagnea, St´ephanie, Briancon, and Hatem, Fessi (2007). Preparation of redispersible dry nanocapsules by means of spray-drying: Development and characterization. *European Journal of Pharmaceutical Sciences* 3 0, 124–135.

Pikal-Cleland, K. A., Rodriguez-Hornedo, N., Amidon, G. L., and Carpenter, J. F. (2000). Protein denaturation during freezing and thawing in phosphate buffer systems: Monomeric and tetrameric galactosidase. *Archives of Biochemistry and Biophysics* 384, 398–406.

Platz, R. M., Patton, J. S., Foster, L., and Eljamal, M. (2002). Methods of spray-drying a drug and a hydrophobic amino acid. *USA Patent* 6, 372, 258.

Randolph, T. W. (1997). Phase separation of excipients during lyophilization: Effects on protein stability. *Journal of Pharmaceutical Sciences* 86(11), 1198–1203.

Reinhard, Vehringa, Willard, R. Fossb1, and David, Lechuga-Ballesterosb (2007). Particle formation in spray drying. *Journal of Aerosol Science* 38 728–746.

Rosenberg, M., Kopelman, I. J., and Talmon, Y. (1990). Factors affecting retention in spray-drying microencapsulation of volatile materials. *Journal of Agricultural and Food Chemistry* 38, 1288–1294.

Satoshi, Ohtakea, Russell, A. Martina, Luisa, Yeea, Dexiang, Chenb, Debra, D. Kristensenb, David Lechuga-Ballesterosa, and Vu, Truong-Lea (2010). Heat-stable measles vaccine produced by spray drying. *Vaccine* 28, 1275–1284.

Serajuddin, A. T. M. (1999). Solid dispersions of poorly water-soluble drugs: Early promises, subsequent problems, and recent breakthroughs. *J. Pharm. Sci.* 88, 1058–1066.

Seville, P. C., Li, H., and Learoyd, T. P. (2007). Spray dried powders for pulmonary drug delivery. *Crit. Rev. Ther. Drug Carrier Sys.* 24(4), 307360.

Shahidi, F. and Han, X. Q. (1993). Encapsulation of food ingredients. *Critical Review in Food Science and Nutrition* **33**, 501–547.

Sie, Huey Lee, Desmond, Henga, Wai, Kiong Ng, Hak-Kim, Chan, and Reginald, B. H. Tana (2011). Nano spray drying: A novel method for preparing protein nanoparticles for protein therapy. *International Journal of Pharmaceutics* **403** 192–200.

Sunkel, J. M. and King, C. J. (1993). Influence of the development of particle morphology upon rates of loss of volatile solutes during drying of drops. *Industrial & Engineering Chemistry Research* **32**, 2357–2364.

Szejtli, J. (1982). *Cyclodextrrns and their Inclusion complexes*. Akademiai Kiado. Budapest.

Tao, Yi, Jiangling, Wan, Huibi Xu, and Xiangliang Yang (2008). A new solid self-microemulsifying formulation prepared by spray-drying to improve the oral bioavailability of poorly water soluble drugs. *European Journal of Pharmaceutics and Biopharmaceutics* **70**, 439–444.

Tanaka, N., Nagai, Y., Kawaguchi, H., Fukami, T., and Hosokawa, T. (2005). *U.S. Patent* 0106240 A1.

Tokumura, T., Tsushima, Y., Tatsuishi, K., Kayano, M., Machida, Y., and Nagai, T. (1985). Preparation of cinnarizine/pcyclodextrin inclusion complex by spray-drying method and the stability of complex in solid state. *Yukuzaiguku* **45**, l6.

Tuleu, C., Newton, J. M., Rose, J., Euler, D., Saklatvala, R., Clarke, A., and Booth S. (2004). Comparative bioavailability study in dogs of a self-emulsifying formulation of progesterone presented in a pellet and liquid form compared with an aqueous suspension of progesterone. *J. Pharm. Sci* **93**, 1495–1502.

Uekama, K. (1981). Pharmaceutical applications of cyclodextrin complexations. *J. Phnrm. Sci. Jpn.* **101.** 857873.

Uekama, K., Uemura, Y., Irie, T., and Otagiri, U. (1983). Analysis of interracial transfer and absorption behavior of drugs following dissolution from cyclodextrin complexes. *Chem. Pharm. Bull* **31**, 36373643.

Vehring, R. (2007). Pharmaceutical particle engineering via spray-drying. *Pharm Res* **25**, 999–1022.

Vidgrén, M. T., Vidgrén, P. A., and Paronen, T. P. (1987). Comparison of physical and inhalation properties of spray-dried and mechanically micronized disodium cromoglycate. *Int. J. Pharm* **35**, 139–144.

Walton, D. E. and Mumford, C. J. (1999). The morphology of spray-dried particles. The effect of process variables upon the morphology of spray-dried particles. *Transactions of the Institution of Chemical Engineers* **77A**, 442–460.

Wan, L. S., Heng, P. W., Chia, C. G., and Cecilia, G. H. (1992). Spray drying as a process for encapsulation and the effect of different coating polymers. *Drug.Dev. Ind. Pharm* **18**(9), 9971011.

Weers, J. G., Schutt, E. G., Dellamary, L. A., Tarara, T. E., and Kabalnov, A. (2001). Stabilized preparations for use in metered dose inhalers. *USA Patent* **6**, 309, 623.

16

Abe, N., Abe, H. et al. (2007). Dumbbell-shaped nanocircular RNAs for RNA interference. *J. Am. Chem. Soc.* **129**(49), 15108–15109.

Afonin, K. A., Bindewald, E. et al. (2010). *In vitro* assembly of cubic RNA-based scaffolds designed in silico. *Nat. Nanotechnol.* **5**(9), 676–682.

Afonin, K. A., Cieply, D. J. et al. (2008). Specific RNA self-assembly with minimal paranemic motifs. *J. Am. Chem. Soc.* **130**(1), 93–102.

Allerson, C. R., Sioufi, N. et al. (2005). Fully 2'-modified oligonucleotide duplexes with improved *in vitro* potency and stability compared to unmodified small interfering RNA. *J. Med. Chem.* **48**(4), 901–904.

Ban, N., Nissen, P. et al. (2000). The complete atomic structure of the large ribosomal subunit at 2.4 A resolution. *Science* **289**(5481), 905–920.

Berman, H. M., Gelbin, A. et al. (1996). Nucleic acid crystallography: A view from the nucleic acid database. *Prog. Biophys. Mol. Biol.* **66**(3), 255–288.

Bindewald, E., Grunewald, C. et al. (2008a). Computational strategies for the automated design of RNA nanoscale structures from building blocks using NanoTiler. *J. Mol. Graph. Model.* **27**(3), 299–308.

Bindewald, E., Hayes, R. et al. (2008b). RNA-Junction: a database of RNA junctions and kissing loops for three-dimensional structural analysis and nanodesign. *Nucleic Acids Res.* **36**(Database issue), D392–397.

Bindewald, E., Kluth, T. et al. (2010). CyloFold: secondary structure prediction including pseudoknots. *Nucleic Acids Res.* **38**(Web Server issue), W368–372.

Breaker, R. R. (2008). Complex riboswitches. *Science* **319**(5871), 1795–1797.

Busi, F., Cayrol, B. et al. (2009). Auto-assembly as a new regulatory mechanism of noncoding RNA. *Cell Cycle* **8**(6), 952–954.

Cate, J. H., Gooding, A. R. et al. (1996). Crystal structure of a group I ribozyme domain: Principles of RNA packing. *Science* **273**(5282), 1678–1685.

Cayrol, B., Geinguenaud, F. et al. (2009a). Auto-assembly of *E. coli* DsrA small noncoding RNA: Molecular characteristics and functional consequences. *RNA Biol.* **6**(4), 434–445.

Cayrol, B., Nogues, C. et al. (2009b). A nanostructure made of a bacterial noncoding RNA. *J. Am. Chem. Soc.* **131**(47), 17270–17276.

Cech, T. R., Zaug, A. J. et al. (1981). *In vitro* splicing of the ribosomal RNA precursor of Tetrahymena: Involvement of a guanosine nucleotide in the excision of the intervening sequence. *Cell* **27**(3 Pt 2), 487–496.

Chen, J. H. and Seeman, N. C. (1991). Synthesis from DNA of a molecule with the connectivity of a cube. *Nature* **350**(6319), 631–633.

Chen, X., Dudgeon, N. et al. (2005). Chemical modification of gene silencing oligonucleotides for drug discovery and development. *Drug Discov. Today* **10**(8), 587–593.

Choung, S., Kim, Y. J. et al. (2006). Chemical modification of siRNAs to improve serum stability without loss of efficacy. *Biochem. Biophys. Res. Commun.* **342**(3), 919–927.

Chworos, A. and Jaeger, L. (2007). Nucleic acid foldamers: Design, engineering and selection of programmable bio-materials with recognition, catalytic and self-assembly properties. In *Foldamers: Structure, Properties, and Applications.* S. Hecht and I. Huc (Eds.). Weinheim, Germany, Wiley-VCH.

Chworos, A., Severcan, I. et al. (2004). Building programmable jigsaw puzzles with RNA. *Science* **306**(5704), 2068–2072.

Davis, J. H., Tonelli, M. et al. (2005). RNA helical packing in solution: NMR structure of a 30 kDa GAAA tetraloop-receptor complex. *J. Mol. Biol.* **351**(2), 371–382.

Davis, M. E., Zuckerman, J. E. et al. (2010). Evidence of RNAi in humans from systemically administered siRNA via targeted nanoparticles. *Nature* **464**(7291), 1067–1070.

Diestra, E., Fontana, J. et al. (2009). Visualization of proteins in intact cells with a clonable tag for electron microscopy. *J. Struct. Biol.* **165**(3), 157–168.

Eddy, S. R. (2001). Non-coding RNA genes and the modern RNA world. *Nat. Rev. Genet.* **2**(12), 919–929.

Feng, S., Li, H. et al. (2011). Alternate rRNA secondary structures as regulators of translation. *Nat. Struct. Mol. Biol.* **18**(2), 169–176.

Flamm, C., Hofacker, I. L. et al. (2001). Design of multistable RNA molecules. *Rna.* **7**(2), 254–265.

Frank, J. (2009). Single-particle reconstruction of biological macromolecules in electron microscopy—30 years. *Q. Rev. Biophys.* **42**(3), 139–158.

Geary, C., Chworos, A. et al. (2011). Promoting RNA helical stacking via A-minor junctions. *Nucleic Acids Res.* **39**(3), 1066–1080.

Grabow, W. W., Zakrevsky, P. et al. (2011). Self-assembling RNA nanorings based on RNAI/II inverse kissing complexes. *Nano. Lett.* **11**(2), 878–887.

Guo, P. (2010). The emerging field of RNA nanotechnology. *Nat. Nanotechnol.* **5**(12), 833–842.

Guo, P., Coban, O. et al. (2010). Engineering RNA for targeted siRNA delivery and medical application. *Adv. Drug. Deliv. Rev.* **62**(6), 650–666.

Guo, S., Tschammer, N. et al. (2005). Specific delivery of therapeutic RNAs to cancer cells via the dimerization mechanism of phi29 motor pRNA. *Hum. Gene. Ther.* **16**(9), 1097–1109.

Heidel, J. D. and Davis, M. E. (2011). Clinical developments in nanotechnology for cancer therapy. *Pharm. Res.* **28**(2), 187–199.

Jaeger, L. and Chworos, A. (2006). The architectonics of programmable RNA and DNA nanostructures. *Curr. Opin. Struct. Biol.* **16**(4), 531–543.

Jaeger, L. and Leontis, N. B. (2000). TectoRNA: One-dimensional Self-assembly through Tertiary Interactions. *Angew. Chemie. Int. Ed.* **14**, 2521–2524.

Jaeger, L., Verzemnieks, E. J. et al. (2009). The UA_handle: A versatile submotif in stable RNA architectures. *Nucleic Acids Res.* **37**(1), 215–230.

Jaeger, L., Westhof, E. et al. (2001). TectoRNA: Modular assembly units for the construction of RNA nano-objects. *Nucleic Acids Res.* **29**(2), 455–463.

Jomaa, A., Stewart, G. et al. (2011). Understanding ribosome assembly: The structure of *in vivo* assembled immature 30S subunits revealed by cryo-electron microscopy. *Rna.* **17**(4), 697–709.

Jossinet, F., Ludwig, T. E. et al. (2010). Assemble: An interactive graphical tool to analyze and build RNA architectures at the 2D and 3D levels. *Bioinformatics.* **26**(16), 2057–2059.

Kasprzak, W., Bindewald, E. et al. (2011). Use of RNA structure flexibility data in nanostructure modeling. *Methods* **54**, 239–250.

Khaled, A., Guo, S. et al. (2005). Controllable self-assembly of nanoparticles for specific delivery of multiple therapeutic molecules to cancer cells using RNA nanotechnology. *Nano. Lett.* **5**(9), 1797–1808.

Klosterman, P. S., Tamura, M. et al. (2002). SCOR: A Structural Classification of RNA database. *Nucleic Acids Res.* **30**(1), 392–394.

Laing, C. and Schlick, T. (2011). Computational approaches to RNA structure prediction, analysis, and design. *Curr. Opin. Struct. Biol.* **21**(3), 306–318.

Levy-Nissenbaum, E., Radovic-Moreno, A. F. et al. (2008). Nanotechnology and aptamers: applications in drug delivery. *Trends Biotechnol.* **26**(8), 442–449.

Limbach, P. A., Crain, P. F. et al. (1994). Summary: the modified nucleosides of RNA. *Nucleic Acids Res.* **22**(12), 2183–2196.

Liu, J., Guo, S. et al. (2011). Fabrication of stable and RNase-resistant RNA nanoparticles active in gearing the nanomotors for viral DNA packaging. *ACS Nano.* **5**(1), 237–246.

Mahendran, R., Spottswood, M. S. et al. (1994). Editing of the mitochondrial small subunit rRNA in Physarum polycephalum. *Embo. J.* **13**(1), 232–240.

Mallardo, M., Poltronieri, P. et al. (2008). Non-protein coding RNA biomarkers and differential expression in cancers: A review. *J. Exp. Clin. Cancer. Res.* **27**, 19.

Mandal, M. and Breaker, R. R. (2004). Adenine riboswitches and gene activation by disruption of a transcription terminator. *Nat. Struct. Mol. Biol.* **11**(1), 29–35.

Martinez, H. M., Maizel, J. V. Jr., et al. (2008). RNA2D3D: A program for generating, viewing, and comparing 3-dimensional models of RNA. *J. Biomol. Struct. Dyn.* **25**(6), 669–683.

Morais, M. C., Koti, J. S. et al. (2008). Defining molecular and domain boundaries in the bacteriophage phi29 DNA packaging motor. *Structure* **16**(8), 1267–1274.

Nasalean, L., Baudrey, S. et al. (2006). Controlling RNA self-assembly to form filaments. *Nucleic Acids Res.* **34**(5), 1381–1392.

Nissen, P., Hansen, J. et al. (2000). The structural basis of ribosome activity in peptide bond synthesis. *Science* **289**(5481), 920–930.

Ohi, M. D., Ren, L. et al. (2007). Structural characterization of the fission yeast U5.U2/U6 spliceosome complex. *Proc. Natl. Acad. Sci. USA* **104**(9), 3195–3200.

Paliy, M., Melnik, R. et al. (2009). Molecular dynamics study of the RNA ring nanostructure: a phenomenon of self-stabilization. *Phys. Biol.* **6**(4), 046003.

Przybyla, J. A. and Watts, V. J. (2010). Ligand-induced regulation and localization of cannabinoid CB1 and dopamine D2L receptor heterodimers. *J. Pharmacol. Exp. Ther.* **332**(3), 710–719.

Ramakrishnan, V. (2010). Unraveling the structure of the ribosome (Nobel Lecture). *Angew. Chem. Int. Ed. Engl.* **49**(26), 4355–4380.

Reeder, J., Steffen, P. et al. (2007). Pknotsrg: RNA pseudoknot folding including near-optimal structures and sliding windows. *Nucleic Acids Res.* **35**(Web Server issue), W320–324.

Rivas, E. and Eddy, S. R. (1999). A dynamic programming algorithm for RNA structure prediction including pseudoknots. *J. Mol. Biol.* **285**(5), 2053–2068.

Rothemund, P. W. (2006). Folding DNA to create nanoscale shapes and patterns. *Nature* **440**(7082), 297–302.

Sander, B., Golas, M. M. et al. (2006). Organization of core spliceosomal components U5 snRNA loop I and U4/U6 Di-snRNP within U4/U6.U5 Tri-snRNP as revealed by electron cryomicroscopy. *Mol. Cell.* **24**(2), 267–278.

Schifferer, M. and Griesbeck, O. (2009). Application of aptamers and autofluorescent proteins for RNA visualization. *Integr. Biol.* (Camb) **1**(8–9), 499–505.

Severcan, I., Geary, C. et al. (2010). A polyhedron made of tRNAs. *Nat. Chem.* **2**(9), 772–779.

Severcan, I., Geary, C. et al. (2009a). Computational and Experimental RNA Nanoparticle Design. *Automation in genomics and proteomics: An engineering case based approach*. G. Alterovitz, M. Ramoni, and R. Mary Benson (Eds.). Wiley, New York, pp. 193–220.

Severcan, I., Geary, C. et al. (2009b). Square-shaped RNA particles from different RNA folds. *Nano. Lett.* **9**(3), 1270–1277.

Shapiro, B. A., Yingling, Y. G. et al. (2007). Bridging the gap in RNA structure prediction. *Curr. Opin. Struct. Biol.* **17**(2), 157–165.

Shu, X., Lev-Ram, V. et al. (2011b). A genetically encoded tag for correlated light and electron microscopy of intact cells, tissues, and organisms. *PLoS Biol.* **9**(4), e1001041.

Shu, Y., Cinier, M. et al. (2011a). Assembly of multifunctional phi29 pRNA nanoparticles for specific delivery of siRNA and other therapeutics to targeted cells. *Methods* **11**(2), 878–887.

Shukla, G. C., Haque, F. et al. (2011). A Boost for the Emerging Field of RNA Nanotechnology. *ACS Nano.* **5**(5), 3405–3418.

Simpson, A. A., Tao, Y. et al. (2000). Structure of the bacteriophage phi29 DNA packaging motor. *Nature* **408**(6813), 745–750.

Steitz, J. A. and Tycowski, K. T. (1995). Small RNA chaperones for ribosome biogenesis. *Science* **270**(5242), 1626–1627.

Steitz, T. A. (2010). From the structure and function of the ribosome to new antibiotics (Nobel Lecture). *Angew. Chem. Int. Ed. Engl.* **49**(26), 4381–4398.

Tamura, M., Hendrix, D. K. et al. (2004). SCOR: Structural Classification of RNA, version 2.0. *Nucleic Acids Res.* **32**(Database issue), D182–184.

Tarapore, P., Shu, Y. et al. (2011). Application of phi29 motor pRNA for targeted therapeutic delivery of siRNA silencing metallothionein-IIA and survivin in ovarian cancers. *Mol. Ther.* **19**(2), 386–394.

Tuschl, T. (2001). RNA interference and small interfering RNAs. *Chembiochem* **2**(4), 239–245.

Valencia-Burton, M., McCullough, R. M. et al. (2007). RNA visualization in live bacterial cells using fluorescent protein complementation. *Nat. Methods.* **4**(5), 421–427.

Venkataraman, S., Dirks, R. M. et al. (2010). Selective cell death mediated by small conditional RNAs. *Proc. Natl. Acad. Sci. USA* **107**(39), 16777–16782.

Winkler, W., Nahvi, A. et al. (2002). Thiamine derivatives bind messenger RNAs directly to regulate bacterial gene expression. *Nature* **419**(6910), 952–956.

Woodson, S. A. (2010). Compact intermediates in RNA folding. *Annu. Rev. Biophys.* **39**, 61–77.

Xayaphoummine, A., Bucher, T. et al. (2005). Kinefold web server for RNA/DNA folding path and structure prediction including pseudoknots and knots. *Nucleic Acids Res.* **33**(Web Server issue), W605–610.

Xia, Z., Gardner, D. P. et al. (2010). Coarse-grained model for simulation of RNA three-dimensional structures. *J. Phys. Chem. B.* **114**(42), 13497–13506.

Yin, P., Choi, H. M. et al. (2008a). Programming biomolecular self-assembly pathways. *Nature* **451**(7176), 318–322.

Yin, P., Hariadi, R. F. et al. (2008b). Programming DNA tube circumferences. *Science* **321**(5890), 824–826.

Yingling, Y. G. and Shapiro, B. A. (2007). Computational design of an RNA hexagonal nanoring and an RNA nanotube. *Nano. Lett.* **7**(8), 2328–2334.

Yiu, H. W., Demidov, V. V. et al. (2011). RNA Detection in Live Bacterial Cells Using Fluorescent Protein Complementation Triggered by Interaction of Two RNA Aptamers with Two RNA-Binding Peptides. *Pharmaceuticals* **4**(3), 494–508.

Yonath, A. (2010). Polar bears, antibiotics, and the evolving ribosome (Nobel Lecture). *Angew. Chem. Int. Ed. Engl.* **49**(26), 4341–4354.

Yusupov, M. M., Yusupova, G. Z. et al. (2001). Crystal structure of the ribosome at 5.5 A resolution. *Science* **292**(5518), 883–896.

Index

M

Milton Keynes UK
Ingram Content Group UK Ltd.
UKHW031143141024
449569UK00024B/1097

9 781774 632352